T0134429

Advances in Intelligent Systems and Computing

Volume 914

Series editor

Janusz Kacprzyk, Systems Research Institute, Polish Academy of Sciences, Warsaw, Poland
e-mail: kacprzyk@ibspan.waw.pl

The series "Advances in Intelligent Systems and Computing" contains publications on theory, applications, and design methods of Intelligent Systems and Intelligent Computing. Virtually all disciplines such as engineering, natural sciences, computer and information science, ICT, economics, business, e-commerce, environment, healthcare, life science are covered. The list of topics spans all the areas of modern intelligent systems and computing such as: computational intelligence, soft computing including neural networks, fuzzy systems, evolutionary computing and the fusion of these paradigms, social intelligence, ambient intelligence, computational neuroscience, artificial life, virtual worlds and society, cognitive science and systems, Perception and Vision, DNA and immune based systems, self-organizing and adaptive systems, e-Learning and teaching, human-centered and human-centric computing, recommender systems, intelligent control, robotics and mechatronics including human-machine teaming, knowledge-based paradigms, learning paradigms, machine ethics, intelligent data analysis, knowledge management, intelligent agents, intelligent decision making and support, intelligent network security, trust management, interactive entertainment, Web intelligence and multimedia.

The publications within "Advances in Intelligent Systems and Computing" are primarily proceedings of important conferences, symposia and congresses. They cover significant recent developments in the field, both of a foundational and applicable character. An important characteristic feature of the series is the short publication time and world-wide distribution. This permits a rapid and broad dissemination of research results.

More information about this series at http://www.springer.com/series/11156

Mostafa Ezziyyani
Editor

Advanced Intelligent Systems for Sustainable Development (AI2SD'2018)

Vol 4: Advanced Intelligent Systems Applied to Health

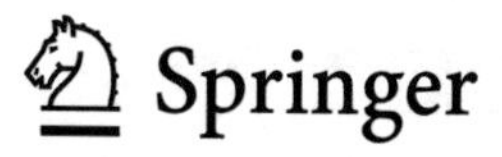

Editor
Mostafa Ezziyyani
Computer Sciences Department,
Faculty of Sciences and Techniques
of Tangier
Abdelmalek Essaâdi University
Souani Tangier, Morocco

ISSN 2194-5357 ISSN 2194-5365 (electronic)
Advances in Intelligent Systems and Computing
ISBN 978-3-030-11883-9 ISBN 978-3-030-11884-6 (eBook)
https://doi.org/10.1007/978-3-030-11884-6

Library of Congress Control Number: 2019930141

This Springer imprint is published by the registered company Springer Nature Switzerland AG
The registered company address is: Gewerbestrasse 11, 6330 Cham, Switzerland

Preface

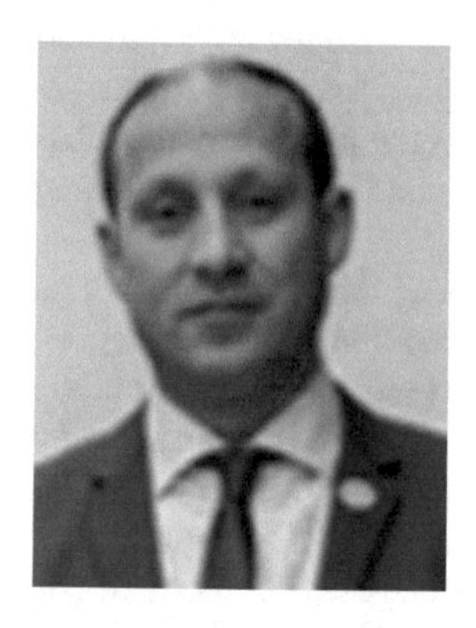

Overview

The purpose of this volume is to honour myself and all colleagues around the world that we have been able to collaborate closely for extensive research contributions which have enriched the field of Applied Computer Science. Applied Computer Science presents a appropriate research approach for developing a high-level skill that will encourage various researchers with relevant topics from a variety of disciplines, encourage their natural creativity, and prepare them for independent research projects. We think this volume is a testament to the benefits and future possibilities of this kind of collaboration, the framework for which has been put in place.

About the Editor

Prof. Dr. **Mostafa Ezziyyani,** IEEE and ASTF Member, received the "Licence en Informatique" degree, the "Diplôme de Cycle Supérieur en Informatique" degree and the PhD "Doctorat (1)" degree in Information System Engineering, respectively, in 1994, 1996 and 1999, from Mohammed V University in Rabat, Morocco. Also, he received the second PhD degree "Doctorat (2)" in 2006, from Abdelmalek Essaadi University in Distributed Systems and Web Technologies. In 2008, he received a Researcher Professor **Ability Grade. In 2015, he receives a PES grade —the highest degree at Morocco University.** Now he is a Professor of Computer Engineering and Information System in Faculty of Science and Technologies of Abdelmalek Essaadi University since 1996.

His research activities focus on the modelling databases and integration of heterogeneous and distributed systems (with the various developments to the big data, data sciences, data analytics, system decision support, knowledge management, object DB, active DB, multi-system agents, distributed systems and mediation). This research is at the crossroads of databases, artificial intelligence, software engineering and programming.

Professor at Computer Science Department, Member MA laboratory and responsible of the research direction Information Systems and Technologies, he formed a research team that works around this theme and more particularly in the area of integration of heterogeneous systems and decision support systems using WSN as technology for communication.

He received the first WSIS prize 2018 for the Category C7: ICT applications: E-environment, First prize: MtG—ICC in the regional contest IEEE - London UK Project: "World Talk", The qualification to the final (Teachers-Researchers Category): Business Plan Challenger 2015, EVARECH UAE Morocco. Project: «Lavabo Intégré avec Robinet à Circuit Intelligent pour la préservation de l'eau», First prize: Intel Business, Challenge Middle East and North Africa—IBC-MENA. Project: «Système Intelligent Préventif Pour le Contrôle et le Suivie en temps réel des Plantes Médicinale En cours de Croissance (PCS: Plants Control System)», Best Paper: International Conference on Software Engineering and New Technologies ICSENT'2012, Hammamat-Tunis. Paper: «Disaster Emergency System Application Case Study: Flood Disaster».

He has authored three patents: (1) device and learning process of orchestra conducting (e-Orchestra), (2) built-in washbasin with intelligent circuit tap for water preservation. (LIRCI) (3) Device and method for assisting the driving of vehicles for individuals with hearing loss.

He is the editor and coordinator of several projects with Ministry of Higher Education and Scientific Research and others as international project; he has been involved in several collaborative research projects in the context of ERANETMED3/PRIMA/H2020/FP7 framework programmes including project management activities in the topic modelling of distributed information systems reseed to environment, Health, energy and agriculture. The first project aims to propose an adaptive system for flood evacuation. This system gives the best decisions to be taken in this emergency situation to minimize damages. The second project aims to develop a research dynamic process of the itinerary in an events graph for blind and partially signet users. Moreover, he has been the principal investigator and the project manager for several research projects dealing with several topics concerned with his research interests mentioned above.

He was an invited professor for several countries in the world (France, Spain Belgium, Holland, USA and Tunisia). He is member of USA-J1 programme for TCI Morocco Delegation in 2007. He creates strong collaborations with research centres in databases and telecommunications for students' exchange: LIP6, Valencia, Poitier, Boston, Houston, China.

He is the author of more than 100 papers which appeared in refereed specialized journals and symposia. He was also the editor of the book "New Trends in Biomedical Engineering", AEU Publications, 2004. He was a member of the Organizing and the Scientific Committees of several symposia and conferences dealing with topics related to computer sciences, distributed databases and web technology. He has been actively involved in the research community by serving as reviewer for technical, and as an organizer/co-organizer of numerous international and national conferences and workshops. In addition, he served as a programme committee member for international conferences and workshops.

He was responsible for the formation cycle "Maîtrise de Génie Informatique" in the Faculty of Sciences and Technologies in Tangier since 2006. He is responsible too and coordinator of Tow Master "DCESS - Systèmes Informatique pour Management des Entreprise" and "DCESS - Systèmes Informatique pour Management des Enterprise". He is the coordinator of the computer science modules and responsible for the graduation projects and external relations of the Engineers Cycle "Statistique et Informatique Décisionnelle" in Mathematics Department of the Faculty of Sciences and Technologies in Tangier since 2007. He participates also in the Telecommunications Systems DESA/Masters, "Bio-Informatique" Masters and "Qualité des logiciels" Masters in the Faculty of Science in Tetuan since 2002.

He is also the founder and the current chair of the blinds and partially signet people association. His activity interests focus mainly on the software to help the blinds and partially signet people to use the ICT, specifically in Arabic countries. He is the founder of the private centre of training and education in advanced technologies AC-ETAT, in Tangier since 2000.

Mostafa Ezziyyani

Contents

Towards an Intelligent Data Analysis System for Decision Making in Medical Diagnostics

El Khatir Haimoudi[1(✉)], Otman Abdoun[1], and Mostafa Ezziyyani[2]

[1] Polydisciplinary Faculty, University UAE, Larache, Morocco
helkhatir@gmail.com
[2] Faculty of Science and Technics, University UAE, Tangier, Morocco

Abstract. Artificial neural networks (ANN) are currently massively used in different fields, especially for very complex problems. In this work we propose an approach to use these systems, and in particular the paradigm of the self-organizing map (SOM) in the medical field. The idea is to use this paradigm to develop an intelligent system able of learning to analyze, classify, and visualize multi-parameter objects in a reduced two-dimensional space in the form of object maps. This approach allows for the visual analysis and interpretation of data to reveal the most informative indicators for decision making. The application in the medical field aims to help make a very good diagnosis to make the most relevant decisions in order to provide appropriate treatment depending on the patient's state.

Keywords: Data analysis · Artificial neural networks · Self-organizing map · Learning · Classification · Visually interpreting · Medical Information Systems · Medical diagnostics · Decision making

1 Introduction

In the medical field it is very important to look for new approaches for the treatment of the results obtained, this need is conditioned by the intensive development of medical science, the widening of deepening possibilities of the etiology, the pathogenesis of disease, the increase in data on markers of various pathologies. In order to make the right decision, which can affect the prediction, evolution and outcome of the disease, doctors are forced to perform a rapid analysis of a large amount of data, and this is impossible to do manually. In this regard, the solution adopted is the use of information technology (IT), and in the context of medicine, it is possible to speak of Medical Information Systems (MIS) [1]. These systems are realized for various purposes in the form of individual automated medical diagnostic devices, among which are modern expert systems (ES). ES are computer programs that perform analysis based on some initial data; they are designed to help specialists in specific areas of knowledge to achieve meaningful results [2]. The use of ES MIS solves various problems, such as prediction of disease development risks, complications and effectiveness of treatment, early diagnosis, treatment planning, monitoring of patient health, automated analysis and statistical processing of clinical material. MIS Expert considerably simplifies the work in situations where it is impossible to represent the problem in numerical form,

M. Ezziyyani (Ed.): AI2SD 2018, AISC 914, pp. 1–13, 2019.
https://doi.org/10.1007/978-3-030-11884-6_1

there is no certainty or precision in the parameters studied, or there is no unambiguous algorithm to solve the problems [3]. These features are suitable for the resolution of medical problems, which represent a large volume of multidimensional, complex and sometimes conflicting clinical data obtained through censored observations. Currently, the use of statistical methods of data processing prevails in medical research. The descriptive methods most commonly used, in traditional statistical studies are survival analysis and multidimensional complex analysis (Discriminant, Clustering, Factorial and Correlation) [4–7]. Recent ES used in medicine, such as data mining methods and artificial neural networks, allowing to solve problems of diagnosis and prediction of various diseases, as well as to choose treatment and prevention tactics [8]. In this work, we base on artificial neural networks to develop an intelligent system for Multiparameter Data Analysis and Visualization. Our approach provides for the classification and clustering of data before their visualizations in a professional manner on two-dimensional maps, allowing the user to easily interpret them in order to make relevant diagnosis and prediction decisions. In the next works we aim at the application of the developed system, in the medical field, for decision making in medical diagnosis. The data that will be used in the future work were prepared by Dr. Dentist I.S. Denego, professor of the National University of Medicine DanyloGalytsky of Lviv, in his research work the doctor divided the patients into 5 groups, this distribution was based on immunological parameters and according to the state of patients affected by the generalized periodontal. The objective of our research is: to classify patients in generalized periodontal period on groups based on hymnological data, and to visualize the sample points of a specific population of patients in weak spaces, and reveal clinical parameters most indicative to use as state indicators.

2 The Application of ANN in Data Analysis

The classical data analysis tools are well known and used in different fields such as finance, biology, medicine and others, among these methods we mention: analysis of variance, typological analysis, principal components analysis, etc. The task of analysis is to reveal causalities, typologies, and features that facilitate the specification of explanatory models, including explicitly formulating a model and estimating it. The Neurocomputing is the part of artificial intelligence that deals with the study of neural networks (RN).

2.1 Architecture and Functioning of RNA

Two concepts underlie this phenomenon: brain structure and learning processes. When considering the structure of the brain, the key element is the concepts of the simplest element of the brain - the "neuron", in this case we are talking about a formal neuron (See Fig. 1).

The standard formal neuron consists of an adder at the input, a nonlinear transformer, and a branch point at the output. The most important element of the neuron is the adaptive adder, which calculates the scalar product of the input vector X and the vector of the adjustable parameters W (connection weight). The nonlinear transformer is an activation function applied to transform the calculated sum t (x, w) into a signal φ (t), several mathematical functions are used the best known among them are: Signedoux, Gaussian Function and Tangent Hyperbolic. The branch point serves to broadcast the output signal to the neuron inputs of the next layer.

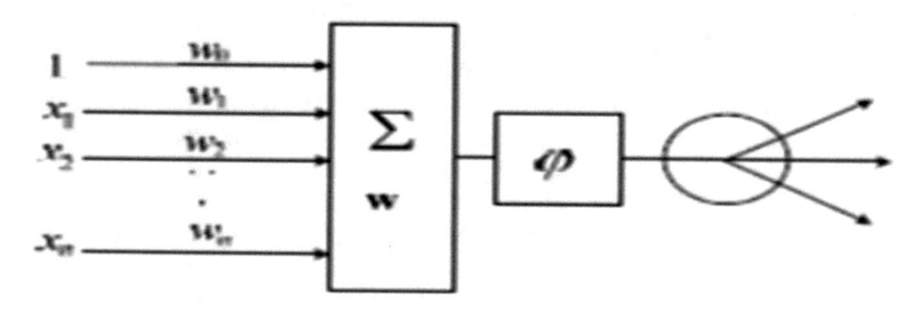

Fig. 1. Formal neuron structure.

The second consideration is based on the possibility of forming connections between neurons, so that many neurons can solve a particular problem; this ability is imitated from the brain of living beings.

A neural network is generally composed of a succession of layers, where each of them consists of a set of neurons, these elements are connected together by synaptic weights, forming a certain architecture, in the figures below are presented some examples (Fig. 2).

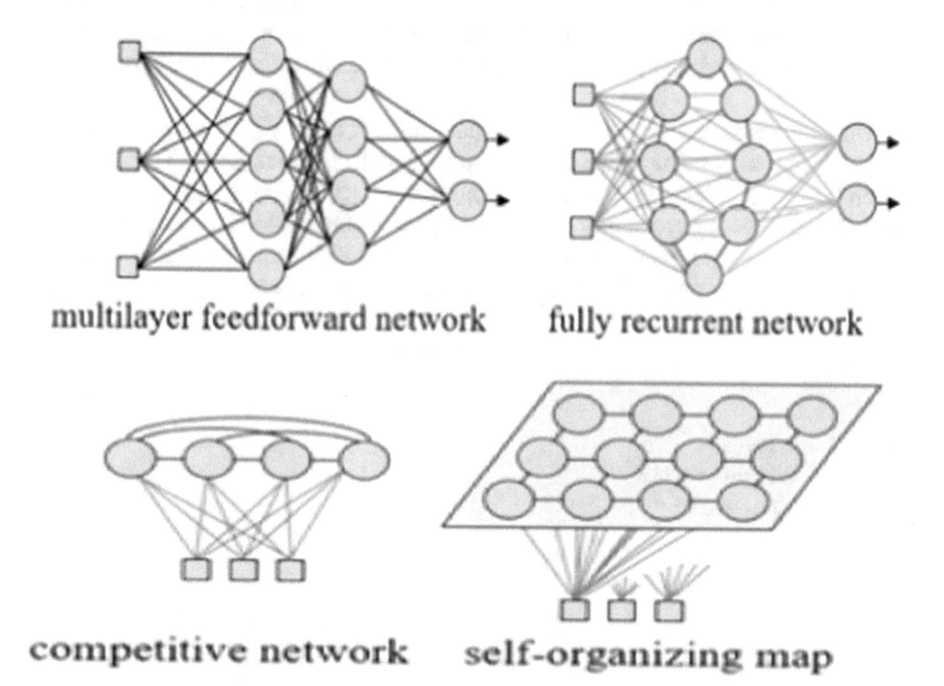

Fig. 2. Exemples d'architectures des réseaux de neurones

Two types of architectures are used in neural networks: layered networks and fully connected networks. In the first type, the neurons are located in several layers. The neurons of the first layer receive the input signals and calculate their outputs, and the branch point diffuses these outputs to the neurons of the next layer. The signals in the network propagate to the output layer where the neurons calculate the outputs of the network. In the first type, the neurons are located in several layers. The neurons of the first layer receive the input signals and calculate their outputs, and the branch point diffuses these outputs to the neurons of the next layer. The signals in the network propagate to the output layer where the neurons calculate the outputs of the network. But in the second type all the neurons are linked together, where the outputs of the neurons are diffused via the connection point to all the neurons of the network.

RNAs are able to learn how to solve problems; the learning process begins with the successive presentation of the observations of the learning multitude, and for each of them the network calculates the error value. This error represents the difference between the input element and that of the desired output for the so-called supervised learning algorithms, or the connection weight vector in the case of unsupervised learning, at the next step the network adjusts the connection weights to gradually degrade this error. The network learns continues for all learning objects until the minimum average error is refined, indicating network stabilization. There are two types of learning algorithms: supervised and unsupervised.

The supervised learning method uses a learning base in the form of input/output pairs (x_n, y_n) où $x_n \in X$ et $y_n \in Y$. In this case the network must learn to determine a compact representation of *f* in *g*, this operation is called indistinctly prediction function, hypothesis or model. It associates to a new entry x an output g (x). The purpose of a supervised learning algorithm is therefore to generalize for unknown inputs what it has been able to learn from the data already processed by experts, this in a reasonable way. It is said that the prediction function learned must have good guarantees in generalization.

Unsupervised learning relies on input data, and for every object presented, neurons compete to be active. They have binary outputs, and they are active when their output is 1. While in other rules several neuron outputs can be active simultaneously, in the case of competitive learning, a single neuron is active at a given time. Each output neuron is specialized to detect a sequence of similar shapes and then becomes a feature detector. For each example a neuron is determined winner on the base of the following function.

$$h = b - dist(W, X) \tag{1}$$

Où: b – le seuil;
W – Weights vector;
X – Input vector.

The winner neuron is the one for which h is the maximum, but if the thresholds are identical, the winner is the one whose weights is closest to the inputs and his output will be set to 1, while the outputs of the other neurons will be set to 0. A neuron learns by moving its weight to the inputs that stimulate it, to increase its chances of winning. If a neuron does not respond to an input, no weight adjustment occurs. If a neuron wins, a portion of the weights of all inputs is redistributed to the weights of the active inputs. Among the neural networks that use unsupervised learning is the self-organizing map.

2.2 The Self-organizing Map (SOM)

The approach proposed in this work is based on artificial neural networks, in particular the self-organizing map (SOM) [9]. These systems are intelligent and able to learn how to classify quantitative multi-parameter data with an unsupervised learning algorithm, thus visualizing the results in a low space often two dimensional with reservation of topological relationships between the initial data (See Fig. 3).

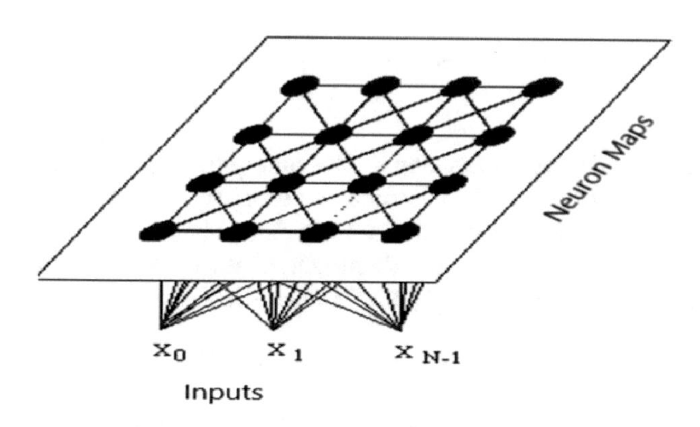

Fig. 3. Two-dimensional self-organizing map

During the learning process, the Kohonen network performs a data analysis of the learning multitude in order to reveal the topological interrelationships between the observations and to identify the winner neuron for each similar objects set, and its neighboring neurons. All these neurons form a cluster with a neighborhood diameter whose center is the winner neurons, in this case we take advantage of two maps, the first one is used to interpret the winner neurons that respond to the particular cases, and the second to Cluster visualization that groups neighboring neurons that respond to nearby cases. The learning data are organized in the form of an array whose dimension is NxM, where N is the numbers of lines that represent the observations in the form of the vectors of M components (See Fig. 4).

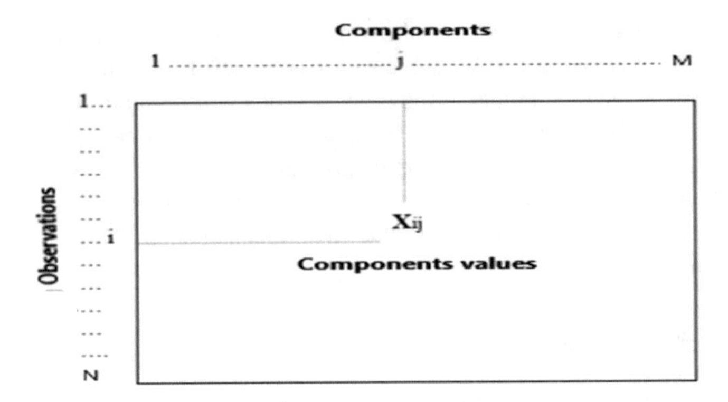

Fig. 4. Learning data table.

The learning procedure begins with a preliminary data processing which provides scaling of the vectors lengths according to the following formula.

$$x_i = x_i \Bigg/ \sqrt{\sum_{j=0}^{n-1} x_j^2} \tag{2}$$

This data normalizations speeds up the learning process by compressing the realization space [10]. After the initialization of the connection weights, the learning vectors are presented at the input of the network randomly one after the other, for each observation vectors, the learning algorithm determines the winner neuron using the metric of the distance Euclidean [11] see formula below.

$$k : \|\mathbf{w}_k - \mathbf{x}\| \leq \|\mathbf{w}_o - \mathbf{x}\| \quad \forall o \tag{3}$$

Subsequently, the algorithm proceeds to adjust the connecting weights of the winner neuron and its neighbors [12] see formula below.

$$w_{ij}(t+1) = w_{ij}(t) + \alpha_i(t)h(d,t) \cdot \left[y_i - w_{ij}(t)\right] \tag{4}$$

The objective of this adjustment is to bring the vectors closer to the connection weights of these neurons to the observation vectors in the space of the realization. The both functions h and α, make it possible to control the convergence as a function of the distance and the learning rate (Number of iterations) [13]. The learning procedure will hold for all observations until the stabilization of the network, which is controlled by the average error calculated at the base of the distances between the vectors of observations and the vectors of the corresponding winner neurons in the realization space.

2.3 The SOM Application Peculiarities

Kohonen's self-organizing map is one of the networks using competitive learning, and its particularity is that during the learning process its algorithm predicts the modification of not only the connecting weights of the winner neuron, but also those of neighboring neurons, only at a slower step. For this type of RNA, the neurons of the output layer are ordered in a single or two-dimensional space, which makes it possible to efficiently visualize the multidimensional data. The neurons that are located in the nodes of the map are the vectors of the connection weights having the same lengths of the training data vectors. Despite the advantages mentioned above, we will perform experimental tests to reveal the disadvantages and ambiguities of its application in multi-parametric data analysis and classification.

In this part the assessment of the learning process includes the total number of iterations, the average distance between the input object vectors and the connection weight vectors during the learning period, as well as the distance between each input object and the corresponding winning neuron. The learning outcome is determined by the number of winning neurons and their distribution on the topographic map, as well as their membership in a particular group (Cluster).

Three tests were done. The first test provides the use of the network for the approximation of the XOR logic function. The learning outcomes are shown in the table and topographic maps below (Fig. 5).

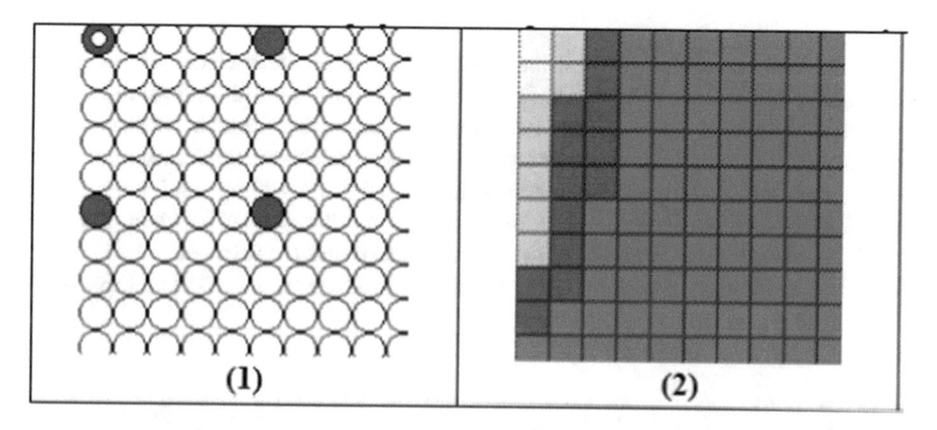

Fig. 5. Topographic maps, approximation results of the XOR function. 1: winner neurons map, 2: clusters map

The learning results of this test show that the network has correctly classified the objects on four winning neurons, and four Clusters have been defined via the neighborhood rule. But on the other hand we find that the result varied according to the number of neurons in the output layer according to the data shown in the table below (Table 1).

Table 1. Input data and the results: example. 1

	Example 1	
	Test. 1	Test. 2
Learning data	(1, 0) (0, 1) (−1, 0) (0, −1)	
Neurons number	10	17
Iteration rate	500	500
Learning rate	0.3	0.3
Initial neighborhood	5	5
Learning period	3	1
Initial weights	0.2	0.2
Medium error	2.879	1.393
Error at the last iteration	2.828	1.339
Error at the last iteration for one object	0.707	0.335
Winner neurons	0, 6, 6, 0	16, 12, 6, 0

In the second example we test the impact of the three parameters on the learning process: the relevance of the result, the learning rate and the initial neighborhood.

The multitude of learning data has three vectors, each of which consists of two components. To complicate the learning process two vectors among them are linear and having regularities between their components. The results show that the network considers the two linear vectors as similar objects and has defined for them the same winning neuron. We also note that the learning speed and the relevance of the results depend on the initial parameters tested in this example see the table below (Fig. 6 and Table 2).

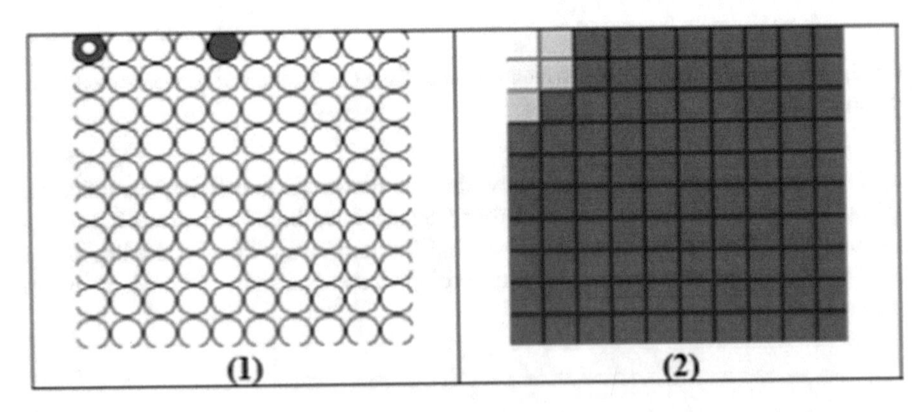

Fig. 6. Topographic maps, the results of the second test. 1: winner neurons map, 2: clusters map

Table 2. Input data and the results: example. 2

	Example 2	
	Test. 1	Test. 2
Learning data	(0.30, 0.40) (0.40, 0.31) (0.91, 1.20)	
Neurons number	10	10
Iteration rate	30	62
Learning rate	0.3	0.1
Initial neighborhood	5	2
Learning period	3	1
Initial weights	0.2	0.2
Medium error	0.227	0.254
Error at the last iteration	0.118	0.149
Error at the last iteration for one object	0.039	0.05
Winner neurons	0, 6, 0	0, 3, 0

In the third example the network was used for Latin alphabet recognition, in our test we limited ourselves to five letters A, X, H, B and I, each letter is presented as a matrix of pixels with a dimension of 5 × 7 see the figure below (Fig. 7).

```
00100
01010
10001
10001
11111
10001
10001
```

Fig. 7. Example of presentation of the letter A

The lit pixels are 1, the others are 0, and the lines of the matrix are concatenated with each other to form a vector of 35 components. The five vectors of the letters proposed for our test constituting the multitude of learning see the figure below.

A: 00100010101000110001111111000110001

X: 10001010100010000100001000101010001

H: 10001100011000111111100011000110001

B: 11111100011000111111100011000111111

I: 00100001000010000100001000010000100

Fig. 8. Learning's multitude for the recognition test of the five letters

The results show that the network has classified the objects into five classes, which is approved by the number of winner's neurons on the first map, the number of clusters on the second map, as well as the data in the table, see figures below.

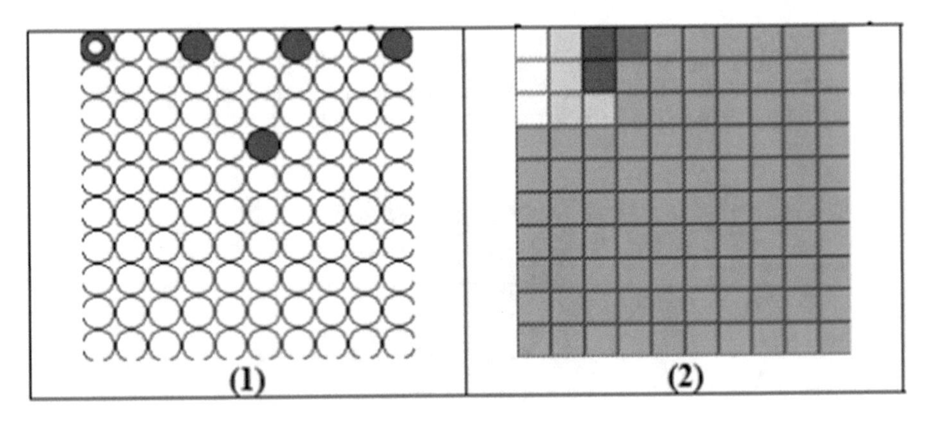

Fig. 9. Topographic maps, the results of the third test. 1: the map of winning neurons, 2: the map of clusters

Note that for this test, the results also depend on the initial parameters such as the learning rate, the initial neighborhood and the number of neurons in the Kohonen layer, see the table below (Table 3).

Based on tests performed in this section, we can say that the self-organizing map is an intelligent tool able to learn how to analyze and classify multi-parametric objects, with the possibility of projection of these data in a small space. The means of visualization used makes it possible to better interpret the results and to reveal the interrelationships between the objects. Some disadvantages and ambiguities have been detected; their elimination can increase the chance of using this paradigm of neural networks in different domains. Our perspective is to develop an approach to a multi-parametric object data analysis and classification system for decision making and its application in medical diagnostics.

Table 3. Input data and the results: example. 2

	Example 2	
	Test. 1	Test. 2
Learning data	See Figs. 8 and 9	
Neurons number	100	100
Iteration rate	500	500
Learning rate	0.3	0.1
Initial neighborhood	5	7
Learning period	3	1
Initial weights	0.2	0.2
Medium error	0.227	0.254
Error at the last iteration	0.118	0.149
Error at the last iteration for one object	0.039	0.05
Winner neurons	0, 6, 0	0, 3, 0

3 The Using Approach of SOM for Data Analysis and Decision Making in Medical Diagnostics

In the medical field the computer tools have brought enough skills to facilitate the task of diagnosis that requires the analysis of a massive complex clinical data. In this work we aim at the realization of a system at the base of an RNA paradigm able to learn to analyze and classify the patients who are affected by the generalized periodontal by presenting the results on three types of cards: the winner neurons map, the cluster map and the map of indicators (See Figs. 3 and 10).

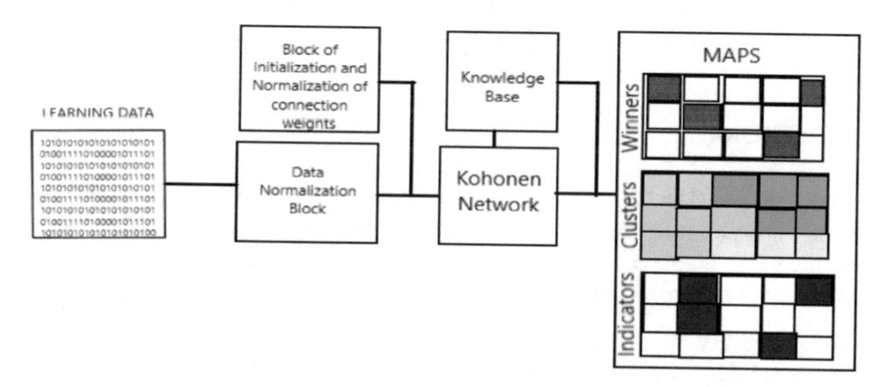

Fig. 10. The proposed system diagram.

The visualization phase begins with the drawing of the three maps according to the given dimension and the knowledge base obtained after the learning processes, the neurons are presented in the form of small rectangles respecting their order in the Kohonen layer of the network. A coloring method is used to give a special color to the winner neurons and a particular color for each of the clusters, as well as the neurons responding to certain chosen indicator. This means of presentation using the three maps allows the user to visually interpret the results of learning data analysis, as well as the classification of patients and their grouping.

The use of the proposed system relies on the type of the map and the information that can carry. For the card of the winning neurons, it visualizes the result of the patients' classification where each winner neuron carries the clinical data of a set of patients having the same hymnological parameters. After the learning step the presentation of a patient's observation stimulates the corresponding neuron giving the doctor a vision of the category to which he belongs, in order to make the necessary decisions.

The cluster map groups the winning neuron with the set of neighboring neurons, the neighborhood metric is the distance between the winner and the other neurons, and it degrades proportionally to the number of iterations. At the end of the learning, the winner neurons become the centers of the Clusters, where each one of them contains the neurons having almost the same characteristics of the winner. In this case we can say that this type of card carries information on the generalization of patient states, and during the interpretation the doctor can easily determine the category to which a new patient belongs, as long as we know the Cluster and its center.

The indicators in our task are the hymnological parameters; the indicator map stimulates the neurons corresponding to the selected indicator. The use of this map will allow the doctor to determine the most informative indicators for each category of patients. The indicator map must be used at the same time with the other two maps. The comparison between the three maps, allow reveals the Clusters and neurons winners corresponding to stimulated neurons in the indicators map.

4 Conclusion

The work proposed in this paper deals with the possibility of using the self-organizing map to realize a smart data analysis system for decision-making, as an example of application was proposed medical diagnosis. The proposed approach takes advantage of some network capabilities not found in other ways such as:

- The possibility of learning.
- The possibility of multi-parametric data projection in a small space.
- The ability to visualize the analysis results in readable and easy form for interpretation.
- The possibility of visual analysis of the results and reveals the most informative parameters.

Our perspective is to develop at the base of our approach a smart data analysis application for decision making in a concrete task in medical diagnosis.

References

1. Nazarenko, G.I., Guliyev, Ya.I., Ermakov, D.E.: Medical Information Systems Theory and Practice. Fizmatlit, Moscow (2005)
2. Abu-Nasser, B.: Medical Expert Systems Survey. Int. J. Eng. Inf. Syst. **1**(7), 218–224 (2017)
3. Андрейчиков, А.В., Андрейчикова, О.Н.: Интеллектуальные информационные системы. Финансы и статистика, Moscow (2004)
4. Румянцев, П.О., Саенко, В.А.: Статистические методы анализа в клинической практике. ГУ РМНЦ РАМН, Обнинск (2009)
5. Liang, W., Shen, G., Zhang, Y.: Development and validation of a nomogram for predicting the survival of patients with non-metastatic nasopharyngeal carcinoma after curative treatment. Chin. J. Cancer **1**, 98–106 (2016)
6. Бокерия, О.Л., Базарсадаева, Т.С., Шварц, В.А., Ахобеков, А.А.: Эффективность статинотерапии в профилактике фибрилляциипред сердий у пациентов после аортокоронарногошунтирования Анналыаритмологии. АННАЛЫ АРИТМОЛОГИИ **11**(3), 161–169 (2014)
7. Aigelsreiter, A., Neumann, J., Pichler, M.: Hepatocellular carcinomas with intracellular hyaline bodies have a poor prognosis. Liver Int. **37**(4), 600–610 (2017)
8. Чубукова, И.А.: Data Mining. М ИНТУИТ БИНОМ Лаборатория знаний, 384 (2008)
9. Aggarwal, V., Ahlawat, A.K., Pandey, B.N.: A weight initialization approach for training self organizing maps for clustering applications. In: Proceedings of 3rd International Conference on Advance Computing Conference (IACC) (2013)
10. Balabin, M.R., Lomakina, I.E.: Neural network approach to quantum-chemistry data: accurate prediction of density functional theory energies. J. Chem. Phys. **131**(7) (2009)
11. Abaei, G., Selamat, A., Fujita, H.: An empirical study based on semi-supervised hybrid self-organizing map for software defect forecast. Knowl.-Based Syst. **74**, 28–39 (2015)
12. Shah-Hosseini, H.: Binary tree time adaptive self-organizing map. Neurocomputing **74**(11), 1823–1839 (2011)
13. El Khatir, H., Fakhouri, H., Cherrat, L., Ezziyyani, M.: Towards a new approach to improve the classification accuracy of the kohonen's self-organizing map during learning process. Int. J. Adv. Comput. Sci. Appl. **7**(3), 224–229 (2016)

Omnet++ Simulation of Facial Nerve Monitoring in Real Time Neurosurgery Based on WBAN

Asma Ammari[1,2](✉) and Rachida Saouli[1]

[1] Department of Computer Science, University of Biskra, Biskra, Algeria
asmaammari902@hotmail.com, rachida.saouli@esiee.fr
[2] National Engineering School of Sfax (ENIS), University of Sfax, Sfax, Tunisia

Abstract. Neurosurgery is one of the most critical medical fields. The neurosurgeons deal with nerves sensitive situations such as paralysis. For the sake of avoiding those risks, the neurosurgeon operates while the patient is partly awake. We are interested in this paper to handle the case of the facial nerve which can be altered during an intervention at the ponto-cerebellar angle specialty of a neurosurgeon expert [1]. In this case wired systems, based on electromyography "EMG" technology, were used in parallel with visual monitoring. However, we have proposed a model of automated system based on Wireless Body Area Networks "WBAN" for facial nerves intraoperative monitoring. Our model is based on active synchronized stimulations. For the aim of assuming the patient comfort also, to add more flexibility to the neurosurgery our proposed model benefits from wireless communication instead of wired connections. We distinguish four scenarios deployed according to the facial muscles anatomy and simulated using OMNet++. The results, obtained by comparing the four scenarios, allowed us to define the optimal scenario according to a set of criteria (the system delivery time, the communication time, the energy consumed, and data processing time).

Keywords: Neurosurgery · Facial nerve monitoring · WBAN · OMNet++

1 Introduction

Neurosurgery is the surgical specialty that treats diseases and disorders of the brain and spinal cord. In neurosurgery, there is an increased risk of nerve damage and infections that can lead to paralysis [2].

It is the case of the facial nerve which can be altered by an intervention at the ponto-cerebellar angle, specialty of [1]. The first approach applied to monitor nerves is visually to observe any movements of its innervated muscles. In the other hand, to reduce the risk of facial paralysis, wired systems based on electromyography "EMG" technology were used in parallel with visual monitoring [3].

However, the current advanced development of wireless communication technologies [4–6] and the advancement in Micro Electro-Mechanical Systems "MEMS" have helped the development of smart sensors and the emergence of Wireless Sensor Networks "WSNs". These networks are made up of small, low power, and low-cost

M. Ezziyyani (Ed.): AI2SD 2018, AISC 914, pp. 14–26, 2019.
https://doi.org/10.1007/978-3-030-11884-6_2

devices that include processing, detection, radio communication, minimal configuration, and fast deployment [7]. Because of these characteristics, WSNs have been used in different fields. Particularly, the Wireless Body Area Networks "WBANs" that have been developed and used to design several Health Monitoring Systems "HMS" with the aim of assuming low cost and efficient data delivery. WBANs have distinguished themselves from wired alternatives, including: ease of the use, reduced infection risk, reduced failure risk, reduced patient discomfort, and low cost of providing care [8].

Inspired and motivated by the advances and the developments of wireless sensors technologies in the medical fields, the ultimate goal of our work is to improve the quality of the neurosurgery at the ponto-cerebellar angle as it is performed by the expert (Boublata in [1]). Thus, our contribution in this paper is designing a simulated model of a WSN based system that allows automated facial nerve intraoperative monitoring without having the patient under frustration from being awakened during the operation time.

The objectives pursued in our work are successively: first, to design a model of our proposed monitoring system. Secondly, implementing several basic modules needed using Omnet++ to be used then for the simulation of our different scenarios. Finally, extracting results.

The aim of our model is to improve the quality of facial nerves monitoring using a specific kind of biosensors called "EMG" sensors. This kind of sensors supposed to be able to: detect, process, and forward if needed EMG signals. In our model the following tasks are assumed:

- Monitoring the facial muscles area using a number of surface "EMGs" wireless sensors that cover the whole facial area and based on automatic electric stimulations to detect any injury appearance.
- Allowing the facial nerve identification using a direct stimulation made by the surgeon according to surgical task needs.

The paper is organized as follows:

- Section 2: presents some related work.
- Section 3: details our proposed model of facial nerve monitoring system, considering four proposed scenarios.
- Section 4: presents the simulation of the proposed system behavior.
- Section 5: provides an analysis of the obtained results.
- Section 6: conclusion and future works are given in.

2 Related Work

This section deals with the presentation of some work and advances related to WBAN and sensors technologies. Many researches have proposed to exploit the WSN in medical fields. In [9], a wireless system was proposed for ambulatory health status monitoring by using multiple sensor nodes to monitor body motion and heart activity. The system consists of a network coordinator and a personal server running on a personal digital assistant "PDA" or a personal computer. Another ambulatory patient monitoring system proposed in [10] was based on arrhythmia detection. The simulation of this model focuses on acquisition, retrieval, and communication of cardiovascular monitoring signals. WSNs are also used in hospitals for patients multi-monitoring [11]. In [12], an enhanced ant colony optimization approach for the travelling salesman problem has been proposed to insure the remote healthcare from health providers, and to balance the distribution of emergency messages in the WBANs. This approach allows determining the shortest path for sending emergency message to the doctor destination through sensor nodes when the patient needs any critical care or any other medical issue arises. In [13], remote patient monitoring systems have been used for the detection of epileptic seizure based on accelerometer sensors. The aim of this system is to improve the quality of the patient's life by determining the location of the patient when a seizure is detected.

Also, WSNs were used to improve surgical performances such as the Body Sensor Network "BSN" glove prototype. It has been developed in [14] to follow the surgeon movement and tasks, during a laparoscopic operation, in order to build training systems for resident students in medicine. In [15], a wireless-fully-passive neuro-sensing system has been proposed. This system is based on implantable sensors and BAN, to enable continuous and unobtrusive monitoring of electrocorticography "ECoG" signals with minimum impact to the individual's activity.

To respond to several requirements needed for the proposed medical applications and systems, many advanced medical biosensors have been designed to improve the quality of medical services especially for neurological uses. Recently, implantable neural dust wireless sensors have been designed in the university of California Berkeley in 2016 [16, 17]. In this case, the aim was to reduce the risk of infections by wiring using ultrasounds. Also, a new nanotechnology skin electrode (called tattoo) has been developed by a group of researchers from Tel Aviv University in 2016 [18]. This tattoo is an alternative to the old EMG systems and can map emotions and monitor facial muscles activities.

3 Our Proposed Model

In this section we present the anatomy of facial nerves and muscles. Then we present the conception details of our proposed system.

According to the expert's indications [1], in the operations that concern the ponto-cerebellar angle the facial nerve injury is the most serious complication which leads to facial paralysis which affects the life quality of the patient. Thus, to monitor facial nerve, we have to carry out facial muscles monitoring. The study of facial nerves and muscles anatomy is required and essential step to determine the deployment of the WSN.

Facial nerve originates in the lateral part of the ponto-bulbary (bulbo-protuberantial) furrow then penetrates the parotid gland, to be distributed at that part essentially by two branches. Each one is divided into several branches as it's illustrated in "Fig. 1" part (a) [19]. The different facial muscles innerved by these ramifications are shown in "Fig. 1" part (b). Our monitoring model is designed to use a number of EMG sensors deployed over the whole facial area following the anatomy illustrated previously. To ensure active monitoring, two wearable stimulation pads supposed to be fixed on the parotid gland part where the principle branch of facial nerve is situated “Fig. 1” part (a). The general schema of our proposed model is shown in “Fig. 2” illustrating the deployment of different components.

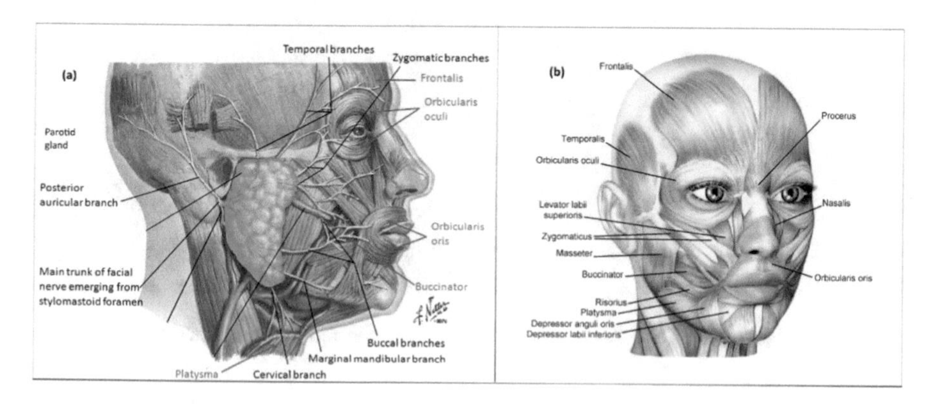

Fig. 1. (a) Facial nerve anatomy. (b) Facial muscules anatomy.

We distinguish different components used in the monitoring system as follows:

- EMG sensor: The facial part is particularly sensitive. Thus, sensors required in our model are based on EMG surface technology and must be miniaturized, flexible, with a processing and storage capacity.
- A coordinator: Is a wireless device with a limited size, situated close to the patient.
- Two stimulation pads: Capable of providing stimulation based on a defined current.
- Base station: Used to display necessary information.
- Surgical stimulator: A regular stimulator to be used, on-demand, by the surgeon directly on the nerve.
- A wearable warning bracelet: Used by the surgeon to tell when the facial nerve is identified.

To analyze our monitoring system, we have proposed four scenarios:

Scenario 1: The functionality of this scenario follows the sequence of steps presented in “Fig. 3” part (a). As a first configuration phase:

(1) The coordinator activates the left and right stimulators to synchronize the monitoring.
(2) Each stimulator initiates a first stimulation.
(3) The EMGs sensors detect an electromyogram signal and each one saves its normal signal information.

Then the second phase will be periodic during the operation following these steps:

(4) Periodically, the coordinator activates both stimulators.
(5) Stimulators stimulate both facial nerve branches.

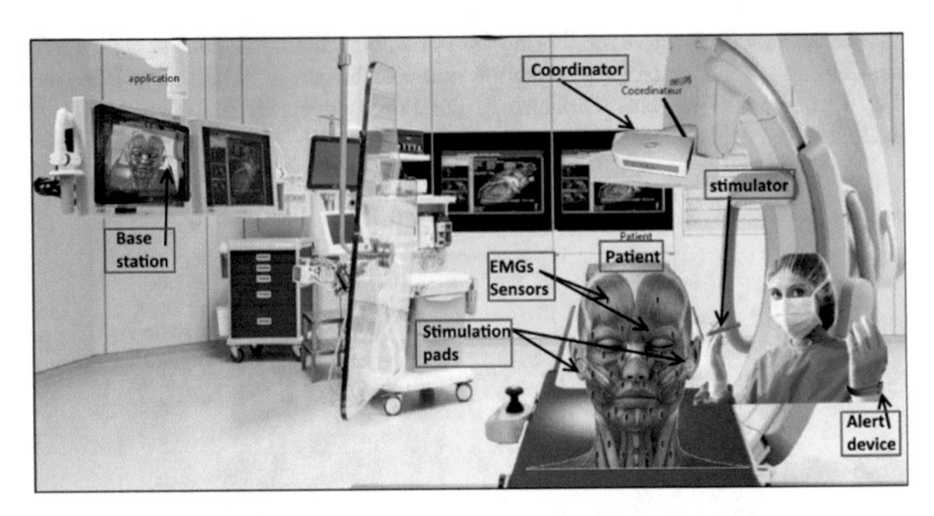

Fig. 2. General deployment of wireless facial monitoring network.

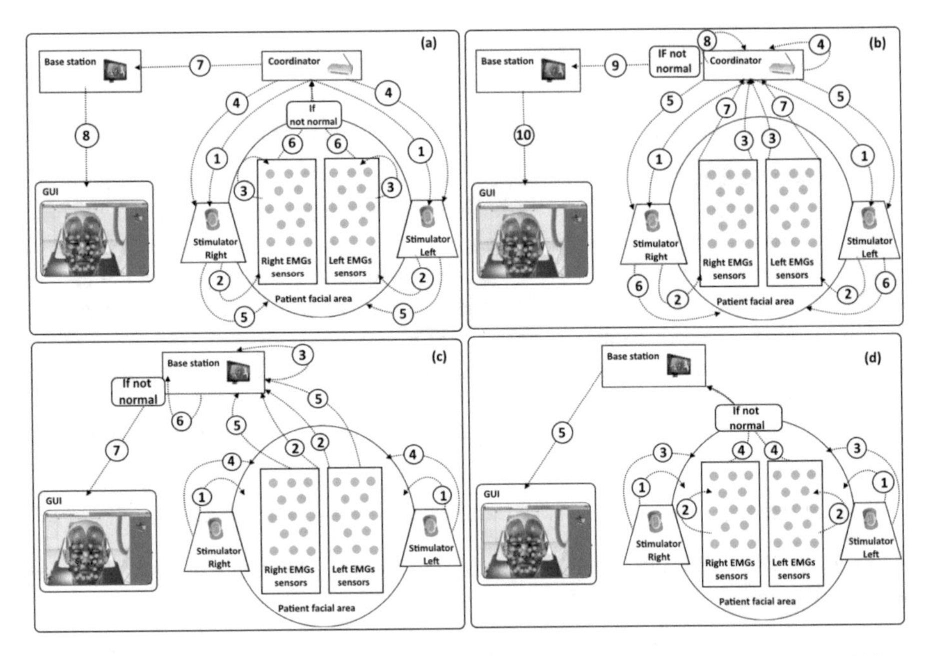

Fig. 3. The functioning of: scenario 1(a), scenario 2(b), scenario 3(c), and scenario 4(d).

(6) The EMG sensors detect the electromyogram signals and do the necessary processing themselves, to tell if the detected signal is normal or not. In the abnormal case, it sends the necessary information to the coordinator.

(7) The coordinator receives the anomaly messages from the EMGs sensors and accumulates them together in a single message to transmit it to the base station.

(8) The base station displays necessary information with an illustration that shows the anomaly location on the GUI.

Scenario 2: In this scenario, the functioning follows the sequence of steps presented in "Fig. 3" part (b). For the first configuration phase:

(1) The coordinator activates the left and right stimulators.
(2) Each stimulator stimulates facial nerve branch.
(3) The EMGs sensors, after detecting the EMG signal, send electromyograms to the coordinator.
(4) The coordinator saves the signals, according to the corresponding source EMG sensor, to consider them as normal signals.

In the next phase, and periodically:

(5) The coordinator activates the left and right stimulators.
(6) Each stimulator stimulates facial nerve branch.
(7) The EMGs sensors detect the EMG signal and send it to the coordinator.
(8) The coordinator processes it, based on the normative signals saved from the previous phase.
(9) If it finds abnormal signals, it will assemble them and send them to the base station.
(10) The base station displays the results and the locations of the detected anomalies.

Scenario 3: In this scenario we proposed that the interaction is direct, between the EMG sensors deployed on the facial part and the base station. Then, with the absence of the coordinator in this case, the left and right stimulation must be programmed to initiate periodic stimulation, regularly and automatically. The functioning of this scenario is shown in the schema of "Fig. 3" part (c). For the first phase:

(1) The stimulators, left and right, stimulate the main branches of the facial nerve.
(2) EMG sensors detect and send signals to the base station.
(3) The base station saves them as normal signals.

Then, periodically, after the stimulation the base station receives the electromyograms and applies necessary processing to know the abnormal signals. And finally, an illustration of the results will be displayed in the graphical interface of the application.

Scenario 4: This scenario requires the same deployment of the third scenario but its functionality follows the steps shown in "Fig. 3" part (d). In the first configuration phase:

(1) Left and right stimulators initiate a first stimulation.
(2) The EMGs sensors detect an electromyogram and each saves its normal signal information.

Then the second phase will be periodic throughout the operation, where periodically:

(3) Both stimulators stimulate the two branches of the facial nerve.

(4) The EMG sensors themselves perform processing to determine whether the detected signal is normal or not. In the abnormal case, the EMG sensor sends the necessary information to the base station.
(5) The base station presents the necessary illustrated information of the anomaly.

Simultaneously with the previous scenarios, and on-demand, the surgeon may use a surgical stimulator to identify the facial nerve while performing a sensitive task as it is shown in "Fig. 4" below.

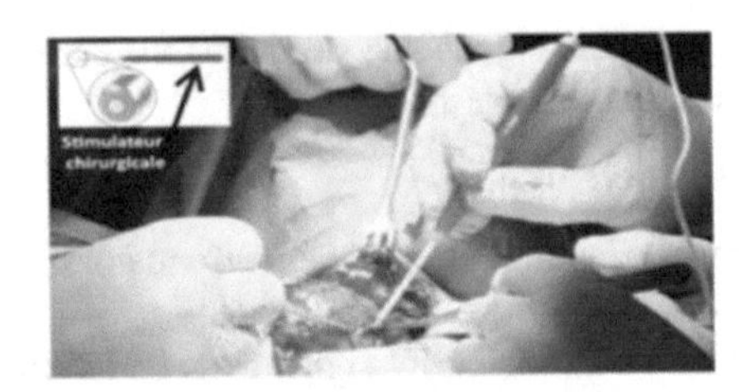

Fig. 4. Using surgical stimulator.

4 Our Proposed System Simulation

The deployment and the analysis of sensors-based network systems require the use of network simulator to ensure lower cost of the prototype presentation. OMNET++ simulator is an open source application developed under GNU license based on C++ language. It is fully programmable, configurable and modular. Because its flexible and generic architecture, it has been used successfully in various domains like the medical field [8–10] … etc. That's why we were motivated to choose OMNeT++ as a network simulator for our monitoring system.

We have implemented our simulation on ASUS computer with the following configurations and software environment: I7 processor, 8 GB for memory, and 1 TB for the hard disk. Using Windows 10 Operating system 64 bits, along with the Framework OMNET++ 4.6.

The main components in our monitoring system are the coordinator, the base station, and EMGs sensors. Therefore, to represent each component we propose the following models:

- The EMGs sensor model: is presented in "Fig. 5" part (a). The model is composed of a sensing unit, small battery, and WSN layers: « application layer, network layer, MAC layer, and Physical layer » .
- The coordinator model: is presented in "Fig. 5" part (b). The model is composed of a small battery, and WSN layers: « application layer, network layer, MAC layer, and Physical layer » .
- The base station model « application interface » : is presented in "Fig. 5" part (c). The model is composed of a notification manager, graphical interface, and the different layers.

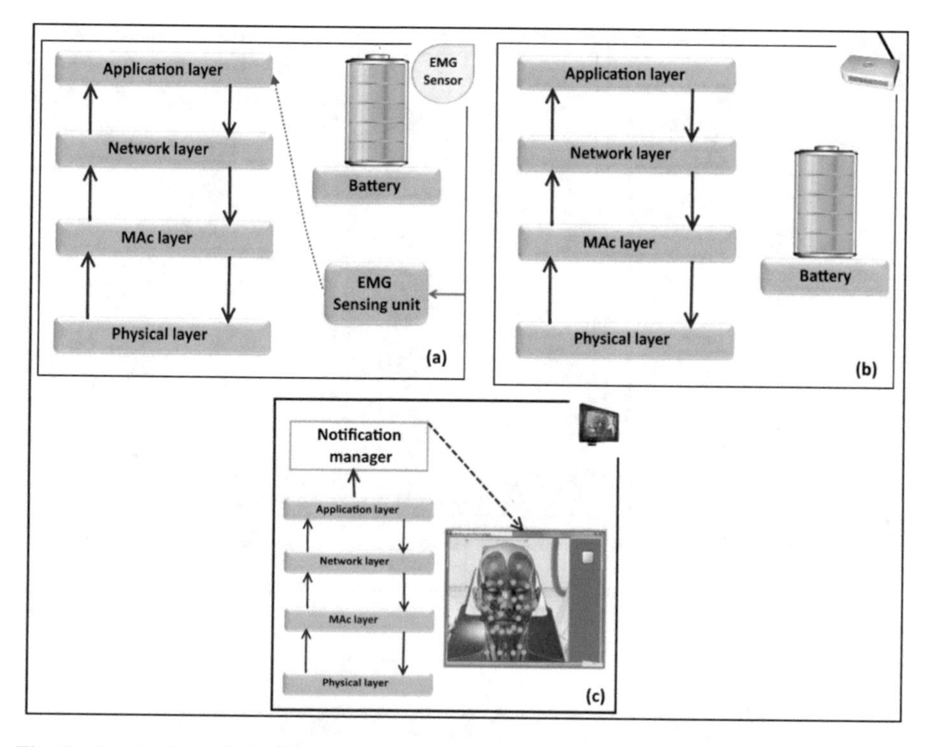

Fig. 5. (a) Modulated EMG sensor architecture. (b) Modulated coordinator architecture. (c) Modulated base station architecture.

When it comes to the implementation phase, we've implemented the different layers, the battery, the sensing unit, as well as the other stimulators and facial nerves, as simple modules. Based on these simple modules, we've created our compound modules following the models presented above. The "Fig. 6" shows: (a): an EMGs sensor module, (b) a coordinator module, and (c) the base station module. The compound module of the application interface is shown in "Fig. 7".

5 Analysis and Results Discussion

To compare the four proposed scenarios, we have selected the following criteria: EMG sensors processing time, the communication time, the energy consumed by the EMG sensor, and the responding time. Then we have discussed them according to four graphics generated according to the simulation results as follows:

The EMG Sensor Processing Time Criterion. According to "Fig. 8", in the case of the first and the fourth scenarios, we distinguish the increase of the EMG processing time. This refers to the functioning of these two scenarios; where EMG sensors are concerned by the processing of EMG signals. However, in the case of the second and

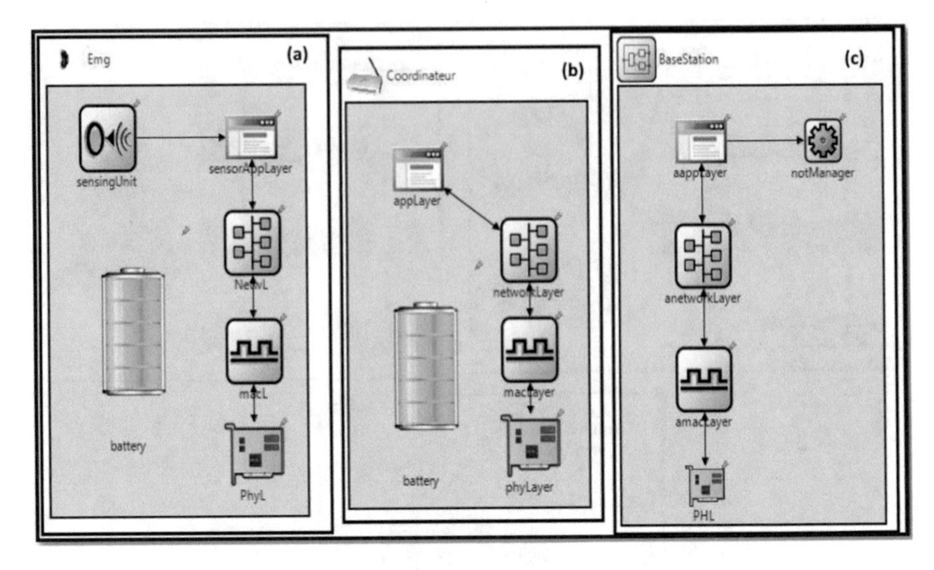

Fig. 6. The simulation models of: (a) the EMG sensors, (b) coordinator, and (c) the base station.

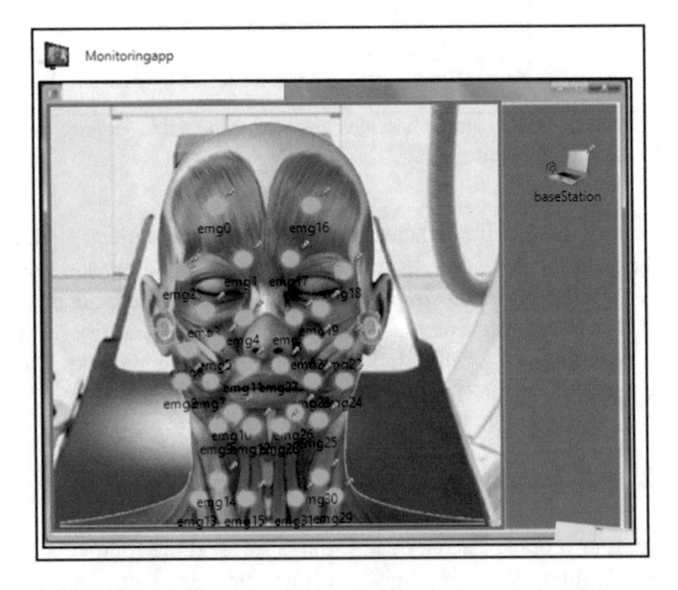

Fig. 7. The simulation model of the interface of the application.

the third scenarios, the transmission of EMG signals is direct without processing which is shown in "Fig. 8" by the decrease of processing time in the EMG sensors.

The Communication Time. In the "Fig. 9", we notice that the time of communications is decreased for the first and the fourth scenarios. This refers to the previous criterion, where the EMG sensors are in charge of reducing the time of communications

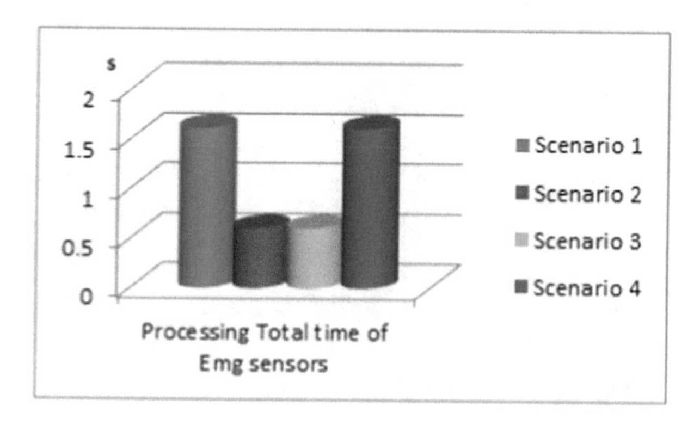

Fig. 8. The EMG sensor processing total time.

by allowing a local decisional processing. In the other hand, the second and the third scenarios showed that the communications time is increased. This is translated by the fact that sensors, in these both scenarios, send EMG signals directly to either the coordinator, the case of the second scenario, or to the base station. Transmission time in the case of the third scenario is higher than the second scenario, which refers to the deployment and the way of handling the transmitted packets.

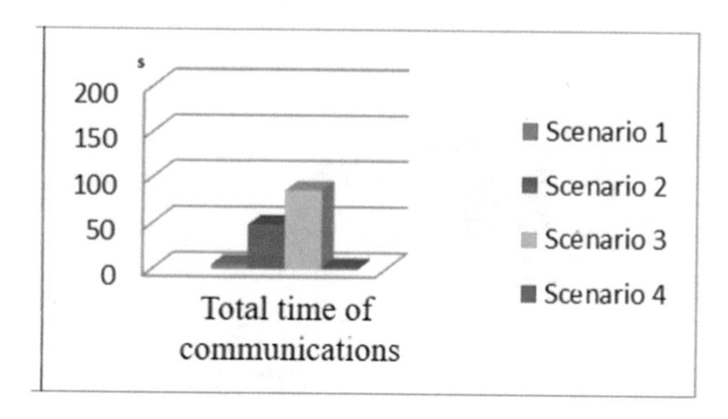

Fig. 9. The number of communication and its duration.

The Energy Consumption Criterion for the EMG Sensor. This criterion depends on the two criteria cited above, because processing doesn't consume energy as much as the case of transmissions. As a consequence, and according to the "Fig. 10", we notice that:

- For the first and the fourth scenarios: The increase of the processing along time with the decrease of the time of transmissions implies energy optimization, as in the "Fig. 10".
- For the second and third scenarios: According to the "Fig. 10", an increase in the energy consumption is noticed, which refers to the increase of the time of transmissions observed in "Fig. 9".

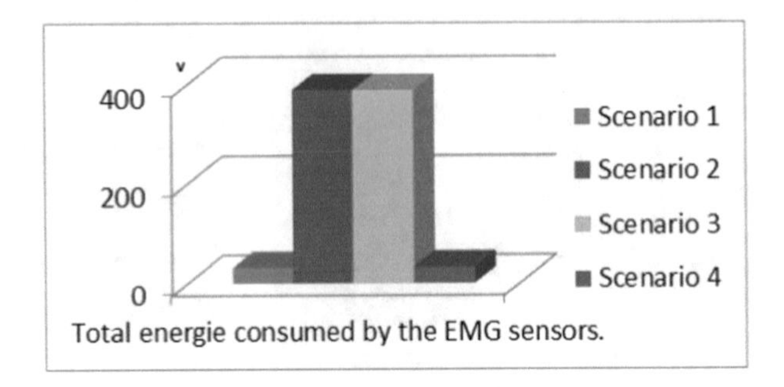

Fig. 10. The energy consumption for the EMG sensor.

The Notification Time Criterion per Period. The time required, to receive notifications at the base station, is different between the fourth scenarios. This depends on the processing time, the communication time, the deployment, and the functioning followed by each scenario as well. According to the "Fig. 11", the response time for the first scenario is the most decreased time, which is assumed by the increase of processing time in parallel with the decrease of transmission time, shown in the previous Figs. 8 and 9.

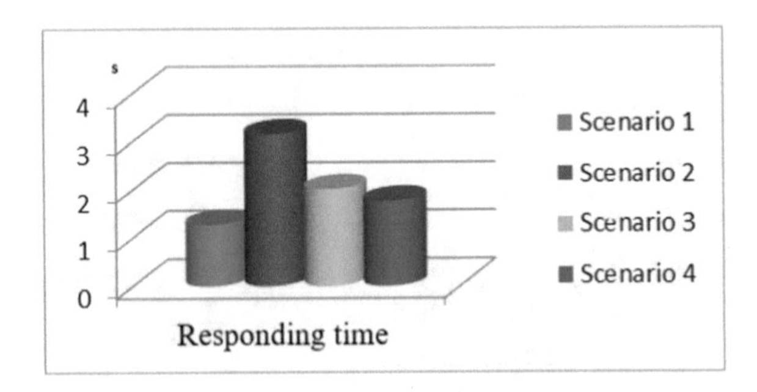

Fig. 11. The notification time criterion.

Finally, according to these observations and these results, we deduce that the first scenario is the optimal scenario. Therefore, this scenario assumes an optimal reduced responding time, and optimizes the energy consumption in the monitoring system as well.

6 Conclusion

WBANs provide new opportunities to the medical applications specifically for patient monitoring. In this paper, we proposed and presented the design of our simulated monitoring system based on wireless body area network. Considering the anatomy of the facial muscles, we specified the deployment and the monitoring functioning according to four scenarios. Then we implemented our simulation and all the corresponding modules under BAN, using the OMNeT++ Framework. To compare our scenarios, we analyzed their functioning according to the following criteria: response time, energy consumption, communication time, and processing time. The discussion of the obtained results showed that the first scenario assumes a better functioning model by optimizing energy consumption and reducing the responding time. As a perspective, firstly, we aim to allow the entire body nerves monitoring; for brain neurosurgeries, using WBANs. In the other hand, we hope that this monitoring model allows real experimentation in the future.

References

1. Boublata, L.: La fonction du nerf facial et la qualité de l'exérèse des schwannomes vestibulaires géants et larges opérés par voie rétrosigmoide transméatale.. Key note lecture congrès WFNS Rome (2015)
2. "Neurosurgery" Spine-health. https://www.spine-health.com/glossary/neurosurgery. Accessed 09 Aug 2018
3. Guntinas-Lichius, O., Eisele, D.W.: Facial nerve monitoring. Adv. Otorhinolaryngol. **78**, 46–52 (2016)
4. Val, T., Campo, E., Van Den Bosschz, A.: Technologie ZigBee/802.15.4 : Protocoles, topologies et domaines d'application. Techniques de l'Ingenieur **TE7508**, 8 (2008)
5. Kurunathan, J.H.: Study and overview on WBAN under IEEE 802.15.6. U. Porto J. Eng. **1** (1), 11–21 (2015)
6. El Chaoui, N.E., Bouayad, A., El Ghazi, M., Bekkali, M.: Modeling and simulation of a wireless body area network for monitoring sick patient remotely. Int. J. Comput. Sci. Inf. Technol. **6**(1), 580–585 (2015)
7. Shobha, G., Chittal, R.R., Kumar, K.: Medical applications of wireless networks. In: Second International Conference on IEEE Systems and Networks Communications, ICSNC, p. 82, August 2007
8. Ngoc, T.V.: Medical Applications of Wireless Networks, April 2008
9. Otto, C., Milenkovic, A., Sanders, C., Jovanov, E.: System architecture of a wireless body area sensor network for ubiquitous health monitoring. J. Mobile Multimed. **1**, 307–326 (2006)
10. Singh, G.D., Saini, D.S.: Arrogyam: arrhythmia detection for ambulatory patient monitoring. In: Contemporary Computing, pp. 168–180 (2010)
11. Aminian, M., Naji, H.R.: A hospital healthcare monitoring system using wireless sensor networks. J. Health Med. Inform. **4**(2), 1–6 (2013)
12. Latha, R., Vetrivelan, P., Jagannath, M.: Balancing emergency message dissemination and network lifetime in wireless body area network using ant colony optimization and Bayesian game formulation. Inf. Med. Unlocked **8**, 60–65 (2017)
13. Borujeny, G.T., Yazdi, M., Keshavarz-Haddad, A., Borujeny, A.R.: Detection of epileptic seizure using wireless sensor networks. J. Med. Signals Sens. **3**(2), 63–68 (2013)
14. King, R.C., Atallah, L., Lo, B.P., Yang, G.-Z.: Development of a wireless sensor glove for surgical skills assessment. IEEE Trans. Inf. Technol. Biomed. **13**(5), 673–679 (2009). Publ. IEEE Eng. Med. Biol. Soc.

15. Kiourti, A., Wang, Z., Lee, C., Scwerdt, H., Chae, J., Volakis, J.L.: A wireless neurosensing system for remote monitoring of brain signals. In: The 8th European Conference on Antennas and Propagation (EuCAP 2014), pp. 3452–3453 (2014)
16. Choi, C.Q.: Wireless 'Neural Dust' Could Monitor Your Brain. https://www.popsci.com/tiny-wireless-implants-could-monitor-your-brain. Accessed 09 June 2018
17. Maharbiz, M.M., Seo, D.J., Alon, E., Carmena, J., Rabaey, J.: Tutorial_BioCAS2014_slides Neural Dust (2014)
18. Staff, I.: Nanotech tattoo maps emotions and monitors muscle activity. http://www.israel21c.org/nanotech-tattoo-maps-emotions-and-monitors-muscle-activity/. Accessed 09 June 2018
19. Boulacel, A.: Facial nerve and Wrisberg Intermediate Nerve - Le NERF FACIAL et nerf intermédiaire. Course Wrisberg Laboratory of Human Anatomy dz, Second year Medicine (2017)

Statistical and Predictive Analytics of Chronic Kidney Disease

Safae Sossi Alaoui(✉), Brahim Aksasse, and Yousef Farhaoui

Faculty of Sciences and Techniques, Department of Computer Science, M2I Laboratory, ASIA Team, Moulay Ismail University, BP 509 Boutalamine, 52000 Errachidia, Morocco
sossialaouisafae@gmail.com, baksasse@yahoo.com, youseffarhaoui@gmail.com

Abstract. Currently, health problems increasingly intrigue the curiosity of data scientists. In fact, data analytics as a rapidly evolving area can be the right solution to manage, detect and predict diseases which threaten human life and cause a high economic cost to health systems. This paper seeks to establish a statistical and predictive analysis of an available dataset related to chronic kidney disease (CKD) by employing the widely used software package called IBM SPSS. Indeed, we manage to create a 100% accurate model based on XGBoost linear machine learning algorithm for successful classification of patients into; affected by CKD or not affected.

Keywords: Chronic kidney disease · Statistics · Predictive analytics · IBM SPSS · Machine learning · Classification

1 Introduction

According to a recent study [1] between 8 and 10% of people worldwide are suffering from a kind of damage in their kidney and due to the complications of chronic kidney disease, death among affected people increases progressively every year.

Chronic kidney disease (CKD), also known as chronic kidney failure; is a syndrome characterized by a continuous loss of kidney function [2]. The two kidneys organs in the renal system perform several essential functions namely removing wastes products from the blood, keeping the balance of fluid levels and generating hormones to produce red blood cells.

The causes of chronic kidney disease can be related to multiple health problems such as diabetes, high blood pressure, high cholesterol, kidney infections, and blockages in the flow of urine and so on [3].

In general there are no symptoms of kidney disease in the early stages. However, when it reaches a more advanced stage symptoms can appear as nausea, loss of appetite, tiredness and weakness, hypertension, sleep problems, edema, blood in urine and decreased mental alertness [2].

Because there is no cure for chronic kidney disease, it is necessary to have regular checks in order to get treatment which can help relieve the symptoms and stop it getting worse.

M. Ezziyyani (Ed.): AI2SD 2018, AISC 914, pp. 27–38, 2019.
https://doi.org/10.1007/978-3-030-11884-6_3

Statistical and predictive analytics in health care can also play a major role in saving life of patients. By exploiting the available data, models can be built and trained to predict several outcomes of interest.

The paper is organized as follows: the next section emphasizes the literature review of analyzing health care datasets using data analytics, Sect. 3 describes the approaches used namely the statistical analytics, the predictive analytics and the selected tools, while Sect. 4 depicts the methodology of work which based on several steps including data collection, data cleaning, data exploration, feature selection, modeling and evaluation. This is followed by a discussion of the results obtained in Sect. 5. Finally, the paper closes with a conclusion.

2 Related Works

Lots of research has been published discussing the efficient application of the tasks of data science in health care.

First of all, Pontillo et al. [4] tried to predict CKD273 which is a urinary biomarker and an advanced chronic kidney disease stage 3 by analyzing 2087 individuals using SAS system for database management and statistical analysis. They take into consideration many factors mainly cohort, sex, age, mean arterial pressure, diabetes, and eGFR. Indeed, they demonstrate that CKD273 can be a predictor of early estimated glomerular filtration rate (eGFR).

Moreover, Chen et al. [5] utilized both types of data particularly structured and unstructured data, in the context of healthcare big data analytics. Effectively, using datasets gathered from hospital related to chronic disease outbreak, they propose a new convolutional neural network based on multimodal disease risk prediction (CNN-MDRP) algorithm which reaches 94.8% of prediction accuracy and it speeds less time than CNN-based unimodal disease risk prediction (CNNUDRP) algorithm.

Also, Gunarathne et al. [6] have analyzed and predicted the patients 'status of being CKD or not CKD using 14 attributes related to chronic kidney disease and some classification algorithms including Multiclass Decision Forest, Multiclass Decision Jungle, Multiclass Logistic Regression and Multiclass Neural Network. The results obtained show that the Multiclass Decision Forest algorithm has the highest accuracy of 99.1% than Multiclass Decision Jungle with 96.6%, after that Multiclass Logistic Regression with 95.0% and finally Multiclass Neural Network with 97.5%.

3 Approaches

In this section, we provide an overview of the two types of data analytics [7], namely statistical and predictive analytics, used to understand our dataset as well as to gain actionable insights from it, in order to make the right decisions about chronic kidney disease. Also, this section depicts the two tools used mainly; SPSS Statistics and SPSS Modeler, created by IBM, the American multinational technology company.

3.1 Statistical Analytics

Statistical analytics can be defined as a component of data analytics utilizes extensively in science [8], from physics to the social sciences. It deals with the collection, the exploration and presentation of large amounts of data for a clear understanding of it. In fact, each company or organization around the world rely on statistics to get useful information from their data. In addition, statistics can provide an approximation for an unknown phenomenon that is difficult or impossible to measure by testing hypotheses.

3.2 Predictive Analytics

Predictive analytics [9] combines many field including data mining, machine learning, artificial intelligence, and statistical modeling, which aim at analyzing historical data so as to identify unknown outcomes and to make future predictions. It allows organizations to become more active and forward looking about future events and to benefit from the provided predictions to anticipate the appropriate actions.

3.3 Selected Tools

In this work, we have selected, SPSS Statistics and SPSS Modeler because these tools are among the most frequently used tools for real projects [10].

Hence, the arguments of choosing SPSS Statistics in this paper are several:

- Being the Leader in the market.
- Handling complex statistical data analysis.
- Creating complex tables by using excellent options.
- Providing highly specialized functionality.

While, SPSS Modeler provides multiple advantages in comparison with other data mining technologies:

- A graphical interface easy to use.
- Analyzing almost all data.
- Saving time through "Automated modeling" which selects the technique that is best suited to solve a problem.
- Allowing flexible deployment.

3.4 Tools Description

SPSS Statistics is a widely used statistical software for solving research and business problems linked to the market, healthcare, government, education, and others. Organizations use SPSS Statistics to understand data, analyze trends, forecast and plan to validate assumptions and drive accurate conclusions.

Statistics integrated in SPSS Statistics:

- Descriptive statistics
- Bivariate statistics

- Geo spatial analysis
- Simulation
- Forecasting
- R extension (GUI).

SPSS Modeler is graphical data science and predictive analytics platform used to build models based on a variety of data mining and machine learning algorithms. SPSS Modeler encompasses the entire data science cycle from data understanding to deployment. Also, it has more advanced functionalities such as text analytics, geospatial analysis and optimization. Table 1 outlines the description of selected tools.

Table 1. Tools description

Tools properties	SPSS statistics	SPSS modeler
Developers	IBM Corporation	IBM Corporation
Year initial release	1968	1994
Operating systems	Windows Linux on z Systems Linux and Unix Mac OS X	Windows Linux Unix Mac OS X
Type	Statistical analysis Data mining Text analysis Data collection	Data mining Predictive analysis
Platform	Java	Java
License	Trial ware or SaaS	Proprietary software
Stable release	25.0/August 8, 2017	18.1/June 2017
Link	https://www.ibm.com/products/spss-statistics	https://www.ibm.com/products/spss-modeler

4 Methodology

During the research study, we have maintained the methodological framework shown in Fig. 1, which mentions the most important steps followed to generate our model including data collection, data cleaning, data exploration, feature selection, modeling and evaluation.

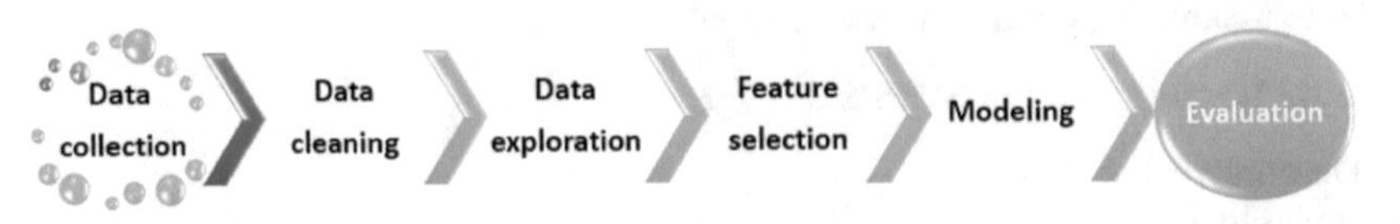

Fig. 1. Methodological framework

4.1 Data Collection

Once the approaches have been chosen, we have selected one dataset related to chronic kidney disease and downloaded from the UCI repository [11]. The chosen dataset was created in 2015 and it has 400 patients as a number of stored instances. Table 2 depicts the selected dataset by the names of 26 attributes and their types; whether they are numerical or nominal and the values of nominal variables.

Table 2. Attributes description

Name of attributes	Type	Nominal values
Patient ID	Numerical	–
Age in years	Numerical	–
Blood pressure in mm/Hg	Numerical	–
Specific gravity	Nominal	(1.005, 1.010, 1.015, 1.020, 1.025)
Albumin	Nominal	(0, 1, 2, 3, 4, 5)
Sugar	Nominal	(0, 1, 2, 3, 4, 5)
Red blood cells	Nominal	(normal, abnormal)
Pus cell	Nominal	(normal, abnormal)
Pus cell clumps	Nominal	(present, notpresent)
Bacteria	Nominal	(present, notpresent)
Blood glucose random in mgs/dl	Numerical	–
Blood urea in mgs/dl	Numerical	–
Serum creatinine in mgs/dl	Numerical	–
Sodium in mEq/L	Numerical	–
Potassium in mEq/L	Numerical	–
Hemoglobin in gms	Numerical	–
Packed cell volume	Numerical	–
White blood cell count in cells/cumm	Numerical	–
Red blood cell count in millions/cmm	Numerical	–
Hypertension	Nominal	(yes, no)
Diabetes mellitus	Nominal	(yes, no)
Coronary artery disease	Nominal	(yes, no)
Appetite	Nominal	(good, poor)
Pedal edema	Nominal	(yes, no)
Anemia	Nominal	(yes, no)
Class	Nominal	(CKD, notCKD)

4.2 Data Cleaning

Data cleaning, is an important part of statistical analysis. In practice, it usually spends more time than the statistical analysis itself. In fact, reading files into SPSS statistic directly is difficult without some sort of preprocessing. In fact, we must verify names, types, labels, and the role of each attribute; either it is an input or a target or both of them.

To simplify the management of our dataset, we transform all attributes into Numeric type by coding nominal attributes. Consequently, this way will increase the accuracy of our model (Fig. 2).

Name	Type	W...	...	Label	...	...	...	...	Measure	Role
ID	Numeric	8	0	Patient ID	...	...	8		Scale	Input
Age	Numeric	8	0	Age in years	...	...	8		Scale	Input
BloodPressure	Numeric	8	0	Blood Pressu...	...	...	8		Scale	Input
SpecificGravity	Numeric	8	3	Specific Gravity	...	...	8		Scale	Input
Albumin	Numeric	8	0		...	...	8		Ordinal	Input
Sugar	Numeric	8	0		...	...	8		Ordinal	Input
RedBloodCells	Numeric	8	0	Red Blood C...	...	...	8		Nominal	Input
PusCell	Numeric	8	1	Pus Cell	...	...	8		Nominal	Input
PusCellclumps	Numeric	8	0	Pus Cell clu...	...	...	8		Nominal	Input
Bacteria	Numeric	8	0		...	...	8		Nominal	Input
BloodGlucoseRandom	Numeric	8	0	Blood Glucos...	...	...	8		Scale	Input
BloodUrea	Numeric	8	1	Blood Urea in...	...	...	8		Scale	Input
SerumCreatinine	Numeric	8	1	Serum Creati...	...	...	8		Scale	Input
Sodium	Numeric	8	0	Sodium in m...	...	...	8		Scale	Input
Potassium	Numeric	8	1	Potassium in...	...	...	8		Scale	Input
Hemoglobin	Numeric	8	1	Hemoglobin i...	...	...	8		Scale	Input
PackedCellVolume	Numeric	8	0	Packed Cell ...	...	...	8		Ordinal	Input
WhiteBloodCellCount	Numeric	8	0	White Blood ...	...	...	8		Scale	Input
RedBloodCellCount	Numeric	8	1	Red Blood C...	...	...	8		Scale	Input
Hypertension	Numeric	8	0		...	...	8		Nominal	Input
DiabetesMellitus	Numeric	8	0		...	...	8		Nominal	Input
CoronaryArteryDisea...	Numeric	8	0	Coronary Art...	...	...	8		Nominal	Input
Appetite	Numeric	8	0		...	...	8		Nominal	Input
PedalEdema	Numeric	8	0	Pedal Edema	...	...	8		Nominal	Input

Fig. 2. Variables view in SPSS statistics

Our chronic kidney disease dataset contains missing values as a common occurrence of all datasets. SPSS Statistics can handle missing values by using different policies. To see a summary of incomplete data, we refer to "Analyze → Missing Values Analysis" in SPSS statistic interface (Fig. 3).

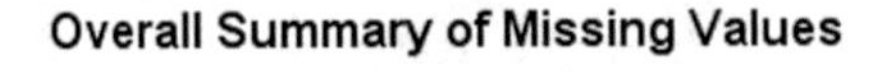

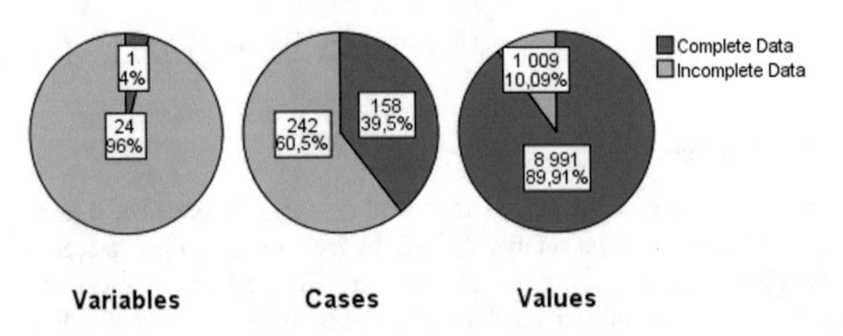

Fig. 3. Overall summary of missing values

4.3 Data Exploration

Data exploration is an initial data analysis in which we can understand the characteristics of the data and the behavior of other features toward the target variable which is Class in our case. In fact, we use a special type of table called a cross-tabulation or crosstab to describe the relationship between two categorical variables.

Table 3. Cross tables for qualitative variables

		Class	
		Not chronic kidney disease	Chronic kidney disease
		Row N %	Row N %
Red blood cells	Normal	70,6%	29,4%
	Abnormal	0,0%	100,0%
Pus cell	Normal	54,4%	45,6%
	Abnormal	1,3%	98,7%
Pus cell clumps	Notpresent	41,5%	58,5%
	Present	2,4%	97,6%
Bacteria	Notpresent	39,6%	60,4%
	Present	0,0%	100,0%
Hypertension	Yes	1,4%	98,6%
	No	59,4%	40,6%
Diabetes mellitus	Yes	1,4%	98,6%
	No	57,1%	42,9%
Coronary artery disease	yes	0,0%	100,0%
	No	42,3%	57,7%
Appetite	Poor	2,4%	97,6%
	Good	47,3%	52,7%
Pedal edema	Yes	0,0%	100,0%
	No	46,6%	53,4%
Anemia	Yes	1,6%	98,4%
	No	44,4%	55,6%
Sugar	0	50,3%	49,7%
	1	0,0%	100,0%
	2	0,0%	100,0%
	3	0,0%	100,0%
	4	0,0%	100,0%
	5	0,0%	100,0%
Albumin	0	72,9%	27,1%
	1	0,0%	100,0%
	2	2,3%	97,7%
	3	0,0%	100,0%
	4	0,0%	100,0%
	5	0,0%	100,0%

Table 3 presents crosstabs between the Class variable and all qualitative variables based on the row percentage which will determine the denominator of the percentage computations. For example, the proportion of patients who have abnormal Red Blood Cells are 100% affected by chronic kidney disease.

Compare Means is the best way to compare multiple numeric variables with respect to one or more categorical variables. It is especially advantageous for summarizing numeric variables simultaneously across multiple factors.

Table 4 shows a group of statistics of quantitative variables across the two categories of class, where the value 0 represents not chronic kidney disease and 1 is chronic kidney disease.

Table 4. Compare means for quantitative variables

Group statistics					
	Class	N	Mean	Std. deviation	Std. error mean
Age in years	0	151	46,81	15,735	1,281
	1	240	54,43	17,411	1,124
Hemoglobin in gms	0	145	15,150	1,3522	,1123
	1	203	10,652	2,1902	,1537
Blood pressure in mm/Hg	0	150	71,33	8,566	,699
	1	238	79,71	15,245	,988
Specific gravity	0	146	1,02233	,002701	,000224
	1	207	1,01394	,004630	,000322
Albumin	0	146	,01	,166	,014
	1	208	1,72	1,376	,095
Blood glucose random in mgs/dl	0	146	108,50	19,854	1,643
	1	210	175,52	92,476	6,381
Blood urea in mgs/dl	0	146	32,911	11,7543	,9728
	1	235	72,656	58,7230	3,8307
Serum creatinine in mgs/dl	0	147	,892	,3351	,0276
	1	236	4,431	6,9772	,4542
Sodium in mEq/L	0	147	141,65	4,882	,403
	1	166	133,88	12,462	,967
Potassium in mEq/L	0	147	4,340	,5840	,0482
	1	165	4,883	4,3476	,3385
White blood cell count in cells/cumm	0	145	7712,41	1834,276	152,328
	1	151	8960,93	3724,567	303,101
Red blood cell count in millions/cmm	0	144	5,359	,6406	,0534
	1	127	3,894	,9852	,0874
Packed cell volume	0	147	46,21	4,389	,362
	1	183	32,79	7,601	,562

4.4 Feature Selection

A better understanding of the relationship between features, outcomes, and patients will have a huge impact on model accuracy.

For feature selection, we use the chi-square independence test which is a procedure for testing if two categorical variables are independent or not.

Table 5. Test chi-square for anemia

Pearson Chi-square tests		
		Class
Anemia	Chi-square	40,128
	Df	1
	Sig.	,000*

Results are based on nonempty rows and columns in each innermost subtable.

*. The Chi-square statistic is significant at the ,05 level

Hypothesis Test Summary

Null Hypothesis	Test	Sig.	Decision
The distribution of Sodium in mEq/L is the same across categories of Class.	Independent-Samples Mann-Whitney U Test	,000	Reject the null hypothesis.
The distribution of Potassium in mEq/L is the same across categories of Class.	Independent-Samples Mann-Whitney U Test	,815	Retain the null hypothesis.
The distribution of Hemoglobin in gms is the same across categories of Class.	Independent-Samples Mann-Whitney U Test	,000	Reject the null hypothesis.
The distribution of White Blood Cell Count in cells/cumm is the same across categories of Class.	Independent-Samples Mann-Whitney U Test	,002	Reject the null hypothesis.
The distribution of Red Blood Cell Count in millions/cmm is the same across categories of Class.	Independent-Samples Mann-Whitney U Test	,000	Reject the null hypothesis.

Fig. 4. Hypothesis test summary of some quantitative variables

For our case the Chi-square statistic is significant at the 0,05 level for all qualitative variables. Indeed, we reject the null hypothesis (H_0); which estimates that the two categorical variables are independent in some population, and we accept the alternative hypothesis (H_1); which assumes that the two variables depend on each other. For instance, Anemia and the class (CKD, not CKD) are dependent as shown in Table 5.

For quantitative variables, we use non parametric tests which are suitable to determine if the distribution of quantitative variable is the same across categories of Class. In fact, we find as shown in Fig. 4 that for only Potassium variable we retain the null hypothesis (H_0) and we reject it for the others.

Finally, we keep 23 features among 26 as inputs to generate the model; these selected features are all qualitative and quantitative variables except Potassium variable, Patient ID, and the Class which is the target.

4.5 Modeling and Evaluation

Machine learning (ML) is an evolving term introduced first in 1959 by Arthur Samuel [12], describing a branch of computer science which enables computers to learn from data without being explicitly programmed.

Recently, machine learning become a driven technology in different fields; including financial trading, heath care, data security, marketing, online search…etc. Also, it has many algorithms such as decision trees, neural networks, K-NN, Bayes, support vector machines [12] and so on.

In the context of data analytics, machine learning techniques are used to create predictive models allowing data scientists to uncover hidden patterns from historical data and to get consequently the right decision making for the future data.

Building a well-represented model necessitates to choose the most performance algorithm among many machine learning techniques, which can be done by using evaluation metrics [13]. Indeed, in this paper we focuses on comparing the selected classification methods using the Overall accuracy metric which represents the weighted average of sensitivity and specificity [14] and measures the overall probability that a patient will be correctly classified into affected by chronic kidney disease or not.

5 Results

Generally speaking, when dealing with predictive modeling it is observed that there is no machine learning algorithm suitable for every problem. This statement goes hand in hand with “No Free Lunch” theorem for supervised machine learning methods [15]. Hence, we should try several algorithms depending on the size and structure of data as well as the kind of the problem wanted to solve.

In practice, SPSS Modeler relies on the provided SPSS machine learning library of algorithms in order to help users to pick the right machine learning algorithm for predictive analytics solutions.

Using SPSS Modeler, we create the snapshot shown in Fig. 5 which presents the dataset used related to chronic kidney disease, connected to the Type gadget which facilitates the dealing with attributes types and their formats, and the auto classifier

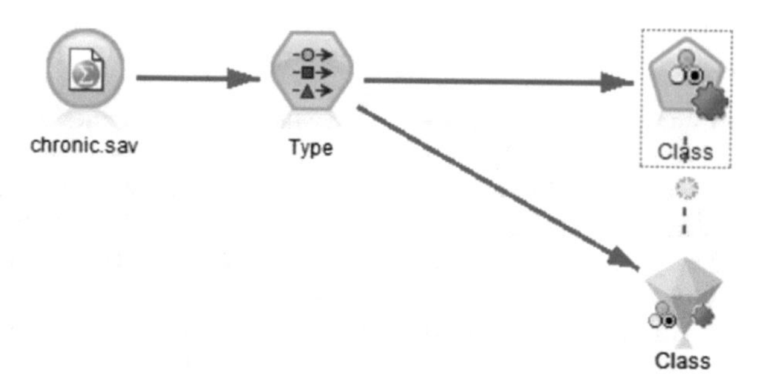

Fig. 5. Snapshot generated by SPSS modeler

gadget which runs all machine learning algorithms implemented in SPSS Modeler and reserved for classification task [16].

In a nutshell, SPSS Modeler gives the appropriate classification algorithm XGBoost Linear which proves its high percentage of accuracy with 100% to assign the correct class of either being chronic kidney disease (CKD) or not CKD to the new patients based on 23 features.

Table 6 shows the first ten models with overall accuracy, build time and the number of features used to generate the model.

Table 6. SPSS modeler results

Model	Overall accuracy	Build time (min)	Number of field used
XGBoost linear	100%	1	23
XGBoost tree	99,75%	1	23
LSVM	99.5%	<1	23
C&R tree	99,25%	1	14
CHAID	98,5%	1	6
Quest	98,25%	1	15
C5	98%	1	4
Random trees	96,528%	<1	23
Tree-AS	90,5%	<1	1
Discriminant	88,5%	1	10

6 Conclusion

To manage the high-risk condition of CKD affecting millions of people around the world. This paper tried to analyze chronic kidney disease dataset using two important types of data analytics, statistical and predictive analytics in order to create a 100% accurate model based on machine learning algorithm. The results obtained can be a key for gaining insights from the dataset, forecasting the CKD status of the new patients and adopting good strategies for improving the safety, efficiency, and quality of the care processes toward CKD disease.

References

1. Chronic Kidney Disease. http://www.worldkidneyday.org/faqs/chronic-kidney-disease/
2. Romagnani, P., Remuzzi, G., Glassock, R., Levin, A., Jager, K.J., Tonelli, M., Massy, Z., Wanner, C., Anders, H.-J.: Chronic kidney disease. Nat. Rev. Dis. Primer. **3**, 17088 (2017)
3. Levey, A.S., Coresh, J.: Chronic kidney disease. Lancet **379**, 165–180 (2012)
4. Pontillo, C., Zhang, Z.-Y., Schanstra, J.P., Jacobs, L., Zürbig, P., Thijs, L., Ramírez-Torres, A., Heerspink, H.J.L., Lindhardt, M., Klein, R., Orchard, T., Porta, M., Bilous, R.W., Charturvedi, N., Rossing, P., Vlahou, A., Schepers, E., Glorieux, G., Mullen, W., Delles, C., Verhamme, P., Vanholder, R., Staessen, J.A., Mischak, H., Jankowski, J.: Prediction of chronic kidney disease stage 3 by CKD273, a urinary proteomic biomarker. Kidney Int. Rep. **2**, 1066–1075 (2017)
5. Chen, M., Hao, Y., Hwang, K., Wang, L., Wang, L.: Disease prediction by machine learning over big data from healthcare communities. IEEE Access. **5**, 8869–8879 (2017)
6. Gunarathne, W., Perera, K.D.M., Kahandawaarachchi, K.: Performance evaluation on machine learning classification techniques for disease classification and forecasting through data analytics for Chronic Kidney Disease (CKD). In: 2017 IEEE 17th International Conference on Bioinformatics and Bioengineering (BIBE), pp. 291–296. IEEE (2017)
7. Ghasemaghaei, M., Ebrahimi, S., Hassanein, K.: Data analytics competency for improving firm decision making performance. J. Strateg. Inf. Syst. **27**, 101–113 (2018)
8. Kestin, I.: Statistics in medicine (2018)
9. Ryu, S.: Book Review: Predictive Analytics: The Power to Predict Who Will Click, Buy, Lie or Die. Healthc. Inform. Res. **19**, 63 (2013)
10. Mikut, R., Reischl, M.: Data mining tools: data mining tools. Rev. Data Min. Knowl. Discov. **1**, 431–443 (2011)
11. UCI Machine Learning Repository: Chronic_Kidney_Disease Data Set. https://archive.ics.uci.edu/ml/datasets/Chronic_Kidney_Disease
12. Sossi Alaoui, S., Farhaoui, Y., Aksasse, B.: A comparative study of the four well-known classification algorithms in data mining. In: Advanced Information Technology, Services and Systems, pp. 362–373. Springer, Cham (2017)
13. Zhu, W., Zeng, N., Wang, N.: Sensitivity, specificity, accuracy, associated confidence interval and ROC analysis with practical SAS implementations. In: NESUG Proceedings Health Care and Life Sciences, Baltimore, Maryland, vol. 19, p. 67 (2010)
14. Alberg, A.J., Park, J.W., Hager, B.W., Brock, M.V., Diener-West, M.: The use of "overall accuracy" to evaluate the validity of screening or diagnostic tests. J. Gen. Intern. Med. **19**, 460–465 (2004)
15. Wolpert, D.H.: The supervised learning no-free-lunch theorems. In: Soft Computing and Industry, pp. 25–42. Springer (2002)
16. Sossi Alaoui, S., Farhaoui, Y., Aksasse, B.: Classification algorithms in data mining. Int. J. Tomogr. SimulationTM **31**, 34–44 (2018)

An Innovative Approach to Involve Students with Learning Disabilities in Intelligent Learning Systems

Fatimaezzahra Benmarrakchi(✉), Nihal Ouherrou, Oussama Elhammoumi, and Jamal El Kafi

Computer Science Department, Chouaib Doukkali University, El Jadida, Morocco
{benmarrakchi.f, ouherrou.n, elhammoumi.o}@ucd.ac.ma, jelkafi@gmail.com

Abstract. Innovations in healthcare education have fostered the development of assistive technologies which have contributed to making the learning environment and information more accessible to learners with learning difficulties. Especially, Intelligent Tutoring Systems (ITS) have proven the benefits of personalized learning. One of the distinctive features of the intelligent system is its Learner Model (LM). In this paper, we propose a LM that takes into consideration individual differences and tends to adapt system parameters for learners with Specific Learning Disabilities (SLDs) before the session begins. The purpose of this research is the development of conceptual bases and a constructional approach of a cognitive LM founded on differentiation. However, developing ITS requires many resources and information about learners as well as it demands a long time to build. To facilitate the design process, we propose a LM, called UPCLEE that takes into account several dimensions of learner's profile. This research demonstrates how the proposed model's levels are taken into account in the design of ITS and how it can be used to provide personalization in computer-based educational systems. In this study, we collected observations, interviews, and surveys and we used a grounded theory approach to develop our LM, then we conducted a user study with 12 students (4 with SLDs) to validate our proposed model.

Keywords: Healthcare education · Information and Communication Technology (ICT) · Specific Learning Disabilities (SLDs) · Intelligent Tutoring System (ITS) · User experience · Learner Model (LM)

1 Introduction

Students with Specific Learning Disabilities (SLDs) often have many kinds of difficulties that lead to academic failure or low achievement. The most common types of learning difficulties involve problems with reading, writing, math, attention, listening, and speaking, such as dyslexia, dyscalculia or dysphasia. SLDs refers to a disorder in one or more of the psychological processes involved in understanding or using spoken

M. Ezziyyani (Ed.): AI2SD 2018, AISC 914, pp. 39–50, 2019.
https://doi.org/10.1007/978-3-030-11884-6_4

or written language. The term SLDs does not involve learning problems that are primary the result of visual, hearing disabilities or mental retardation.

Dyslexia is one of the most common learning disabilities, it is a disorder manifested by difficulties in reading. According to [1], the percentage of dyslexics among the normal population is around 7%.

Recently, studies are focusing on the potential benefits of Information and Communication Technology (ICT) use in healthcare education to improve and develop interactive experiences that can assist and help students with SLDs [2]. For instance the work of [3] about the use of assistive mobile applications for individuals with dyslexia aimed at reeducating and monitoring the learning process, or the work of [4] about the inclusion of individuals with learning difficulties in virtual learning environment.

Although there are a variety of research within the areas of SLDs, ICT use, and a wide range of modeling approaches, there still seems to be a research gap. However, the effectiveness of several applications has not been demonstrated. Plus, there is no unified strategies in designing e-learning systems for individuals with SLDs neither guidance for choosing a model suitable for particular learner. Research is, therefore, needed on the instructional design side of ICT for individuals with SLDs.

LM is a key element in adaptive learning systems. However, the challenge lies in the fact that individuals with SLDs have specific cognitive ability characteristic and different learning needs. Although extensive research has been carried out on learner modeling and intelligent e-learning systems, there have been no studies found that investigate LM for individuals with SLDs. Hence, this present study took the initiative to explore the learning experiences of students with SLDs so as to propose an innovative approach based on differentiation, with the aim to design a LM that takes into account a several dimensions of learner's profile. Therefore, we decided to investigate the possibilities offered by advanced technologies, to develop a conceptual base and a constructional approach of a cognitive user model, which we called UPCLEE.

The rest of this paper is organized as follows. The next section covers related work, followed by our proposed approach in Sects. 3 and 4 presents the user study and conclusion and future work in Sect. 5.

2 Related Work

2.1 Communication Technology for Learners with SLDs

Some researchers have been interested in assistive e-learning systems, for instance the work of [5] that proposed an assistive learning environment to enhance the learning experience of learners with SLDs in their academic life. The aim of this assistive system is to transform the content in an acceptable way by learners with SLDs. The architecture of the framework contains 6 major modules as follows: Content repository, learner profile, assistive learning engine, transformation base, learners' goal and monitoring module. However, the main disadvantages of the system were that it was focused only on one major barrier of dyslexic learners, which is reading activity. Therefore, the system seems to be not useful for all types of dyslexic learners, because it does not differentiate between types of dyslexia.

Related studies [6] about the inclusion of students with learning difficulties in ICT use, proposed an adaptive mobile learning system based on the analysis of dyslexic students' learning style preferences. The outcomes stated that learners with dyslexia have strong preferences for a specific learning style, compared to learners from control group that have mild learning style preferences. Although, research solutions developed by these researchers were significant and adequate, most of them focused only on fundamental literacy skills, weaknesses and difficulties. However, they seem not helpful for all individuals with SLDs. Especially because the degree of their learning disabilities differs. Thus, there is still a lack of integrated tools that provide individuals with learning difficulties with the appropriate set of adjustments according to a diversity of individual learning needs.

2.2 Learner Model (LM)

LM has triggered interest from many researchers. Genetic Graph method [7] is the first approach to a learner-based modeling, the system analyzed the requisite skills for playing a game into atomic components and created links between these components. Recent research work [8] has been done on implicit user modeling based on artificial intelligence. Accordingly, implicit data captured during the interaction with web systems and statistical methods and clustering techniques were performed. The outcomes reveal a strong significant relationship between the users' cognitive styles and preference toward a specific type of learning content.

Many studies have proposed solutions to overcome the literacy barriers of students with learning disabilities. Some researchers have been interested in e-learning systems. One example is [9] who developed a software system for reading and writing called iLearnRW for students with dyslexia. Another example is [10] who proposed a LM technique for individuals with learning difficulties in virtual environments, or the work of [4] who studied the importance of personalized assistive tools for learners with SLDs. However, LM plays a principal role in learning and it has important implications for e-learning systems. LM can be defined as the process of creating a model of the learner to personalize a system. Generally, LM represents essential information about each learner and control her/his goals, the content she/he views, and the manner in which she/he navigates in the virtual environment. According to [11], LM is a representation of static and dynamic information about an individual that is utilized by the adaptive interactive system to provide adaptation effects. LM can be based on explicit or implicit information. Explicit collection of learner's information is provided directly by the learner through Web registration forms or questionnaires, while implicit collection of learner's information is extracted automatically by systems to presume learner's characteristics and it is obtained by tracking the learner's navigation behavior by interacting with the system.

3 Our Proposed Model UPCLEE

Learners are characterized by different learning styles, abilities, and interests. Differentiated instruction is a term that has been defined in the field of education as a teaching theory that implements varied instructional approaches and methods in order to be adapted according to learners of different ages, abilities and learning skills. So as to attain their goals in different ways and also to make learning interesting and engaging [12].

In intelligent learning systems, LM can contain different information depending on what we are trying to model, especially what characterizes our target learners. It represents what the system knows about the learner, this information could be cognitive, behavioral or psychological. LM can relate to one or more aspects of the learner such as: misconceptions, problem-solving speed, motivation, metacognitive aspects and working memory capacity. However, to design LM we should know the characteristics of each learner. Hence, the challenge lies in the fact that individuals with SLDs have specific cognitive ability characteristic and different learning needs. Therefore, our proposed model is founded on differentiation and it tends to analyze and adapt the learning environment that takes into consideration learners characteristics. This model takes into account different dimensions of learner profile. The main objective is to provide a structured learner profile and provide learning systems with relevant information to adapt the learning to the specificities of learners with SLDs. The idea behind this model is to introduce a system that pays attention to the specific needs of learners with SLDs, assesses, diagnoses their problems and provide help.

3.1 Levels of Our Proposed Model UPCLEE

The proposed model addresses different levels that serve to better understand the difficulties of learners with SLDs. UPCLEE (User profile, Preferences Profile, Cognitive Profile, Learning Profile, Errors Profile, and Experience Profile) focuses particularly on 6 levels wish are based on the researched theories in the respective domain as described as follows:

- Level 1 User Profile

Demographic Data: This is a static level that represents demographic information that represents the learner in terms of personal information which includes a set of attributes of identification, such as name, surname, age, gender, etc.

- Level 2 Preference Profile

Learning preference or learning style refers to the preferential way in which the student absorbs, comprehends and retains information. There are numerous learning models and theories that attempt to clarify and explain the learning styles differences, such as Kolb's learning styles model [13], Felder and Silverman [14], and VAK learning style model [15].

Previous work [6], investigated learning styles preferences of students with specific learning disabilities. Researchers administered VAK and Honey & Mumford questionnaires to 28 Moroccan students with ages between 8 and 10 years old, 8 students with dyslexia and 20 students without SLDs to compare student's preferred learning style. The outcomes suggested that individuals with SLDs have strong learning style preference. In the same study they proposed an adaptive m-learning game, which matches directly with students learning styles through the use of advanced digital technology. The study confirmed that when students have an understanding of their learning style dominance, they could be empowered to learn in terms of their strengths. Other study was carried out by [16] to investigate whether teaching to students with dyslexia's preferred learning styles would improve their performance and attainment in both literacy and numeracy, the researcher conducted a user study with seven British students aged between 7 and 8 years, using both qualitative and quantitative methods. The outcomes showed an improvement in performance and attainment in spelling and numeracy. It also indicated that teaching and learning styles influence the quality of learning, assuming that when students with dyslexia are taught to their strengths and given more ownership over their learning, then their whole school experience may be improved.

On the basis of the evidence currently available, it seems fair to suggest that providing an adaptive learning environment that takes into account learners' learning style could positively affect their performance. Further, if it is confirmed that the students are taught using their preferred learning styles, they might improve their attitudes to learning and behavior. Therefore, the objective of this level is to meet the needs of learners and determine their preferences for learning materials.

- Level 3 Cognitive Profile

Prior identification of the learner's needs and cognitive characteristics is an important aspect of the design process of intelligent e-learning systems. Cognitive styles are information processing habits representing the learner's typical style of perceiving, thinking, problem solving and remembering. In fact, each individual has his/her own styles for collecting and organizing information into knowledge [16]. However, to provide systems with this kind of information, at least a user profile is needed to gather user data. In a study conducted by [4], who investigated the use of dyslexic's cognitive styles and learning preferences as determinant factors for personalization. The authors used the interactions between cognitive traits model (CTM) [17], Felder-Silverman learning style (FSLSM) [13] dimensions, the dual coding theory [18] and VAK learning style model [15] to reveal some possible links between dyslexic's cognitive styles and learning preferences. The outcomes showed that the use of the cognitive style mapping for students with SLDs represent an important element in LM.

In other study carried out by [19] to investigate the benefits of incorporating learning styles and cognitive traits in virtual educational systems. The researchers conducted an experiment with 297 students was performed to improve student modeling, relationships between learning styles and Working Memory Capacity (WMC). The results showed the existence of a relationship between learning styles and cognitive traits.

Therefore, in this current investigation we add the cognitive profile level that represents cognitive style of learners with SLDs. This level emphasizes the importance of individual cognitive characteristics such as WMC, inductive reasoning skill, and associative learning skill.

- Level 4 Learning Profile

This level focuses on defining learning objects (LO) according to the learner's state of knowledge in order to provide optimal conditions for learning. LO is a small reusable group of contents to provide tutorials to the learner. There are numerous specifications and standards to develop LO such as IEEE LOM, IMS Learning Resource, and IMS CP.

In a study conducted by [19] they developed a personalized e-learning system for students with SLDs. It is an assessment model for alphabet learning with learning objects that includes: (i) Assessment model (ii) Ontologies and architecture and (iii) Knowledge-base and learning object. The researchers claimed that this system is useful for students who face dyslexia in elementary school mainly in the age group of 6 and 9 years old. The outcomes indicate the effectiveness of the use of e-learning methods, such as cognitive trait, ontologies and LO.

- Level 5 Errors Profile

Our approach assumes that each learner is unique, in that, the virtual learning environment must encourage and support individual differences [20]. This level identifies the particular errors of each learner. The phonological awareness that can encircle errors during reading and writing, errors in problem solving and repetitive errors. Indeed, the identification of the errors specific to learners with SLDs, makes it possible to identify the fields in which the learner has low performance and to propose to her/him aids in the deficit areas. The importance of this level was confirmed by many research studies across different languages and cultures. One example is the work of [21], about spelling errors of adults with dyslexia, the researchers conducted a user study with 100 students with dyslexia and 100 matched control students, all participant had Dutch as mother tongue. The results indicate 3 main error categories: phonological, orthographic, and grammatical errors. They indicate, also that higher-education students with dyslexia made on average twice as many spelling errors as the controls.

Other examples can be found in the study done by [22], who investigated reading and reading-related skills of 15 French-speaking adults with dyslexia compared with chronological-age controls and reading-level controls. The results reveal that adults with dyslexia exhibited lower phonological reading-related skills than control group only and were better than reading-level controls on the rapid automatic naming, also, a deficit in the sub-lexical reading procedure was observed when compared to reading-level controls. Also, the work of [23] about Chinese speaking aphasic patients reveals subtypes of acquired dyslexia and dysgraphia in Chinese, the outcomes assume that the language environment, and specifically the type of script used to read and write, play an important role in determining the phenotype of dyslexia in Chinese. Another similar study is the work of [24], who investigated the experience of Arabic learners (group of 32 students) when reading online text. The outcomes indicate that dyslexic learners made significantly more spelling errors in reading Arabic online text compared to non-dyslexics. This comparison between learners with dyslexia and chronological-age controls has yielded insights into the need to consider features of the Arabic language and the need to provide the appropriate set of adjustments according to the diversity of user differences.

The evidence presented in this level suggests that the identification of learner's errors in reading and writing is very important in learning environment and it should not be ignored.

- Level 6 Experience Profile

This level is interested in adapting the presentation of the knowledge and helping the learner navigates through the graph composed by all the components, taking into account the progress of the learner according to her/his experiences. Learner experience can be defined as an internal state (emotions, motivation, and mood) and sensations about systems' characteristics (complexity, usability, functionality) that learners may experience during their interactions with the learning system. Confirming to [25] the satisfaction of psychological needs such as competence, relatedness, autonomy, meaning, security are the principal sources of positive experience with interactive technologies.

Studies that investigated the experience profile can be found in the work of [26], who designed a model for serious game from a user experience perspective for deaf children experiencing difficulty in literacy learning. The proposed model includes four elements: user profile, learning strategies, serious games and requirements. The researchers conducted a user study with 6 deaf children from Mexico, aged between 12 to 15 and have problems in learning literacy. They used research techniques, including activities, such as observations, interviews with the teachers, and questionnaires so as to discover the needs and level of literacy learning. The researchers claimed that the proposed model might be useful for identifying the relevant needs to support deaf children and their teachers and they assumed that these four elements are important aspects to be considered in designing serious games for children with learning difficulties. Figure 1 illustrates the levels of our proposed model UPCLE.

3.2 UPCLEE Life-Cycle

The initialization of user profile can be considered as a starting point of the life-cycle of users with special needs. This step collects information on users and built a model of the learner based on UPCLEE's levels. Generally, there are two ways to obtain data, so that the system can initialize the learner model: implicit or explicit questions such as tests and questionnaires. Then, the construction of the learner model based on the gathered data. However, there exist numerous models to construct a learner model, for instance, stereotypes, overlay and buggy model.

Stereotypes make it possible to group all learners of an adaptive system into several groups according to certain characteristics that are generally shared. Stereotypes are a set of frequent characteristics of the user they represent a category or group of learners. There are two types of stereotypes; fix and default. In the fix type, the learner is assigned to a predefined stereotype at the abstract level, while the default type is more flexible. First, the learner is assigned to the initial stereotype. This means that the initial stereotype has a default value. Then, the system will observe the learners and gather

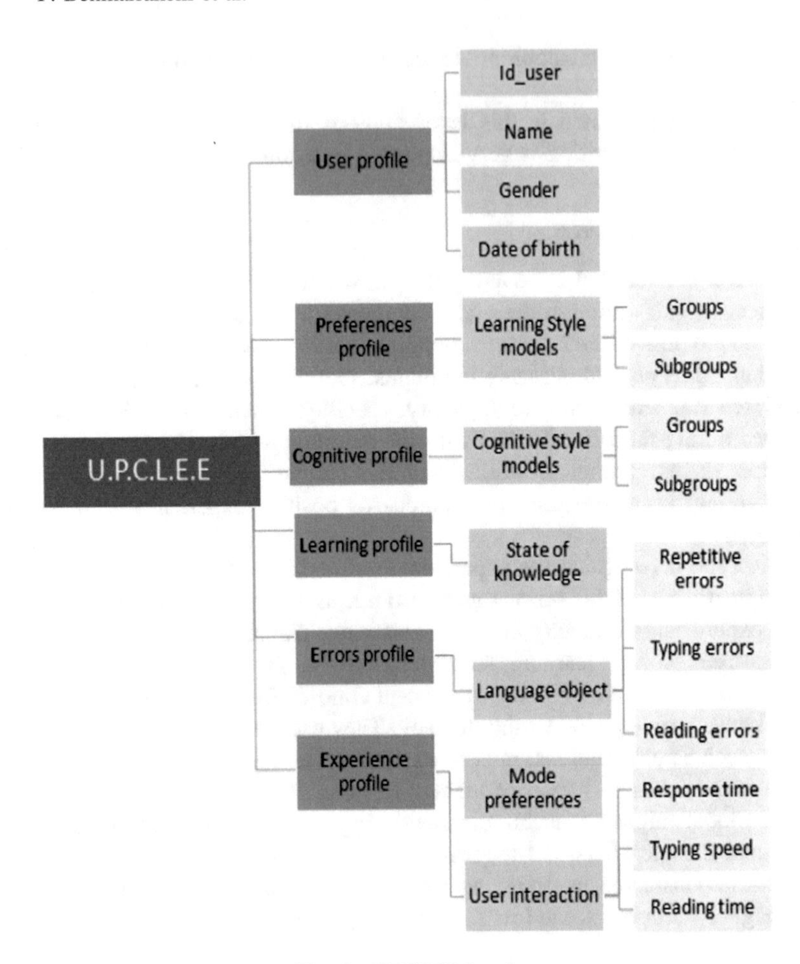

Fig. 1. UPCLEE levels.

their data in learning process. Finally, the system changes the initial stereotype to a new, more precise stereotype.

The overlay model is based on the fact that the learner model is a subset of the domain model. Buggy model is based on a list of potential errors that learners could commit by adding to the knowledge of the expert a library of misconceptions (bug library).

The construction is followed by the exploitation and updates. Finally, the reutilization of profiles that consists in the use of learner profiles to customize the learning activities to come. Figure 2 illustrates the life-cycle of our proposed model UPCLEE and the system prototype.

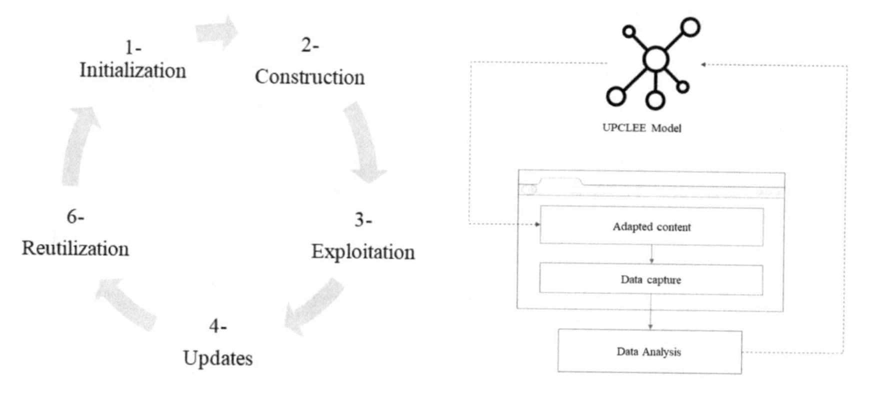

Fig. 2. The proposed adaptive e-learning system (a) UPCLEE life-cycle (b) System prototype.

4 User Study

In order to validate our proposed model, we conducted a user study with 12 students (4 with SLDs) to evaluate the importance of UPCLEE level's. In this present experiment, we focused on two UPCLEE levels, Errors profile and Experience profile. We compared the profile of students with and without SLDs.

Errors profile: the main objective of this level is to collect and identify student with SLDs errors in writing and reading in Arabic, then compare it with the control group. All participants were asked to read an online text and type it, the text contains about 80 words. The score was calculated as follows; how many misspellings per word. It is also possible that one single word contains more than one error; it can have different types of spelling errors.

Experience profile: the main objective of this level is to study the experience of students with SLDs in e-learning environments. For that, we focused on time spending in virtual environments, we used an educational game developed by [5] and we calculated the time spending in the game (seconds).

4.1 Participants

The sample of this study is composed of 12 participants (n = 12) and divided into two groups, the experimental and control group. The experimental group consists of 4 participants aged between 8 and 12 years. They were selected by the head of the phonology department of language-health center - El Jadida Morocco. The control group is composed of 8 children with the same age, they were selected from primary schools from El Jadida city. According to their medical records, they had no prior diagnosis of learning disabilities. All participants were native Arabic speakers. Table 1 presents the distribution of participants in terms of gender and group.

Table 1. Distribution of participants in terms of gender and group

	Experimental group	Control group (NoSLDs)[a]	Total
Girls (n)	01 (with Dyslexia and Dysorthographia)	04	05
Boys (n)	03 (one with Dyslexia and Dysorthographia and two with Dyslexia)	04	07
Total (n)	04	08	12

[a] No Specific Learning Disabilities

4.2 Results

The statistical analysis was performed using R software, version (3.5.0), with condition of $p < 0.05$ for significant results. Table 2 presents results of t-test.

Table 2. Results of t-test and descriptive statistics for errors profile and experience profile by groups.

	Experimental group		Control group (NoSLDs)		95% CI for mean difference		
	M	SD	M	SD	t	df	p
Errors profile							
Reading errors	38.75	09.32	04.75	02.43	7.172	3.20	0.0044**
Writing errors	66.75	11.87	03.62	03.02	10.46	3.19	0.0014**
Experience profile							
Time spending in the game	1005.0	57.44	615.0	146.0	6.59	9.809	<0.001***

* $P < 0.05$
** $P < 0.01$
*** $P < 0.001$

Primary results reveal that students with and without SLDs have different profile which confirms the importance of UPCLEE levels in e-learning environments.

5 Conclusion and Future Work

The growing importance of advanced technologies applied to healthcare education offers to students with various backgrounds the opportunities to develop their learning skills and overcome their difficulties. This work, showed how new initiatives in the field of education at the crossroads of healthcare and technology can be shaped and implemented in practice.

In this study, we proposed a cognitive LM for learners with SLDs, which we called UPCLEE. The model takes into consideration the characteristics of each learner. It collects 6 levels of learner profile: User profile, Preferences Profile, Cognitive Profile, Learning Profile, Errors Profile and Experience Profile. The primary evaluation confirms the importance of UPCLEE levels in e-learning systems.

However, at this stage this kind of initiative can only be achieved through multidisciplinary collaborations with many functional, technical and financial means. Therefore, the exploitation of such a model seems to be the next step, to realize a first functional prototype of our model. Clinical studies can then be carried out to prove the effectiveness of the proposed approach so as to support students with learning disabilities and other neuropsychological disorders.

Acknowledgment. This work was financially supported by an Excellence Grant accorded to Fatimaezzahra Benmarrakchi (2UCD2015), Nihal Ouherrou (3UCD2018) and to Oussama El Hammoumi (11UAE2017) by the National Center of Scientific and Technical Research (CNRST)-Minister of National Education, Higher Education, Staff Training and Scientific Research, Morocco.

The authors are grateful to the children who participated in this study, as well as their parents. The authors would like to acknowledge the president and staff at Speech-Language Pathology Service-Health center, El Jadida Morocco. The authors are also thankful to the speech therapist Ilham ELhousni for her valuable suggestions and recommendations.

References

1. Peterson, R.L., Pennington, B.F.: Developmental dyslexia. Lancet **379**(9830), 1997–2007 (2012). https://doi.org/10.1016/s0140-6736(12)60198-6
2. Kah, A.E., Lakhouaja, A.: Developing effective educative games for Arabic children primarily dyslexics. Educ. Inf. Technol. 1–20 (2018)
3. Madeira, J., Silva, C., Marcelino, L., Ferreira, P.: Assistive mobile applications for dyslexia. Procedia Comput. Sci. **64**, 417–424 (2015)
4. Benmarrakchi, F., Kafi, J.E., Elhore, A.: Supporting dyslexic's learning style preferences in adaptive virtual learning environment. In: 2016 International Conference on Engineering MIS (ICEMIS), pp. 1–6 (2016)
5. Assistive E-Learning System for the Learning Disabled - ScienceDirect. http://www.sciencedirect.com/science/article/pii/S1877050915003750. Accessed 09 Mar 2017
6. Benmarrakchi, F., Kafi, J.E., Elhore, A., Haie, S.: Exploring the use of the ICT in supporting dyslexic students' preferred learning styles: a preliminary evaluation. Educ. Inf. Technol. 1–19 (2016)
7. Goldstein, I.P.: The genetic graph: a representation for the evolution of procedural knowledge. Int. J. Man-Mach. Stud. **11**(1), 51–77 (1979)
8. Papatheocharous, E., Belk, M., Germanakos, P., Samaras, G.: Towards implicit user modeling based on artificial intelligence, cognitive styles and web interaction data. Int. J. Artif. Intell. Tools **23**(02), 1440009 (2014)
9. Cuschieri, T., Khaled, R., Farrugia, V.E., Martinez, H.P., Yannakakis, G.N.: The iLearnRW game: support for students with Dyslexia in class and at home. In: 2014 6th International Conference on Games and Virtual Worlds for Serious Applications (VS-GAMES), pp. 1–2 (2014)

10. Benmarrakchi, F.E., Kafi, J.E., Elhore, A.: User modeling approach for dyslexic students in virtual learning environments. Int. J. Cloud Appl. Comput. IJCAC **7**(2), 1–9 (2017)
11. Frias-Martinez, E., Magoulas, G., Chen, S., Macredie, R.: Modeling human behavior in user-adaptive systems: recent advances using soft computing techniques. Expert Syst. Appl. **29** (2), 320–329 (2005)
12. How to Differentiate Instruction in Mixed-ability Classrooms - Carol A. Tomlinson - Google Livres. https://books.google.co.ma/books?hl=fr&lr=&id=A7zI3_Yq-lMC&oi=fnd&pg=PR5&dq=Tomlinson,+C.+A.+(2001).+How+to+differentiate+instruction+in+mixed-ability+classrooms.+ASCD.&ots=Wlm1GvyQ_n&sig=8VGTDdlBor7IqfVtDgaWoWxj4kE&redir_esc=y#v=onepage&q=Tomlinson%2C%20C.%20A.%20(2001).%20How%20to%20differentiate%20instruction%20in%20mixed-ability%20classrooms.%20ASCD.&f=false. Accessed 15 Mar 2018
13. Kolb, A.Y., Kolb, D.A.: Learning styles and learning spaces: enhancing experiential learning in higher education. Acad. Manag. Learn. Educ. **4**(2), 193–212 (2005)
14. Felder, R.M., Silverman, L.K.: Learning and teaching styles in engineering education. Eng. Educ. **78**(7), 674–681 (1988)
15. Fleming, N.D., Mills, C.: Not another inventory, rather a catalyst for reflection (1992)
16. Exley, S.: The effectiveness of teaching strategies for students with dyslexia based on their preferred learning styles. Br. J. Spec. Educ. **30**(4), 213–220 (2003)
17. Witkin, H.A.: Individual differences in ease of perception of embedded figures*. J. Pers. **19** (1), 1–15 (1950)
18. Lin, T., et al.: Cognitive trait model for persistent student modelling. Presented at the EdMedia: World Conference on Educational Media and Technology, vol. 2003, pp. 2144–2147 (2003)
19. Graf, S., Liu, T.-C., Kinshuk, Chen, N.-S., Yang, S.J.H.: Learning styles and cognitive traits – their relationship and its benefits in web-based educational systems. Comput. Hum. Behav. **25**(6), 1280–1289 (2009)
20. Benmarrakchi, F., Kafi, J.E., Hore, A.E.: A different learning way for pupils with specific learning disabilities. Int. J. Comput. Technol. **14**(10), 6157–6162 (2015)
21. Spelling in Adolescents With Dyslexia: Errors and Modes of Assessment - Wim Tops, Maaike Callens, Evi Bijn, Marc Brysbaert (2014). http://journals.sagepub.com/doi/pdf/10.1177/0022219412468159. Accessed 05 Feb 2018
22. Martin, J., Colé, P., Leuwers, C., Casalis, S., Zorman, M., Sprenger-Charolles, L.: Reading in French-speaking adults with dyslexia. Ann. Dyslexia **60**(2), 238–264 (2010)
23. Yin, W.G., Weekes, B.S.: Dyslexia in Chinese: clues from cognitive neuropsychology. Ann. Dyslexia **53**(1), 255–279 (2003)
24. Benmarrakchi, F., Kafi, J.E., Elhore, A.: Communication technology for users with specific learning disabilities. Procedia Comput. Sci. **110**, 258–265 (2017)
25. Needs, affect, and interactive products – Facets of user experience | Interacting with Computers | Oxford Academic. https://academic.oup.com/iwc/article-abstract/22/5/353/684432. Accessed 08 Feb 2018
26. Cano, S., Arteaga, J.M., Collazos, C.A., Amador, V.B.: Model for analysis of serious games for literacy in deaf children from a user experience approach. In: Proceedings of the XVI International Conference on Human Computer Interaction, New York, NY, USA, pp. 18:1–18:9 (2015)

A New Method Based-Gentle Adaboost and Wavelet Transform for Breast Cancer Classification

Nezha Hamdi[1], Khalid Auhmani[2](✉), Moha Mrabet Hassani[3], and Omar Elkharki[4]

[1] High Institute of Engineering and Business (ISGA), Marrakech, Morocco
[2] Department of Industrial Engineering, National School of Applied Sciences, Cadi Ayyad University, BP 63, 46000 Safi, Morocco
k.auhmani@uca.ma
[3] Department of Physics, Faculty of Sciences Semlalia, Cadi Ayyad University, Marrakech, Morocco
[4] Faculty of Sciences and Technologies, Tangier, Morocco

Abstract. In this paper we have realized a comparative study of mammograms classification accuracy based on a new Gentle Adaboost algorithm for different wavelet transforms and different features. Our proposition deals with the combination of a new Gentle Adaboost based algorithm with three wavelets transforms. In this new algorithm, the main classifier is realized by weighted weak classifiers. These weak classifiers are constructed from the sub-bands of discrete wavelet transform, stationary wavelet transform and double density wavelet transform. Used features are extracted from transformed mammograms. We have investigated the effect of these wavelet transforms combined with the extracted features on the classification accuracy. Receiver Operating Curves (ROC) tool is employed to evaluate the performance of the propositions. Mammograms of MIAS Database are used as samples to classify. True positive rate is plotted versus false positive rate for different types of features and for Gentle Adaboost iterations. Results showed that the best area under curve (AUC), is reached for Zernike moments combined with double density wavelet transform and it is equal to 1 for both t = 10 and t = 50.

Keywords: Artificial intelligence · Image processing · Machine learning · Gentle Adaboost · Wavelet transform · ROC · Feature extraction

1 Introduction

The Boosting approach for classification purposes is an assembly of weak classifiers for final robust classifier [1–4]. The first boosting algorithm used in pattern recognition is AdaBoost (Adaptive Boosting) [1, 5]. The fundamental idea of the AdaBoost algorithm is the combination of weak classifiers to build robust classifier. A “weak classifier” is an elementary classifier which cannot classify accurately the training set. At each iteration of AdaBoost algorithm, we aim to find an optimal weak classifier by computing the classification error. Depending on the error value, we calculate the weight of

M. Ezziyyani (Ed.): AI2SD 2018, AISC 914, pp. 51–63, 2019.
https://doi.org/10.1007/978-3-030-11884-6_5

the weak classifier, and update the data weights (initially equal) so that the weights of misclassified objects are increased and the weights of well classified objects are reduced. This aims to find another weak classifier in the following iteration that classifies better misclassified examples. The final classifier is the hybridation of all selected weak classifiers with their weight. The AdaBoost algorithm is sensitive to noise. An improvement was proposed; it is the Gentle AdaBoost algorithm [6].

Our purpose in this paper is the classification of mammographic images. Gentle AdaBoost algorithm is used with discrete wavelet transform (DWT), double density wavelet transform (DDWT) and stationary wavelet transform (SWT). These wavelet transform are multiresolution analysis tools that have been recently applied to image processing, and various classification systems [7]. They are applied here for feature extraction. Gentle AdaBoost algorithm is used to build a robust classifier by aggregation of weak classifiers. Our approach is implemented in MATLAB. Performances are studied and evaluated on MIAS Database. The rest of sections is as follows. Gentle AdaBoost algorithm, wavelet transforms and different extracted features discussed in Sect. 2.1. In Sect. 2.4 we present the adopted methodology to build the robust classifier. Experimental results are presented in Sect. 3. Conclusion and perspective are presented in Sect. 4.

2 Materials and Methods

2.1 Gentle AdaBoost Approach

The Adaboost algorithm [1], is based on the principle that the opinion of several weak classifiers is better than that of a single complex and robust classifier. In the AdaBoost algorithm is proposed an a priori probability distribution on the learning set in terms of the response to the previous algorithm iteration. The AdaBoost algorithm is sensitive to noise. Propositions have been made to solve this problem like Gentle AdaBoost [6] or BrownBoost [8].

In Gentle AdaBoost, Each feature is considered as a weak classifier. In this context, the weak classifier learning corresponds to the detection of a threshold and a parity that indicates the direction of the inequality symbol that best separate the positive and negative examples. The algorithm selects the n most informative descriptors, give them a weight W and applies a threshold th. This approach is effective because of its stability and robustness when it comes to noisy data [9]. First, in Gentle AdaBoost algorithm [10] authors use a weighting scheme that exploits a function of margins which decreases slower than the exponential function used by AdaBoost. Gentle AdaBoost minimizes the exponential loss function of AdaBoost using Newton steps [11]. Secondly, Gentle AdaBoost is a variation of the Real AdaBoost approach which stimulates performance by applying a regression by the weighted least squares method. Furthermore, Real AdaBoost and Gentle AdaBoost don't normalize all learners weighted in the same way, since the normalization function of Real AdaBoost is given by [10]:

$$F_m(X) = P_W(y = 1|X) - P_W(y = -1|X) \tag{1}$$

Whereas for Gentle AdaBoost, updating the class of weighted probability is given by the following function:

$$f_m(x) = \frac{1}{2}\log\left(\frac{P_W(y=1|X)}{P_W(y=-1|X)}\right) \tag{2}$$

More details about Gentle AdaBoost algorithm can be consulted in [12].

2.2 Wavelet Transform

Wavelet transform is a very interesting tool used in image processing, computer vision, pattern recognition and other fields [13, 14]. Hamdi et al. [15] have used discrete wavelet transform combined with Gentle Adaboost for MIAS mammograms classification. The main reason for Wavelet transform robustness is its great flexibility for choosing bases and the low computational complexity [16]. Three different wavelets transforms are used in this paper; the discrete wavelet transform (DWT), the double density wavelet transform (DDWT) and the stationary wavelet transform (SWT) for feature extraction and weak classifiers generation. Background of DWT is explained in [15].

Stationary Wavelet Transform
The stationary wavelet transform (SWT) has a similar tree structured implementation without any decimation (sub-sampling) step. The main strength of SWT is its time-invariance property [17] which is useful in many applications. The SWT algorithm is slightly different from that of DWT. Figure 1 shows the SWT filter bank for one-level image decomposition. The four sub-bands obtained after the decomposition are approximation (LL) and detail, namely, horizontal (LH), vertical (HL) and diagonal (HH) sub-bands. LL band can be decomposed into a similar filter bank for next level of decomposition. Since, SWT does not include down sampling operations, it is a redundant transform. The size of the sub-bands remains the same for the decomposed image for any levels of decomposition in Stationary Wavelet transform [17, 18].

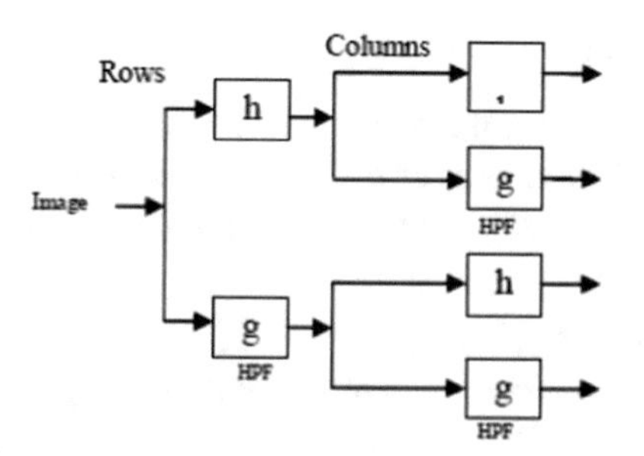

Fig. 1. Stationary wavelets transform filter bank for one-level image decomposition [18]

Double Density Wavelet Transform
The double density wavelet transform provides higher directional selectivity, better peak signal to noise ratio and visual perception than the spatial domain methods and

other frequency domain methods [18, 19]. DDWT is a shift insensitive, directional, complex wavelet transform with a very low redundancy factor of two regardless of the number of scales. Double density wavelets have a single scaling function and two wavelet functions. Figure 2 shows the DDWT scheme [18].

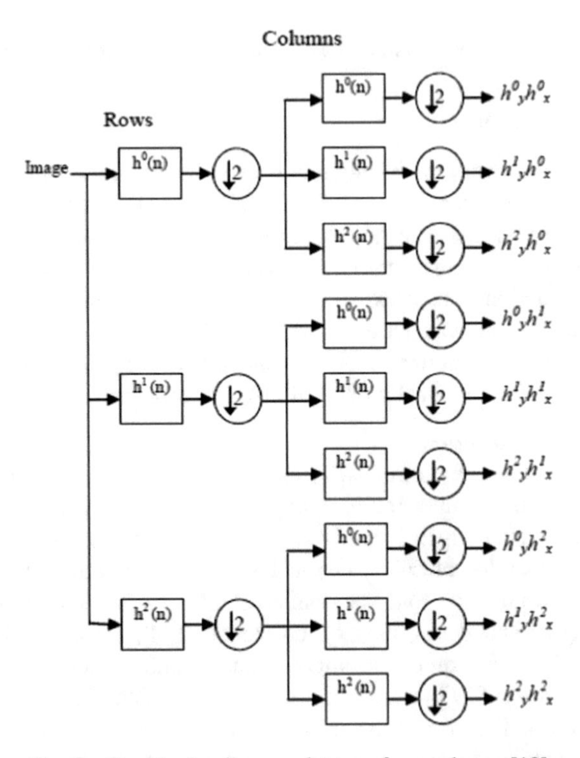

Fig. 2. Double density wavelet transform scheme [18].

2.3 Feature Extraction

Features are calculated to form the feature vector for subsequent learning step. These descriptors are extracted from a set of two classes labelled mammograms (normal and abnormal). After wavelet transformation of each mammogram, these following features are extracted [15, 20–23].

- Energy and the standard deviation.
- Tamura parameters: coarseness, contrast and directionality, histogram of 3 bins on the coarseness. In total, this group of descriptors forms a vector of six texture features.
- Radon's characteristics are calculated for angles 0°, 45°, 90 ° and 135°. We also calculate the histogram of 3 bins for the four series, which gives a vector of 12 features.
- Zernike's moments of order n = 12 are calculated corresponding to 49 features.

2.4 The Proposed Approach

The proposed approach presented in Fig. 3 performs a classifiers aggregation of "decision stump" type. The first classifier (corresponding to the first sub-band) is built using the equal weights. Several boosted classifiers, are cascaded as shown in Fig. 4 to achieve an efficient classification.

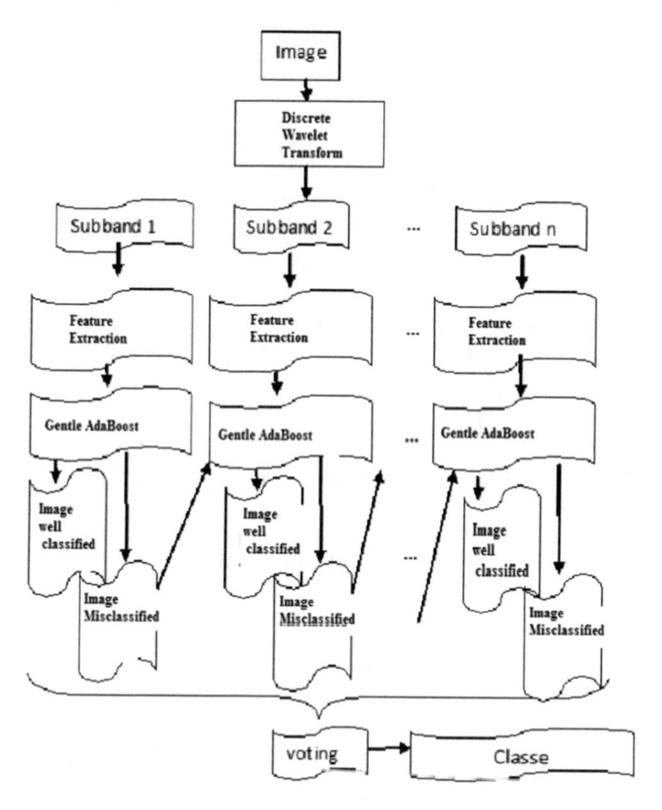

Fig. 3. The proposed approach scheme for mammograms classification based on Gentle AdaBoost and different wavelet transform

At each iteration, the optimal classifier is searched and low classification error is calculated. Depending on the error, we calculate the weight of the weak classifier, and update the data weights (initially equal) so that the weights of misclassified images are increased and the weights of well classified data are reduced (Hamdi et al. 2015). In order to improve the performance evaluation, the samples are sorted in each dimension and the error of stump is updated incrementally during the course in each dimension. The evaluation of the stump is very simple, as you only have to compare the attribute designated by the latter with a threshold calculated also during training. The stump defines an hyperplane orthogonal to an axis and since the number of stump is finite, it is possible to test them all and so find the one that minimizes the error function. The stump will always return the minimum drive error classifier.

The proposed algorithm combining gentle Adaboost and wavelet transform is as following:

The proposed algorithm:Input
Let S the Learning base
$S = \{(x_1, y_1)\ldots,(x_N, y_N)\}$

- Learning set of N= m + l objects, x labels yi, m number of negative objects (y=-1) et l number of positive objects (y = 1).
- Each object x_i is a grayscale image which undergoes :
  - A preprocessing
  - A wavelet transform (DWT or SWT or DDWT)
  - Features extraction
- Let w_t a probability distribution, initialized at 1/N
- Let N_h the number of algorithm steps, corresponding to the number of hypothesis f_t.
- Let L the number of sub-band
- F(x)=0

Output: Powerful classifier

Begin

While m< L Do

for t= 1……N_h

1 – For each feature j, adjust the regression function f_j of the weak classifier to the learning objects associated with their weights w_t by the weighted least square method.

The error associated to the feature is :

$$\varepsilon_j = \sum_i w_t \left| f_j(x) - y \right|$$

2 – Select the weak classifier f_t having the

smallest error ε_t

$$F(x) \leftarrow F(x) + f_t(x)$$

3 - Update weight penalizing the best classified examples by :

$$w_{t+1} = w_t e^{-y f_t(x)}$$

The final boosted classifier is the defined by :

$$F(x) = \sum_{i=1}^{N_h} f_t(x)$$

End

$$m = m + 1; \qquad w_t = w_{t+1}$$

End

3 Results and Discussion

3.1 Dataset

The evaluation of our proposition is carried out on the original mammograms of MIAS database [24]. These images are decomposed into regions of interest (ROI) of size 256 * 256 and applied our method on the ROI. 107 mammograms are used; 56 samples are tumoral and 51 samples are normal. Figure 4 shows an example of original image and a ROI containing Microcalcifications.

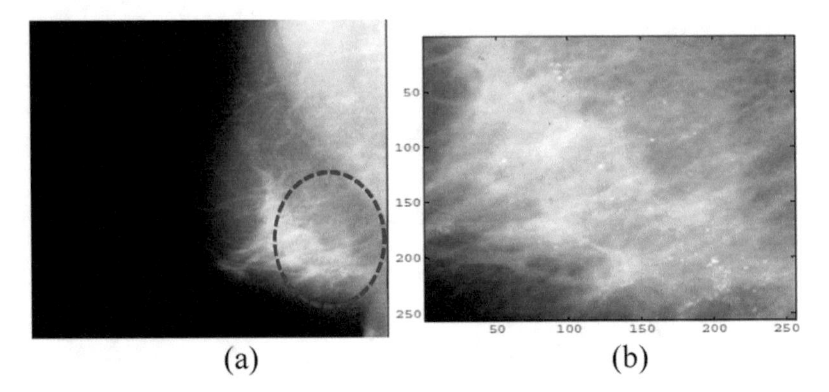

Fig. 4. Sample of the used mammograms: (a) 1024 × 1024 typical breast image (mdb233), (b) 256 × 256 region of interest containing microcalcifications.

3.2 Results

Receiver Operating Curves (ROC) is used to measure the performances of the proposed approach. The area under the ROC curve (AUC) indicates the classification accuracy. It can be interpreted as the probability of assigning a higher score to a positive object when it randomly chooses a positive and a negative object.

Experiments are achieved for two values of iterations $t = 10$ and $t = 50$. Figures 5 and 6 show the ROC curves corresponding to DWT and for $t = 10$ iterations and $t = 50$ iterations respectively. Obtained results show that the first observation that one can make is that Zernike moments provide the best classification rate of mammograms for all used wavelet transforms. For DWT the area under the curve (AUC) is high in both cases $t = 10$ and $t = 50$. The classification accuracy has been improved for $t = 50$ iterations for all feature types. In fact AUC = 0.98 and 0.99 for $t = 10$ and $t = 50$ respectively.

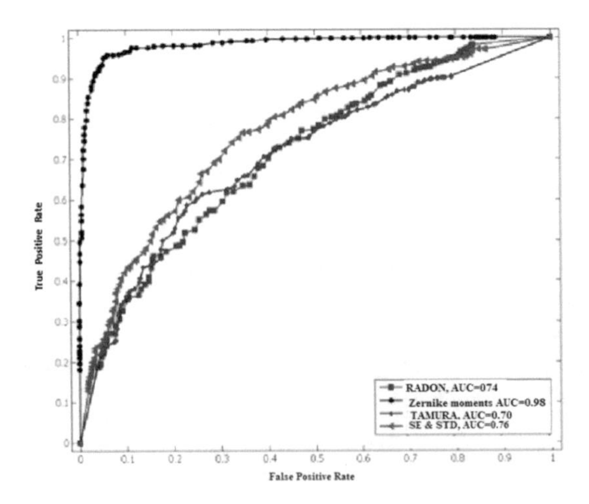

Fig. 5. ROC curves for different features and for t = 10 iterations, features are extracted from DWT sub-bands.

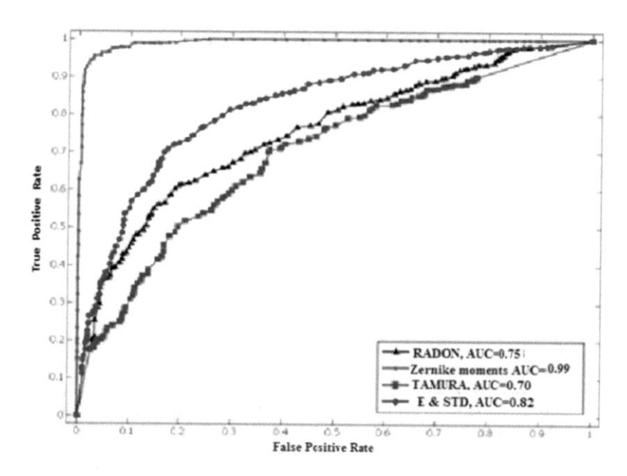

Fig. 6. ROC curves for different features type and for t = 50 iterations, features are extracted from DWT sub-bands.

Figures 7 and 8 show the ROC curves generated for DDWT and for t = 10 iterations and t = 50 iterations respectively. The AUC is equal to 1 and to 0.99 for Zernike moments and RADON features respectively in both cases of iteration number. TAMURA features and Energy and standard deviation provide an AUC around 0.78 without significant improvement versus the iteration number.

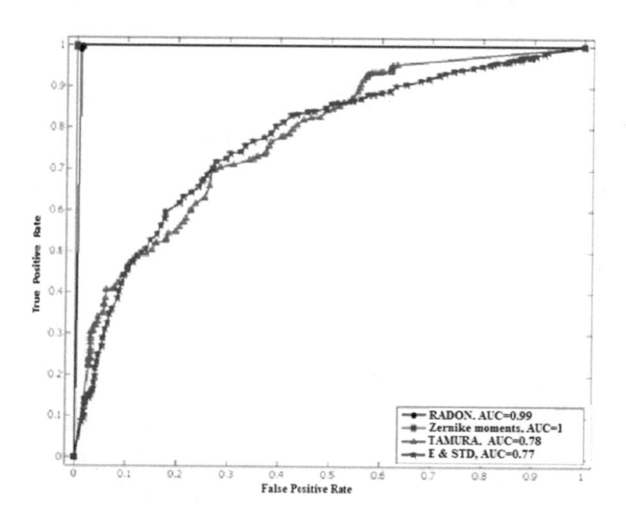

Fig. 7. ROC curves for different features type and for t = 10 iterations, features are extracted from DDWT sub-bands

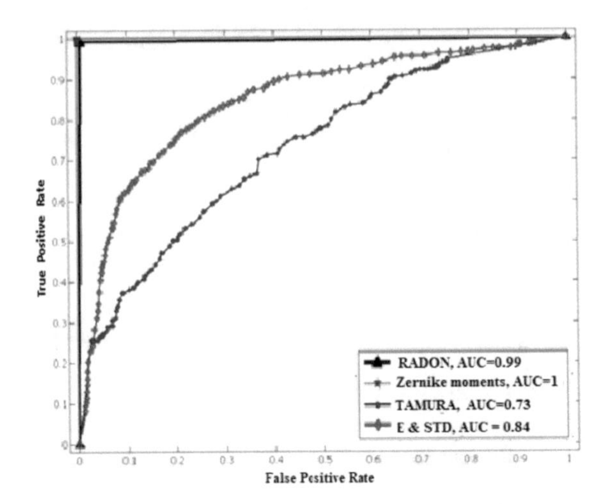

Fig. 8. ROC curves for different features type and for t = 50 iterations, features are extracted from DDWT sub-bands

Figures 9 and 10 show the ROC curves generated for SWT and for t = 10 iterations and t = 50 iterations respectively. The best AUC in this case is equal to 0.99 and to 0.97 for Energy and Standard deviation features t = 50 and t = 10 respectively. For the other features, there is a slight improvement for t = 50 vis-à-vis to t = 10.

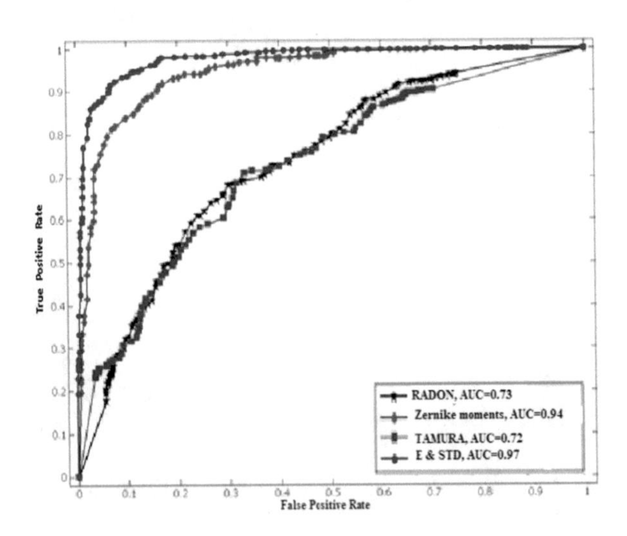

Fig. 9. ROC curves for different features type and for t = 10 iterations, features are extracted from SWT sub-bands.

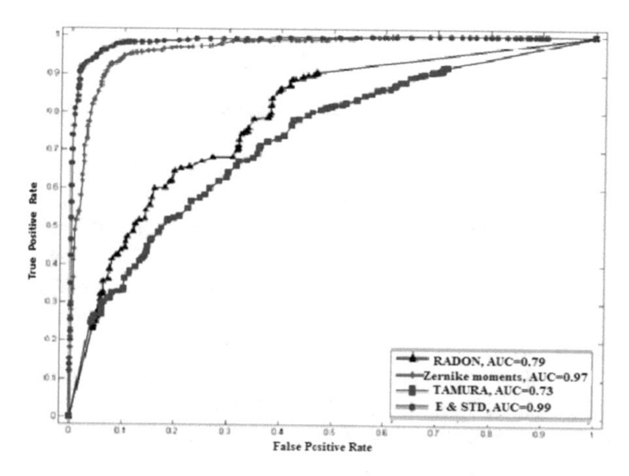

Fig. 10. ROC curves for different features and for t = 50 iterations, features are extracted from SWT sub-bands.

4 Conclusion

This work is dedicated to a comparative study of mammograms classification accuracy based on a new Gentle Adaboost algorithm for different wavelet transforms and for different features. Our main contribution in this study is the combination of a new algorithm based Gentle Adaboost with three wavelets transforms. In this new algorithm, the best classifier is constructed by weighted weak classifiers. The weak classifiers are extracted from the sub-bands of discrete wavelet transform, stationary wavelet transform and double density wavelet transform. Some features are also extracted from transformed mammograms. We have investigated the effect of these wavelet transforms combined with the extracted features on the classification accuracy

Firstly, the mammogram undergoes a wavelet transform after what some features are extracted; Zernike moments, Tamura parameters, Radon characteristics, Energy and standard deviation. These features are grouped in a feature vector to learn the weak classifier. For DWT the area under the curve (AUC) is near to 1 in both cases $t = 10$ and $t = 50$. The classification accuracy has been improved for $t = 50$ iterations for all feature types. For DDWT the AUC is equal to 1 and to 0.99 for Zernike moments and RADON features respectively in both cases of iteration number. TAMURA features and Energy and standard deviation provide an AUC around 0.78 without significant improvement versus the iteration number.In case of SWT, the best AUC is equal to 0.99 and to 0.97 for Energy and Standard deviation features for t = 50 and t = 10 respectively. For the other features, there is a slight improvement for t = 50 vis-à-vis to t = 10. The best obtained result is AUC = 1 for Zernike moments features combined with double density wavelet transform in both cases of the algorithm iteration number.

References

1. Freund, Y.: Boosting a weak learning algorithm by majority. Inf. Comput. **121**(2), 256–285 (1995)
2. Meir, R., Ratsch, G.: An introduction to boosting and leveraging. In: Lecture Notes in Artificial Intelligence, pp. 118–183 (2003)
3. Schapire, R.E.: The strength of weak learnability. Mach. Learn. **5**(2), 197–227 (1990)
4. Schapire, R.E.: The boosting approach to machine learning: an overview. In: Proceedings of the MSRI Workshop on Nonlinear Estimation and Classification (2002)
5. Schapire, R.E., Singer, Y.: Improved boosting algorithms using confidence-rated predictions. Mach. Learn. **37**(3), 297–336 (1999)
6. Hastie, T., Tibshirani, R., Friedman, J.: Elements of Statistical Learning: Data Mining and Inference and Prediction. Springer, New York (2001)
7. Nanni, L., Lumini, A.: Wavelet selection for disease classification by DNA microarray data. Expert Syst. Appl. **38**(1), 990–995 (2011)
8. Freund, Y.: An adaptive version of the boost by majority algorithm. Mach. Learn. **43**(3), 293–318 (2001)
9. Vezhnevets, A.: Modest AdaBoost – teaching AdaBoost to generalize better. In: Paper presented at the Graphicon, Novosibirsk Akademgorodok, Russia, pp. 322–325 (2005)
10. Friedman, J., Hastie, T., Tibshirani, R.: Additive logistic regression: a statistical view of boosting. Annal. Stat. **28**, 337–374 (2000)
11. Culp, M., Johnson, K., Michailidis, F.: ada: an R Package for Stochastic Boosting (2007)
12. Kanade, T., Jain, A., Ratha, N.K.: Audio-and video-based biometric person authentification. In: 5th International Conference, AVBPA 2005, Hilton Rye Town, NY, USA, 20–22 July (2005)
13. Lesecq, S., Gentil, S., Fagarasan, I.: Fault isolation based on wavelet transform. J. Control Eng. Appl. Inform. CEAI **9**(3;4), 51–58 (2007)
14. Cioaca, T., Dumitrescu, B., Stupariu, M.-S.: Lazy wavelet simplication using scale-dependent dense geometric variability descriptors. J. Control Eng. Appl. Inform. CEAI **19** (1), 15–26 (2017)
15. Hamdi, N., Auhmani, K., Hassani, M.M., Elkharki, O.: An efficient gentle adaboost-based approach for mammograms classification. J. Theor. Appl. Inf. Technol. **81**(1) (2015)
16. Zhang, B.L., Zhang, H., Je, S.S.: Face recognition by applying subband representation and kernel associative memory. IEEE Trans. Neural Netw. **15**, 166–177 (2004)
17. Nason, G.P., Silverman, B.W.: The stationary wavelet transform and some statistical applications in Wavelets and Statistics. In: Lecture Notes in Statistics. Springer, New York (1995)
18. Arivazhagan, S., Ganesan, L., Savithri, C.N.: Effective multi-resolution transform identification for characterization and classification of texture groups. ICTACT J. Image Video Processing, **02**(02) (2011)
19. Gopi, V.P., Babu, V.S., Dilna, C.: Image resolution enhancement using undecimated double density wavelet transform. Signal Process. Int. J. (SPIJ) **8**(5), 67 (2014)
20. Tamura, H., Mori, S., Yamawaki, T.: Texture features corresponding to visual perception. IEEE Trans. Syst. Man Cybern. SMC **8**(6), 460–473 (1978)
21. Howarth, P., Rüger, S.: Evaluation of texture features for content-based image retrieval. In: Proceedings of the International Conference on Image and Video Retrieval (CIVR 2004), LNCS, vol. 3115, pp. 326–334, Dublin, Ireland (2004)
22. Deans, S.R.: Hough transform from the radon transform. IEEE Trans. Pattern Anal. Mach. Intell. PAMI **3**(2), 185–188 (1981)

23. Murphy, L.M.: Linear feature detection and enhancement in noisy images via the Radon transform. Pattern Recognit. Lett. **4**, 279–284 (1986)
24. Suckling, J., et al.: The mammographic image analysis society digital mammogram database. In: Exerpta Medica International Congress Series, vol. 1069, pp. 375–378 (1994). http://peipa.essex.ac.uk/info/mias.html

A Conditional Sentiment Analysis Model for the Embedding Patient Self-report Experiences on Social Media

Hanane Grissette(✉) and El Habib Nfaoui

LIIAN Laboratory, Department of Computer Science,
Sidi Mohamed Ben Abdellah University, Fez, Morocco
Hanane.grissette@usmba.ac.ma

Abstract. Getting accurate, honest, reliable and credible minute insight is the most crucial objective of conducting medical and pharmaceutical research on social media. Nowadays, healthcare manufacturing companies use Sentiment Analysis (SA) to identifying the misleading of patients self-report experiences and shared medical information on social media. As a target level of analysis, a set of medical components in each document (post, message, tweet, etc.) have a semantic formalism which, similar to a dependency parse in the whole space of analysis regarding the time axes. However, Time property is been substantially very important allowing more real-time personalization to efficiently detect patient emotional state and what may be suffering from. Specially, when an irregular sentiment towards drugs or set of events may cover. In this paper, we aim at defining a conditional Sentiment Analysis model which summarizes sentiment information looking at the historical data towards dependent entities for yielding short or long-term predictions based on quantifying exactly what change is. This model hybrid an unsupervised biomedical concept extraction with autoregressive time series modelling. This hybridization aims at online updating the model by smoothing and extracting new relevant target features when deals specifically with newly emerged diseases, medical events, Drug issues and potential side effects. The evaluation results on a real pharmaceutical industry and healthcare tweets show that our proposed oriented-context method performs better than existing models.

Keywords: Medical information · Sentiment Analysis · Patient self-report · Social media · Healthcare · Time series modelling

1 Introduction

Nowadays, Sentiment Analysis (SA) is the pioneering approach used to analyze people's opinions about a product or an event to identify breakpoints in public opinion [1] towards a specific target/subject. Specifically, Patients and health consumers are storming intentionally their experiences and their opinions on Social media. However, regarding this daily massive shared patient's experiences, time property is substantially very important at detecting the minute sentiment information covered towards a set of drugs or events. For example, a negative event like chemical therapy or radiation

M. Ezziyyani (Ed.): AI2SD 2018, AISC 914, pp. 64–77, 2019.
https://doi.org/10.1007/978-3-030-11884-6_6

therapy may occur several times with given ADE (Adverse Drug Event) even more time of medication or patient change. Indeed, each time they may appear with an irregular sentiment polarity.

In the context of medical and pharmaceutical industry, the traditional form of clinical notes such as CRFs (Case Report Form) that used to summarize physical examination and details of the medical history of patients' experiences towards specific drugs or events is not credible and less efficient at defining the changeable emotional state of patients through the process of medication. Moreover, the existing methods of SA are less helpful at defining the real quantity of emotion due to the sentiment computation complexity regarding medical text that needs several transformations. Moreover, the major Issue is the inability of such general-purpose SA tools to accurately recognizing and defining the sentiment expressed towards medical components e.g. drugs, side effects or ADE (Adverse Drug Events) and newly emerged medical entities or diseases or treatments/scientific studies at large [2]. Indeed an irregular sentiment is covered towards these items when may appear collectively at a different time of medication.

In this paper, we present a hybrid system based on an unsupervised biomedical concept extraction in a given context with autoregressive time series modelling. In Order to define the daily model by mining and personalizing various changeable emotional state of users towards a specific target (medical entity) or subject (event).

The remainder of the paper is organized as follows. Section 2 gives a view of sentiment analysis approaches and methods in the same research context. Section 3, introduces the aspects of analysis were taken in this study. Section 3, we explained the proposed system and tasks. Section 4 we present the experimentation of baseline method and results of the proposed system applied on twitter microblogs. Section 4.3 summarize the contribution of this paper and outlines research directions towards achieving further advances in this area.

2 Sentiment Analysis

There has been an increased interest in analyses on health social media content. In 2016, Rodrigues et al. [3] develop a Sentiment Analysis tool "SentiHealthCancer (SHC-pt)" that improves the detection of the emotional state of patients in Brazilian online cancer communities. In other studies, Liu et al. [4] develop a framework consists of medical entity extraction for recognizing patient discussions of drug and events. Leaman et al. [5] explored the value of patient intelligence on pharmacovigilance on social media. Rill et al. [6] proposed early detection of the Twitter trend, which was faster than Google Trends. They considered temporal changes in the number of tweets to decide the emerging topic. The polarity of tweets was decided using sentiment lexica like SenticNet3, SWN, etc., where the polarity of novel words was determined by plotting a relational graph of emerging political tweets at different time periods.

Otherwise, there are many general-purpose [7] sentiment analysis tools such as VADER (Valence Aware Dictionary and Sentiment Reasoner) is a lexicon and rule-based sentiment analysis tool that is specifically attuned to sentiments expressed in social media. When those tool miss identifies several specific domain components and does not incorporate specific dictionaries cannot establish the accurate meaning of expressed sentiments toward specific Pharma or medical object/subject. We have tracked those gaps of the existing tools by analyzing Pharma's reviews based on the existing methods [8]. Otherwise, the previous studies are less efficient due to data sparseness, low accuracy due to non-consideration of context, type of text like culture text modifiers, and presence of domain-specific words, as they may result in an inaccurate classification of users' opinions.

3 Proposed System and Aspect of Analysis

Twitter is one of the most well-known online social networks that enjoy extreme popularity in the recent years. Precisely, a millions of patients' messages and reports have been posted each day. Moreover, proposed system aims at detecting real-world sentiment expressed towards a medical components on twitter. It is about analyze and get the latest and the credible survey by identifying embedding relation between patient self-reports. Briefly, it is three aspect based sentiment analysis model.

3.1 Aspects of Analysis

SA is the task of extracting sentiments and detecting attitudes concerning different topics and entities as expressed in textual input. The classical methods of identifying sentiment polarity aim at calculating sentiment' sum of global text based on sentiment dictionaries that are considered as a set of its individual words. Indeed, the amount of positiveness/negativeness is quantified in a binary fashion, which assigned High point to positive polarity and low point to negative polarity [9].

Text Aspect
Nowadays, SA has a big interest in not just identifying sentiment but also perform multi-task analysis based on several aspects of analysis [2]. Specifically, within analysing a sentiment of patients self-report contents. Collectively, these reports contain highly unstructured data combining text, drugs name, emoticons, ADE and unknown issues related to an event or drug that are used in making public aware of various issues [10]. Our system has considered three main aspect. Text aspect is important stage of identity relevant sentiment of patient messages or reports on social media [11], it still complicated due to the form of text that may so limited, informal and ambiguous. In this case, getting processed word-distribution space has big gain to determine opinion words [12]. Indeed, we explore in depth the semantic relation between text items to detect the relevant opinion word as features saving the correlation between them [13].

Entity Aspect

Medical features: The medical text or patient self-report may contain another type of entity as a combination of specific medical components e.g. medical event, side effects or ADE or drugs' name. In order to enhance the accuracy of sentiment classification is been mandatory to analyse sentiment regarding entity aspect of analysis.

In this stage, we attempt to recognize and define irregular medical features. Table 1 below presents some tweets in the medical context that is annotated based on Unified System language System (UMLS) knowledge sources. Thus, it clearly show how the tweet can contain dependent medical components and how can context and target of analysis may be different each time.

Table 1. Annotated tweets based on UMLS knowledge sources.

Tweet	Medical entities
"@nejmkplus: Question of the Week-An 85yo smoker w/mod stage II COPD presents for routine f/u & reports dyspnea http://t.co/4LcTwUj7iX"	T1Disease 52 55 mod T2Symptom-or-Side-Effect 105112 dyspneaR2 Comorbid_Condition Arg1:T1 Arg2:T2
"Weight loss can reduce asthma severity in obese adults http://t.co/pdn86EZ4NH"	T1Disease 24 30 asthma T2 Treatment 1 12 Weight loss T3Person 49 55 adults T4Weight 43 48 obese R1Treated_By Arg1:T1 Arg2:T2R2 Weighs Arg1:T3 Arg2:T4
"More asthma symptoms caused by mouse infestations than cockroach exposure http://t.co/RMj8vmv7qw"	R3 Is_Suffering_From Arg1:T3 Arg2:T1 T1 Risk-Factor 32 50 mouse infestations T2 Disease 6 21 asthma symptoms R1Increases_Likelihood_Of Arg1:T1 Arg2:T2

Real-word annotations are Performed an explicit way for system to recognize and label the topic and target of analysis.

Twitter features: Also, Twitter has specific features e.g. retweet count, hashtags, mentions and form of text. However, Twitter is responsible for popularizing the use of term hashtag as way to group conversations to follow a particular topic or highlight specific entity. Indeed, we go over Slicing and dicing data to analyse hashtags and the other related twitter entities, mentions and retweet count that are interesting to define who are factors can affect relevant daily sentiment appeared towards a specific target. Hashtag aspect can directly pop up a hidden subjectivity of related topic or entity. Table 2 below shows the most informative hashtag of 18992 hashtag appeared in 249581 tweets in many times.

Table 2. The most informative hashtag of 18992 hashtag appeared in 249581.

Hashtag	Frequency
GOT7	1249
갓세븐	1155
Trump	100
Cancer	120
Cancer	135
마크	621
Mark	543
뱀뱀	436
Love	433
BamBam	426
BT21	340

The plot below describes how some hashtags can appear frequently in patient reports. That may refer to an importance of object/subject in real time speaking (Fig. 1).

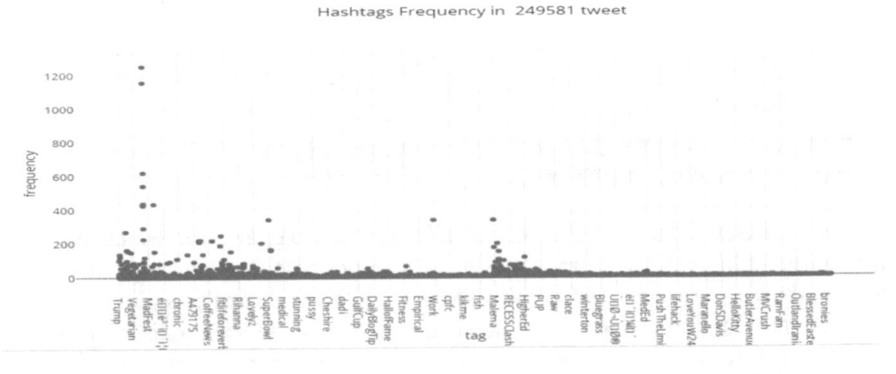

Fig. 1. The 50 most informative hashtag of 18992 hashtag appeared in 249581 tweets.

Regarding the time axes, hashtag frequency vary differently in several time fraction. As shown in the Fig. 2 below.

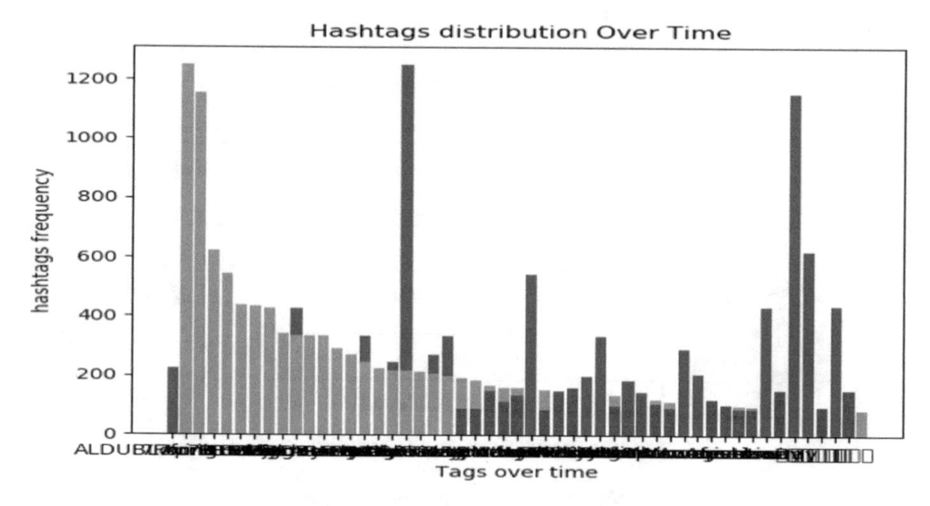

Fig. 2. Example of changeable frequence of hashtag over the time axes.

Time Aspect
Find the "signal from the noised patient report" in real time through the medication period is very interesting in the term of speed responsiveness to detect issues related drugs or treatments e.g. it allows looking at map time of inter-infections components (disease, drug or event).

We mainly concerned with Time series modelling that often suggests time aspect based analysis. Thus, time series generated from uncorrelated report/tweet that is generally motivated by the presumption that correlation between adjacent items in time is best explained in terms of a dependence of the current value on past values. The time domain approach focuses on modelling some future value of a time series as a parametric function of the current and past values.

3.2 Proposed System

Our proposed system present a conditional sentiment analysis to detecting new irregular features based on past features. In the first level, we aim at preparing our space to be as an input of filtering and selecting relevant features. Indeed the selection features was performed based on three aspects of analysis, that is will combine each time to be as an input of Autoregressive learning method. The daily update aims at detecting irregular features based on time series. When our system will able to label emerged entities based on historical data of past irregular features. As shown in the Fig. 3.

Data Streaming: Streaming Data is data that is generated continuously when interacting with Twitter via a REST API, we can search for existing tweets in fact, that is,

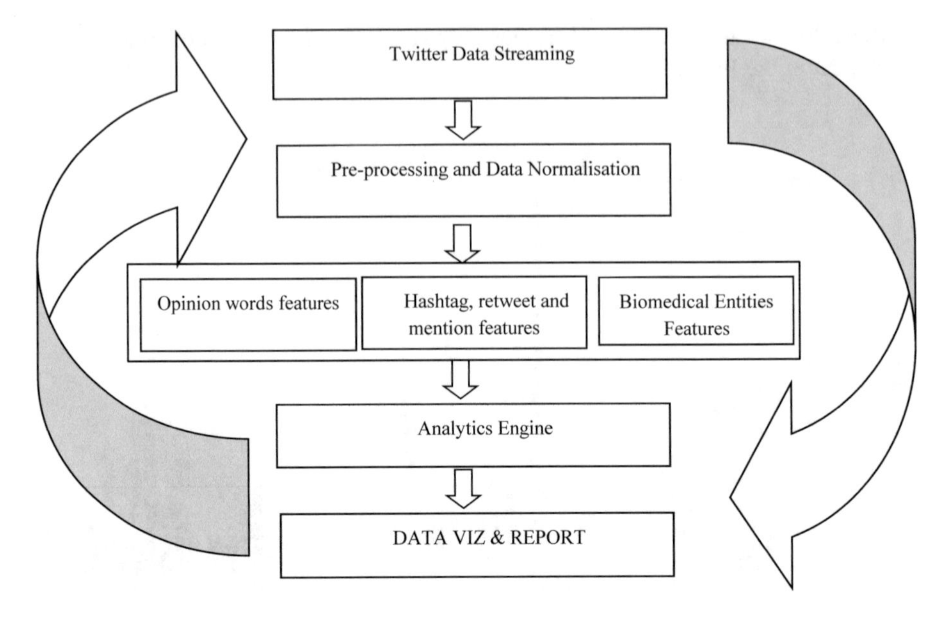

Fig. 3. View of proposed system

tweets that have already been published and made available for search. Often these APIs limit the amount of tweets you can retrieve, not just in terms of rate limits as discussed in the previous section, but also in terms of time span. In fact, it's usually possible to go back in time up to approximately one week, meaning that older tweets are not retrievable. A second aspect to consider about the REST API is that these are usually the best effort, but they are not guaranteed to provide all the tweets published on Twitter, as some tweets could be unavailable to search or simply indexed with a small delay. On the other hand, the Streaming API looks into the future. Once we open a connection, we can keep it open and go forward in time. By keeping the HTTP connection open, we can retrieve all the tweets that match our filter criteria, as they are published.

The Streaming API is, generally speaking, the preferred way of downloading a huge amount of tweets, as the interaction with the platform is limited to keeping one of the connections open. On the downside, collecting tweets in this way can be more time consuming, as we need to wait for the tweets to be published before we can collect them. To summarize, our system use the Streaming API to download and seek the massive amount of tweets in medical and pharmaceutical context.

Preprocessing Data: This step is about prepare collected unstructured data instead, that is, the raw text of the tweet. We'll use text preprocessing method, normalization and we'll perform some statistical analysis on the tweets.

However, the data preprocessing is a crucial step in sentiment analysis [11], since selecting the appropriate preprocessing methods, the correctly classified instances can be increased [12]. In view of the above, our system used combinations of methods:

- Tokenization.
- Emoticons replacement.
- Punctuation marks.
- Word normalization.
- Regular expressions operations.
- Removing other twitter components: URL and slang stuff that is considered as twitter abbreviation like RT (RT is an abbreviation for ReTweet, which is like Repeat).

Features Extraction: Opinion words model is created at first level, n-grams method is used for developing opinion-word features. As mentioned above, a number of additional features that occasionally can enhance our system to be more concisely in calculating real-word expressed sentiment towards drug name, medical event or company name. E.g. hashtags, retweeted count, mentions and medical entities. Medical entities can be diseases, drugs, symptoms, etc. Previously, researchers in the field have used hand crafted features to identify medical entities in medical literature. It has been found that in contrast with semantic approaches which require rich domain-knowledge for rule or pattern construction, statistical approaches are more scalable. Medical Entity Recognition is a crucial step towards efficient medical texts analysis [14]. In recent years, tools such as MetaMap and cTAKES have been widely used for medical concept extraction on medical literature and clinical notes. The Case of QuickUMLS [15] a fast, unsupervised, approximate dictionary matching algorithm for medical concept extraction.

In this study, we extend unsupervised biomedical concept extraction medical entity recognition for tweets based on The UMLS, or Unified Medical Language System, is a set of files and software that brings together many health and biomedical vocabularies and standards to enable interoperability between computer systems. Then, a second medical features model was created based on QuickUMLS. Moreover, we have developed an additional functions of specific twitter setting to seek related features: Hashtags and mentions. As shown in the previous section twitter features like hashtag that may occurred frequently in several patient report will hardly correlated with expressed sentiment behind.

Analytics Engine: Stream learning approach suggest incremental changes to the algorithm basically, its retraining as new record on a new set of tweets come in. the updating process applied on whole space. Our system is based on this stochastic calculation in which future values are estimated based on past values regarding each time at the combination set of features and sentiment.

The supporting new main function of our system:

- Quantify exactly what change is over time and the sentiment behind.
- Tracking the relationship between irregular features from time perspective.

Often Machine learning task operate with a dataset that has a single slice of time or don't consider the time aspect at all. Our system time-dependent is based on classified tweet to get link extracted feature with a given sentiment score. Each time irregular feature appears, sentiment score will be firmly informed and fed into autoregressive algorithm to generate a new model. As the primary objective of time series analysis is to provide a statistical setting for describing the character of data. The case of our system that is defined a collection of random features sentiment-labeled indexed according to the order they are obtained in time. In order to yield the correct class and confident prediction of each new input, we attempt to discretize our extraction model. That means, we make a number of statistical properties repeat constantly over time. In this step we use Kalman Filter for fitting a modified form of continuous time autoregressive model, which can be particularly useful with uncorrelated twitter data as sampled time series. Briefly, Kalman Filter uses a series of measurements observed over time to produce estimate of unknown variable as shown in Fig. 4. The case of our system, when embedded patient report has many unknown components. In a fixed interval a set of irregular features were created when unobserved components Estimation is conditional on the information made available after time t. as shown in the Fig. 4.

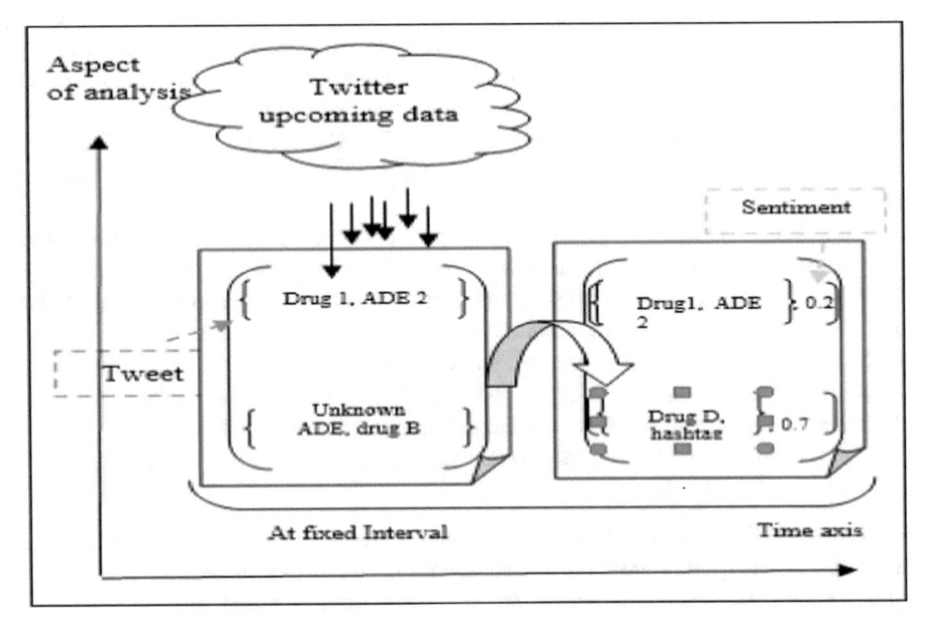

Fig. 4. Describe how connect the values at adjacent time period

4 Experimentation and Discussion

4.1 Dataset

We use sentiment140 (sentiment140, s.d.) dataset in this step, it contains 1,600,000 tweets extracted using the twitter API that were hand-classified. The polarity of the tweet (*0* = negative, *2* = neutral, *4* = positive). In addition, we rescaled sentiment value as range of values from 0 (completely negative) to 1 (completely positive) and assume that values from 0.35 to 0.50w are somewhere in the middle and they are neutral.

4.2 Baseline Model

The baseline model is the well-known model that hybrid lexicon-based approach and Machine learning algorithm. Indeed, it is a static quantification based on TF-IDF vectorization and uses regression learning method. We used Rest API to collect tweets in the context of the pharmaceutical industry. Table 3, in this table the following information, text of tweet, value of sentiment given by the baseline tool.

Table 3. Results of baseline on over 1 M tweets.

Tweet	Medical entity	Sentiment	Polarity
@novartis phrama Asthma plus anxiety plus food is a bad time	Asthma [disease] Anxiety [frequent word on ADE]	0.4794693	Negative
@furlermate Awe I have asthma so I feel your pain	Asthma [disease] Pain [frequent word on ADE]	0.1683138	Negative
Major weight loss decreases risk of asthma attacks http://t.co/6X0NXkH4ij	Asthma attack [effect drug]	0.4999725	
Fr @MyKembangSepatu Common asthma steroids linked to side effects in adrenal glands: After stopping steroids c… http://t.co/QmBrVhEzkm	Asthma [disease] Asthma steroids [ADE] Side effects in adrenal glands [other] Steroids [drug]	0.6101256	Positive
Daniel Radcliffe is one of the God's most unattractive creations since the aardvark	Aardvark [drug] Unattractive [frequent word on ADE]	0.6523491	Positive
Nasal vs throat microbiome diversity with differential risk for asthma. #AAAAI15	Nasa, throat [drugs] Risk for asthma [appeared ADE]	0.6872751	Positive
Philadelphia Zoo mourns death of 23-year-old black bear A 23-year-old Asiatic black bear who had been battling cancer for several months was…	Cancer [disease] Death [frequent word on ADE]	0.6095794	Positive

In the above results, classified tweet have bad estimation, thus the baseline model do not able to adopt the existing relationship between medical entity (asthma steroids), disease (asthma attacks) and ADEs (Common asthma steroids linked to side effects in adrenal glands) that can hardly change the quantified sentiment every time they appeared collectively. Specifically, when speaker's experiences linked to specific healthcare/pharmaceutical firms.

4.3 Results and Output Data from the Study

In the previous section, we highlight how our system can be more concisely to define the hidden sentiment information that correlates temporally with many modalities regarding irregular components.

In what follows, we present the results obtained by applying Kalman filter parameters generated from uncorrelated features as based-model for continuous time series fitting, as described in the previous section. The proposed method is a statistical measure that summarizes sentiment information looking at the historical data towards dependent entities from the time perspective. It deals specifically with newly emerged diseases, events or Drug's ADE. This model will minimize the annotation cost and get dynamic identification of real word entities while maximizing the performance of our sentiment classification Machine Learning based. Whether a public sentiment indicator extracted from daily twitter data. To this end, we have streamed a large number of tweets from the present. Table 4 show some obtained results on a different slice of time. As shown in Fig. 5 many sentiments covered differently over the time. That is clearly described by time series modeling in Fig. 6. On the same day, we have a changeable emotional state ranged from 0, 1 extremely negative to 0, 9 extremely positive towards several medical components (drugs names, medical events), scientific studies or pharmaceutical company name at large. Indeed, medical components may frequently capture varied elements ranging from medical issues, product accessibility issues to potential side effects.

Table 4. Obtained results of experiments on different time interval

Twitter data	Time interval	Positive tweets	Negative tweets	System accuracy
11768 tweet	From [Thu Nov 02 22:55:36 +0000 2017] To [Thu Nov 02 22:59:22 +0000 2017]	120	40	0,85
49993 tweet	From [Fri Jan 05 12:54:01 +0000 2018] To [Jan 05 12:54:01 +0000 2018]	180	111	0,70
32428 tweet	From [Sat Jun 03 21:35:51 +0000 2018] To [Sat Jun 03 21:35:51 +0000 2018]	129	87	0,80
4903 tweet	From [Fri Apr 15 01:57:47 +0000 2018] To [Fri Apr 15 01:59:47 +0000 2018]	210	91	0,77
5993 tweet	From [Sat Jun 03 21:35:51 +0000 2018] To [Sat Jun 03 21:40:01 +0000 2018]	20	60	0,75

When observations are irregular in time space, modifications to the estimators need to be made. Time series problems usually look at four main components:

- Seasonality: it aims at seasonal behavior that assume a series is generated as the sum of trend effect, and error.
- Trends: it aims at noting the gradually increasing underlying trend and the rather regular variation.
- Cycles: It tends to exhibit repetitive behavior, with regularly repeating cycles that are easily visible. This periodic behavior is of interest because underlying processes of interest may be regular and the rate or frequency of oscillation characterizing the behavior of the underlying series would help to identify them.
- Irregular components: regarding time axes in patients life through medication process, several drugs issues are possible, new diseases emerged can appear with unknown ADE.

In Order to prove the efficiency and the ability of our system to detect and solve problems that is change. We should detect a frequency of detected irregular components over seasonality and others components. We can seek another type of setting and specific irregular features in this context of analysis several drugs/events depending seasonality and periodic factors. In the presence of uncertainty caused by noised and emotional state of the speaker, the main objective of proposing Kalman filter as learning algorithm is to combining sentiment information and take advantage of the appeared correlations between past defined components and newly emerged ones based on stream information continuously changing.

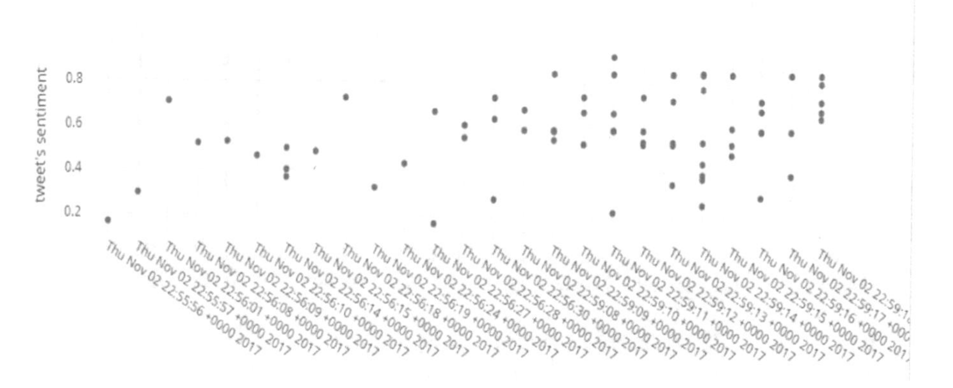

Fig. 5. Describes how connect the values at adjacent time periods

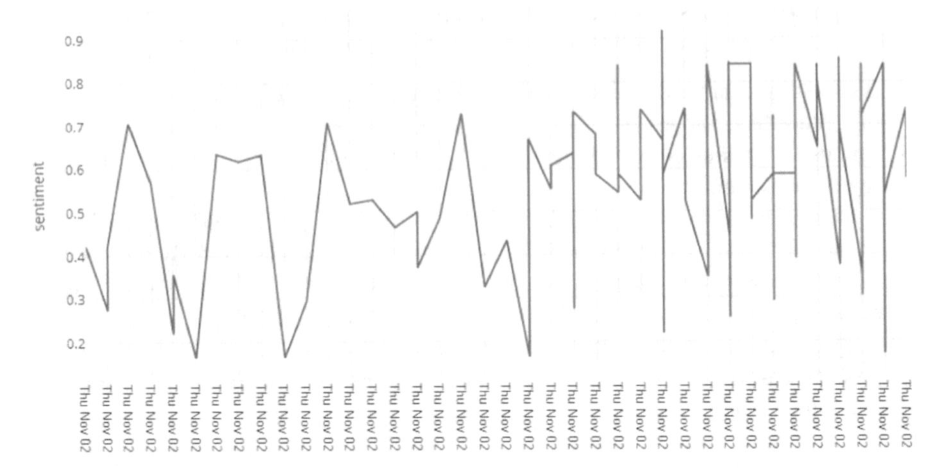

Fig. 6. Covered sentiment over Time of 100 tweet in 60 s on Thu Nov 02 22:55:57:01–60

5 Conclusion

SA is offering real opportunities to obtain fine grain data on patients and their environment that ensures a competitive edge to better understanding patients' experiences shared on social media. Turning patients' opinions into actionable information is having a profound impact on healthcare and pharmaceutical firms. Patients self-reports on social media, frequently capture varied elements ranging from medical issues, product accessibility issues to potential side effects. The case of our system that aim at identifying the embedded relationship between those components over the time axes.

Our perspective study aim at enhancing capabilities' system of better observing patients' physiological signals and helps provide situational awareness to the bedside and have an approximate idea of what the general mood is. Otherwise, from the time perspective, we can reconstruct visually some original hypothesis that may support patient and save lives.

References

1. Akcora, C.G., Bayir, M.A., Demirbas, M., Ferhatosmanoglu, H.: Identifying breakpoints in public opinin. In: SigKDD, Proceedings of the First Workshop on Social Media Analytics (2010)
2. Ravi, K., Ravia, V.: A survey on opinion mining and sentiment analysis: tasks, approaches and applications (2015). https://doi.org/10.1016/j.knosys.2015.06.015
3. Rodrigues, R.G., das Dores, R.M., Camilo-Junior, C.G., Rosa, T.C.: SentiHealth-cancer: a sentiment analysis tool to help detecting mood of patients in online social networks. http://dx.doi.org/10.1016/j.ijmedinf.2015.09.007
4. Liu, X., Chen, H.: A research framework for pharmacovigilance in health social media: identification and evaluation of patient adverse drug event reports

5. Leaman, R., Wojtulewicz, L., Sullivan, R., Skariah, A., Yang, J., Gonzalez, G.: Towards internet-age pharmacovigilance: extracting adverse drug reactions from user posts to health-related social networks. In: Proceedings of the 2010 Workshop on Biomedical Natural Language Processing, Association for Computational Linguistics, pp. 117–125 (2010)
6. Rill, S., Reinel, D., Scheidt, J., Zicari, R.V.: PoliTwi: early detection of emerging political topics on twitter and the impact on concept-level sentiment analysis. Knowl.-Based Syst. **69**, 24–33 (2014)
7. Tang, H., Tan, S., Cheng, X.: A survey on sentiment detection of reviews. Expert Syst. Appl. **36**, 10760–10773 (2009)
8. Grissette, H., Nfaoui, E.H., Bahir, A.: Sentiment analysis tool for pharmaceutical industry & healthcare. Trans. Mach. Learn. Artif. Intell. (2017)
9. Catal, C., Nangir, M.: A sentiment classification model based on multiple classifiers. Elsevier (2017). https://doi.org/10.1016/j.asoc.2016.11.022
10. Jusoh, S., Alfawareh, H.M.: Techniques, applications and challenging issue in text mining. Int. J. Comput. Sci. Issues **9**, 431 (2012)
11. Singh, T., Kumari, M.: Role of text pre-processing in twitter sentiment analysis. **89**, 549–554 (2016). https://doi.org/10.1016/j.procs.2016.06.095. Elsevier
12. Krouska, A., Troussas, C., Virvou, M.: The effect of preprocessing techniques on Twitter sentiment analysis. IEEE (2016). https://doi.org/10.1109/iisa.2016.7785373
13. Wilson, T., Wiebe, J., Hoffmann, P.: Recognizing contextual polarity: an exploration of features for phrase-level sentiment analysis
14. Awachate, P.B., Kshirsagar, V.P.: Improved Twitter sentiment analysis using N gram feature selection and combinations. Int. J. Adv. Res. Comput. Commun. Eng. **5**(9), 154–157 (2016)
15. Soldaini, L., Goharian, N.: QuickUMLS: a fast, unsupervised approach for medical concept extraction (2016)

Clustering and Social Recommendation Applied in Health Community of Practice

Meriem Hafidi(✉), El Hassan Abdelwahed, Sara Qassimi, and Rachid Lamrani

Faculty of Sciences Semlalia Marrakech FSSM, Cadi Ayyad University, Marrakesh, Morocco
{meriem.hafidi, sara.qassimi, rachid.lamrani}@ced.uca.ac.ma, abdelwahed@uca.ac.ma

Abstract. Social networks are increasingly used to exchange information. The social users are the main origin of the shared web resources and contents. However, they are also influenced by these shared data. The exchanges and interactions produced are an important element for defining the profiles of these users. In this paper, we investigate modeling of individuals using a user-centered model, in particular the activity and social pressure features. We propose a user profile enrichment approach based on extracted tags from shared resources. Our goal is to link similar users in order to build sub-networks according to users' profiles. Thus, determining the central and important nodes in the network will establish basis for the web resources recommendation, information diffusion and community resuscitation. Our research will interest doctors' communities to share their knowledge through network. It will teach the most basic health care information to the patients of certain chronic diseases such as diabetes.

Keywords: Social networks · User profile · Dynamic of interactions and communities detection · Recommendation · Collective intelligence · Health community of practice

1 Introduction

A social network is a way of connecting people; it promotes interaction among users. Linked individuals within a social network exchange information such as messages and share resources. One of the first assets of social networks is the speed of information dissemination: a user decides to share the information with his neighbors who could read it, or send it to targeted users through messages. Another interesting example is the recommender systems, which are mainly based on the dissemination of information to well-targeted and selected subsets in the network. This application is observed in the field of digital marketing or also to maintain a dynamic of communities through the resuscitation of information and dead resources. One of the challenges of social networks is to increase the number of users, the detection of communities and the study and analysis of exchanges and interactions between users [1]. These interactions can be of different kinds; either direct exchange of information between the users or via the sharing of resources in a context of collaborative activities.

M. Ezziyyani (Ed.): AI2SD 2018, AISC 914, pp. 78–89, 2019.
https://doi.org/10.1007/978-3-030-11884-6_7

The dynamics of Interactions between users, the sharing of resources and exchanges between them have an impact on the creation of communities within networks and the emergence of collective behavior. The interactions between members of the network reflect the type of their behaviors and activities within the network. In most cases, interactions born from the dissemination and sharing of information. This last idea strongly depends on the attitudes of users within the network to disseminate information. Users have different approaches to sharing content and information [2]. It is crucial to analyze and maintain a dynamic dissemination of information between users in order to ensure effective collaboration between them and the emergence of a collective intelligence. In fact, the dynamicity of information dissemination and so the dynamic of interactions among users depend on the users' interest, their behavior and their positioning within the network.

The determination of user's interest and profile is important for the study of communities within the network. Besides, it promotes the dynamicity of exchanges and the dissemination of information between users as well as the recommendation of relevant resources matching users' needs. Indeed, the ability to share resources (messages, documents, etc.) by a user can influence his neighbors and encourage them to share it in turn: an individual surrounded by broadcasters will tend to rebroadcast information. For example in Twitter it has been shown that diffusion depends on content and hashtags [3].

1.1 Our Motivation and Challenges

The research conducted in our project carries on the dynamics of interactions between individuals, communities' detection and the emergence of global collective behavior. As an application, we focus on health community of practice. Indeed, doctors' communities exchange different information and resources (electronic health records, diagnosis, interpretation reports, etc.) during their medical activities.

In fact, we consider that the health community of practice comprises not only the doctors but also patients and their families. Analyzing and enhancing the dynamic of interaction among members of the health community will emerge the shared knowledge promoting the collective intelligence.

In general, we are interested in different types of interaction relying members of a social network and their dynamics.

In particular, our project aims to realize a knowledge sharing system based on the diffusion of information and exchanges among members of the health community (doctor-doctor, doctor-patient, family-patient, patient-patient, doctor-family).

The Fig. 1 shows a general architecture of our system that ensures an intelligent sharing of knowledge among the users.

The first layer (User Layer) represents the connection of users. It creates space for each user(doctor/patient) with the ability to interact with the community. Each user will have a detailed profile fed from his discussions, shared resources and center of interests. The second layer (Clustering Layer) creates clusters according to the profiles of the users (similar users), their competences as well as their interactions. These clusters will be the object of recommendation of users and resources.

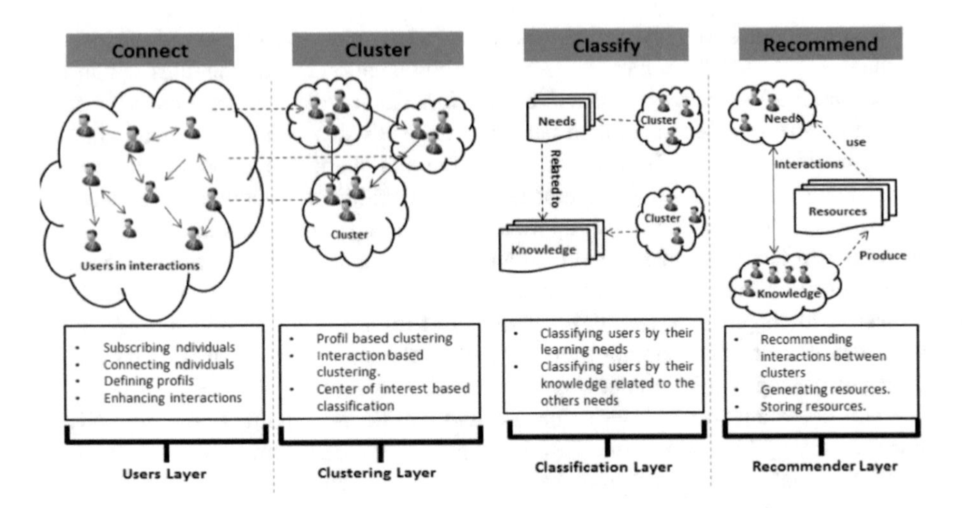

Fig. 1. General architecture of our smart knowledge sharing system

The third layer (Classification Layer) classifies the objects of either learning requests or solving problems sent by the individuals. On the other hand it classifies the sub-networks of users able to create supports or exchange resources related to the previously sorted requests. The fourth layer (Recommender Layer) leads interactions between clusters previously organized for exchanging resources and information related to the listed needs. This layer also saves and capitalizes resources for later use.

In this paper, we focus on the first two layers of our system, namely Users Layer and Clustering Layer. We are interested in studying the characteristics of individuals within the community. We will present the diffusion models specially the threshold model. The diffusion of information keeps a dynamics of interaction between users. We will identify a user-centered model that determines the user's ability to broadcast. This will be an important way to choose a base for a resource recommendation and reactivation of passive communities. The user-centered model includes three factors [4] presented below:

- The correspondence between the content of the information disseminated and the interests of the users;
- The tendency of users to disseminate; if they disseminate little or much information;
- The social pressure applied by the users; it's the number of neighbors who broadcast the content.

We also propose a user profile enrichment approach from resources' tags and content shared or accessed by the user (see Fig. 2). This approach aims to build community of similar users according to their interests, in order to recommend contents to the specific sub-communities. It will enhance the study of probability of resources' dissemination.

This paper is structured as follows. In the first section we give a review of the user's centered concepts by modeling its three characteristics influencing the information's diffusion. The second section describes the proposed approach that enriches the

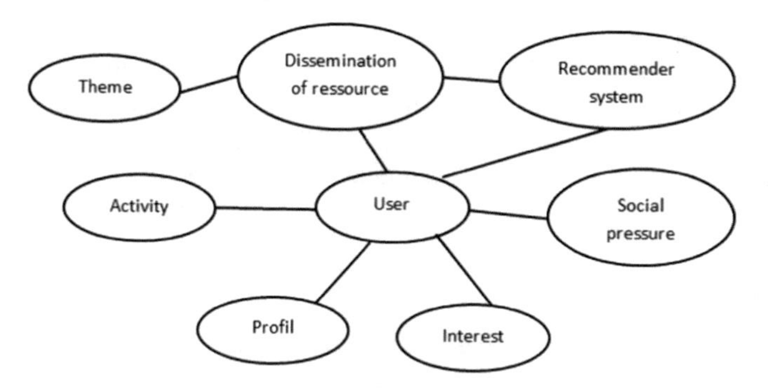

Fig. 2. The discussed concepts map

interests of the users in order to construct sub-communities according to the user interests for a selective recommendation. Finally we conclude with a discussion and analysis of the approach.

2 Literature Review

2.1 Health Community of Practice

The community of practice is a group of individuals who learn and pass on their knowledge to others, including through various collectives [5]. Another definition given to the community of practice is that of Wegner: "A community of practice is a group of individuals who interact, build relationships and through it gradually develop a sense of belonging and mutual commitment" [6]. A community of practice is characterized by a working environment shared by a group of individuals with heterogeneous levels of competence. CoPs (community of practice) are being increasingly used as a tool to improve clinical and public health practices and to facilitate the implementation of evidence based practices. CoPs have been used to [7] delete knowledge boundaries, promote standardization of practice, and create new ideas knowledge and practices. Mainly, the online health CoPs appears to help patients and their families to learn about health best practices, to have a support and to interact with similar individuals in similar circumstances. Many online health communities are being created around the world and are benefiting from crowdsourcing, for example Doccheck, Coliquio, Voxmed, Medcrowd … etc. Those communities are limited to the doctors and not include the patients and their families. Our goal is to build a system that leads interactions between doctors and patients, and allows exchanging information among all users.

2.2 Collective Intelligence

Collective intelligence means the combining of behavior, preferences, or ideas of a group of people to create novel insights. When a group of individuals collaborate or compete with each other, intelligence or behavior that otherwise didn't exist suddenly emerges [8]; the actions of a little group of individuals slowly spread within the community until the actions become the norm for the community; this is commonly known as *collective intelligence (CI)*. There are many ways that collective intelligence can benefit health best practices. In fact CI develops knowledge retention, so using CI approach can record, store, stimulate, innovate and bring available the knowledge across the health CoP [9].

2.3 Community Detection

Community detection has become a major research area in recent years. For example, community detection can help to do viral marketing; it can be used to make the recommendation. A community is defined as a subgraph composed of densely connected nodes and weakly related to other nodes of the graph [10]. Many unsupervised methods of clustering have been developed to extract information from the topology of the networks. From a set of individuals, a graph is built. Then we apply the clustering algorithm. Community detection helps us to identify similar users within the health CoP in order to recommend interactions between them.

2.4 Social Recommendation

Several works have been proposed in the literature for the recommendation in social networks. In general, authors use user-related tags to recommend users who have shared similar tags and/or recommend shared resources. First they build a profile for each user. Then from this profile the authors will be able to recommend resources using the similarity measure between the users. Recently, searches are based on both the history of user tags and resources and their social contacts [11]. Other researchers [12] have proposed tag recommendations in folksonomies based on the most used tags. However, these recommendations are not personalized because the same tags are offered to each user. In other recent approaches offering user profile enrichment from tags [13], the user profile is fed from the resource tags. The recommendation is based on the proximity between the tags and the proposed resource.

2.5 User Behavior

Our goal as presented before is activating interactions within the community by resources' recommendation and the broadcast of those resources. In this section we present three characteristics of the user having an influence on resources' diffusion within a network [4]:

- User activity (active or passive).
- Social pressure.
- The resource topic and user interest.

The user decides to rebroadcast information if he is active and tends to share content and resources, if he belongs to a community of broadcasters and content's creators and of course if the theme of the resource or content to share corresponds to his interests.

User Activity
This characteristic explains the active or passive nature of the individual. It could be drawn from the analysis of user traces.

Social Pressure or Neighbors Pressure
The social pressure represents the number of user's neighbors who shared a resource at a time t; having two broadcaster neighbors increases the probability of diffusion twice. The social pressure calculated by the number of active neighbors around the user who can activate it. This characteristic is much more important than the others. It compensates the non-interest of the user by the resource as well as his willingness to share.

Resource Topic
A user will be more attentive to a resource near to his interests. He will have more tendencies to read it and share it again. In another way the subject of the resource presents a great factor in the propagation of the information [16]. The representation of the relationship between the content and the user is given by the proximity between the profile and the content. The interests of a user u_i and the description of a resource r_k are defined in the same space: $i_i \in R$ and, $r_k \in R$. Then the proximity is defined by the following form:

$$P(u_i, \mathcal{I}, r_k, S_p) = S(i_i, r_k) - S_p \quad (1)$$

Where $S(i_i, r_k)$ is the measure of similarity between the interests and the description of the resource. S_p is thresholds for defining whether the two objects are sufficiently close. If the similarity is greater than the threshold, the proximity will be positive. It will be negative in the opposite case. Subsequently, the proximity defines the probability that a user can broadcast resource or not.

This article focuses on the user's characteristics and proposes an approach to enrich the user profile to be able to refine the calculation of information dissemination probability and push the quality of resource recommendation according to existing profiles. We will present this approach in the next section.

3 Proposed Approach

The user profile is a set of characteristics describing the user, his interests his habits, his preferences… Profile building is done by extracting useful information provided by users or by analyzing their traces [18]. In this paper we propose a dynamic user profile construction approach from the shared resources and contents' tags in order to have a membership in the same space [19]. The profile is composed of three sections; the first one contains the elements given by the user (Last name, first name, age, city …). The second one defines the MBTI (Myers Briggs Type Indicator) preferences of the user and which can also calculate his activity [17], and the last one contains the information that characterize the interests. This approach aims to refine the interests of the user in order to define proximity between his profile and the shared resource. The interests of the user correspond to one of the most important characteristics used in the recommendation systems and also in the probability of diffusion measurement. The interests can be divided into two types, long term and short term interests [20]. The interest is long term if the user is still interested in the theme. It's short term if the user is interested in this topic for a short time or does not tend to share resources related to it. It's important to choose the method of extraction of interests from resources, comments, messages, notation, tags …and assign a score for each interest [21]; this score explains the importance of the tag and its sustainability.

Before exposing our approach, we will give mathematical models for the characteristics of the user (presented above) explaining his behavior and his ability to broadcast resources.

By this way, it can be easy to feed the second section describing the profile.

3.1 User Activity

We propose to define it according to the model (2) below:

$$(u) = \frac{\sum_{k=0}^{n} Shared\ resources}{\sum_{k=0}^{n} seen\ resources + \sum_{k=0}^{n} created\ resources} \tag{2}$$

The user activity of a user u corresponds to the ratio between the number of resources that a user has shared and the resources that has been created and seen.

3.2 Social Pressure

We consider a directed graph of users G = (U, E) composed of a number of users U = {u1…un} with a set of links E between its users. We consider u1 a central user where his degree of centrality is greater than 1 calculated using the equation: $\mathrm{DC(i)} = \sum \mathrm{U/n} - 1$ [14] and initiator at time t = 0. We also consider an inactive user u2 at time t = 0 with V (u2) = 3 (number of incoming neighbors) is also the threshold for it to become active. Figure 3 explains the pressure of the diffuser neighbors applied to the user u2. We denote Pui,uj the pressure applied by ui on uj. We applied the threshold diffusion model for resource diffusion in users' network [15].

The pressure is represented by: algorithm for calculating the number of active neighbors.

$$\mathrm{SP}\,(u_i) = \sum_{i=0}^{n} \text{active broadcaster Users} \tag{3}$$

3.3 Resource Topic

We will give the mathematical presentation of this characteristic in the proposed approach.

Our Approach is divided into 3 steps.

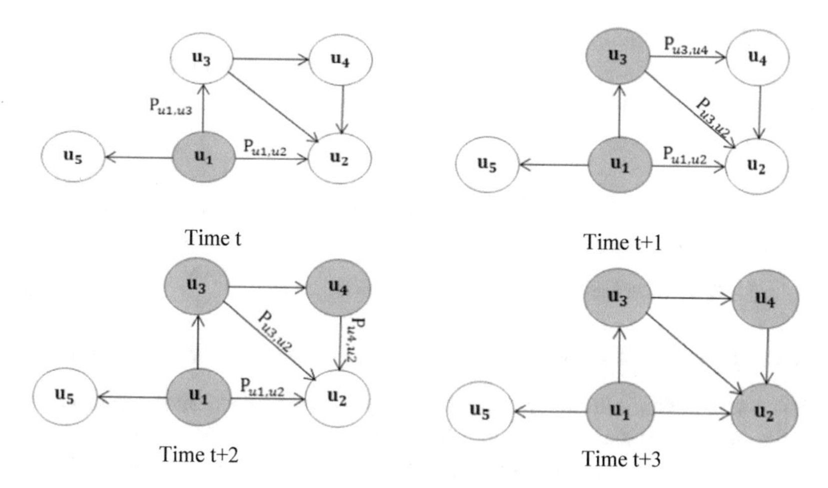

Fig. 3. Pressure of active neighbors in a social network following the threshold diffusion model

First Activity of the User (Cold Start)

In this first step the user is newer, he begins to consult and share content and resources, or exchange messages with his neighbors. This information will be used as a first enrichment of the interests section of the user. Our method exploits the most relevant extracted tags from the shared resources and then enriches the profile with these Tags. In this way the definition of the profiles will be done using the Tags (considered as centers of interest). This operation must be done over time at many times specified in advance.

Refine the User Profile

In this second step, we try to refine the user profile by calculating the importance of the Tag before adding it. This importance is calculated by the formula that we have already proposed in another article [22]:

The importance of the tag is related to its frequency of use (4).
Frequency of the tag t_i to annotate the resource r (5).
Frequency of users who use the tag t_i to annotate the resource r (6).

$$\mathrm{I}(t_i) = F_t(t_i)^* F_u(t_i) \tag{4}$$

$$F_t(t_i) = \frac{Number\ of\ t_i\ annotating\ the\ resource\ r}{\sum_{j=0}^{n} t_j\ annotating\ the\ resource\ r} \tag{5}$$

$$F_u(t_i) = \frac{Number\ of\ users\ who\ use\ t_i\ to\ annotate\ the\ resource\ r}{Number\ of\ users\ who\ annotate\ the\ resource\ r} \tag{6}$$

After calculating the importance of tag, we add it with a high importance to the interests of the user, and we assign it a score that is automatically incremented with the number of resources that the user has used and which are tagged by the same tag.

Calculation of Similarity

This step is divided into two purposes: the first one is the ability to calculate the proximity between profiles and resource themes, the second one is the identification of similar users.

Proximity

The computation of the proximity $P(I_i,r_k)$ represents the number of common characteristics between the interests of a user and the tags of the resource with a comparison threshold S_s. The interests are represented by a tag's vector $\overrightarrow{V}_I$ and the resource is represented by the tag's vector $\overrightarrow{V}_r$, the difference between the two vectors is the angle α. If α is zero then the criteria are similar, if $\alpha = \pi/2$ the two vectors are orthogonal so the profile of the user and the resource are not close. To calculate the similarity we use the cosine function (9), we consider x_p a set of interests with the highest scores that determine the long-term interests for the user (7):

$$\text{Interests} = \{(\text{Tags};\ \text{Score})\}, \tag{7}$$

and y_r set of Resource Tags described as:

$$\text{Description Web Resource} = \{(\text{metadata};\ \text{score})\} \tag{8}$$

$$\text{Cosinus}\,(x, y) = \frac{card(x_p\, y_r)}{\sqrt{card(x_p).card(y_r)}} \tag{9}$$

Graph of Similar Users

To create subnets of similar users that share the same interests, we calculate the weight between each pair of users $W(U_i, U_j)$ (10), (using our approach) this identifies the relationships between individuals according to their preferences.

$$W(U_i, U_j) = \frac{card(x_i\, y_j)}{\sqrt{card(x_i).card(y_j)}} \tag{10}$$

Where x and y are a sets of users' interests.

We can also calculate the weight using the equation below:

$$W(U_i, U_j) = \frac{\sum_{t=1}^{n} Tag_t\ attributed\ by\ U_i\ and\ U_j}{\sum_{t=1}^{n} Tags} * \frac{\sum_{r=1}^{m} Resource_r\ annotated\ by\ U_i\ and\ U_j}{\sum_{r=1}^{m} Resources} \tag{11}$$

In this case if the weight is very high both users will have more similar interests. If the weight is 0 so the users are not linked (Fig. 4).

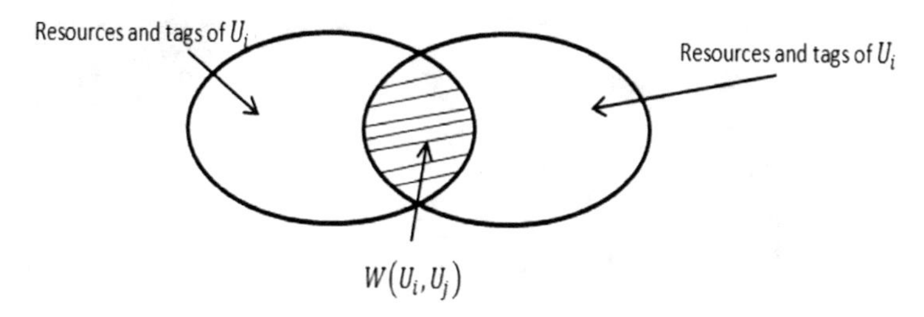

Fig. 4. Weight between two users.

4 Discussion

In this paper, we tried to explain how tag-based user profile enrichment and will make pertinent the recommendation. Also we determined the importance of user profile modeling for the purpose of recommendation and resources diffusion. Therefore, we can combine the 3 characteristics of a user (activity, pressure, proximity), and present the user by the following feature vector:

$$\rho^{u_i,r} = \mu_1 \mathrm{A}(u_i) + \mu_2 \,\mathrm{SP}(u_i) + \mu_3 \,\mathrm{P}(u_i, r) \tag{12}$$

The parameters μ1, μ2, μ3 control the influence of each dimension of the diffusion.

Our approach exceeds the others one by building the user profile from the relevant tags (calculated from their frequency of use and annotation) of the resources that consulted and/or shared that are considered as the user interests with attribution of a score that defines the "long-term" notion of interest. Then the recommendation will be based on the calculation of the proximity between the user and the resource by calculating the similarity between the tags of the profile with high score and the tags of the resource.

As a result of our semantic profile enrichment, we can build sub-communities by grouping similar users according to their interests. Figure 5 re-introduce Fig. 1 and explains the mechanism that links sub-communities built from profile enrichment with recommender systems and resources. The user-centered model allows determining the user who is both broadcaster and central, so it represents an entry for the community. The recommender system is based on the recommendation of the resource that is close to the interests of this selected user. So the targeted resource will be distributed to the entire community for the purpose of its reactivation. For the same purpose that is community reactivation the recommender system recommends the resources shared by users to their neighbors in the same community.

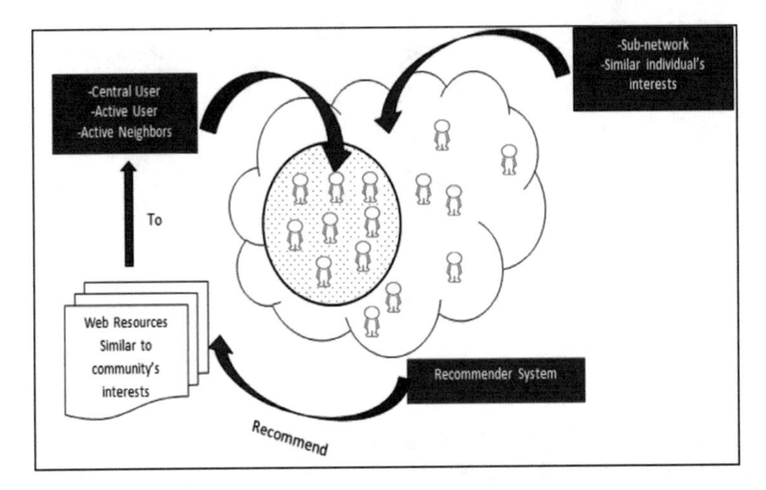

Fig. 5. Resources recommendation to sub-communities of similar individuals

5 Conclusion and Perspectives

We presented in the first section of our paper, a user-centered model based on the study of the user characteristics: the user activity and influence of his neighbors on his resource sharing. In the second section, we proposed a user profile enrichment approach from the resources' tags shared by the user. This method allows us to have an insight on his interests in order to: first calculate the proximity between the profile and the resource we want to recommend to the user to be broadcasted.

In future works, we aim to analyze several algorithms of diffusion models that use the characteristics presented in this article, as well as their use in the prediction of information diffusion in order to choose the best path that can push or cut the diffusion. Our goal is to apply our profile enrichment approach to doctors and patients communities and use their shared documents and sent messages. Before that, the effectiveness of our approach will be attested by the results of an experimental evaluation using an open Dataset (Delicious Social Network) of users' traces.

References

1. Hanneman, R.A., Riddle, M.: Introduction to Social Network Methods. University of California, Berkeley (2005)
2. Boyd, D., Golder, S., Lotan, G.: Tweet, tweet, retweet: conversational aspects of retweeting on twitter. In: Proceedings of the 2010 43rd Hawaii International Conference on System Sciences, HICSS 2010. IEEE Computer Society (2010)
3. Suh, B., Hong, L., Pirolli, P., Chi, E.H.: Want to be retweeted? Large scale analytics on factors impacting retweet in twitter network. In: Proceedings of the 2010 IEEE Second International Conference on Social Computing, SOCIALCOM 2010. IEEE Computer Society (2010)

4. Lagnier, C.: Information Diffusion within the social networks. Diffusion de l'information dans les réseaux sociaux, Intelligence Artificielle. Université de Grenoble (2013)
5. Wenger, E., McDermott, R., Snyder, W.: Cultivating Communities of Practice: A Guide to Managing Knowledge. Harvard Business School Press, Boston (2002). Amy HI Lee received the MBA degree from the University of British Columbia, Canada
6. Wenger, E., McDermott, R., Snyder, W.: A Guide to Managing Knowledge: Cultivating Communities of Practice. Harvard Business School Press, Boston (2002)
7. Ranmuthugala, G., Plumb, J.J., Cunningham, F.C., Georgiou, A., Westbrook, J.I., Braithwaite, J.: How and why are communities of practice established in the healthcare sector? A systematic review of the literature. BMC Health Serv. Res. **11**, 273 (2011)
8. Mačiulienė, M., Skaržauskienė, A.: Emergence of collective intelligence in online communities. J. Bus. Res. **69**, 1718–1724 (2016). Mykolas Romeris University, Lithuania
9. Scarlat, E., Maries, I.: Simulating collective intelligence of communities of practice using agent based methods. In: Agent and Multi-Agent Systems: Technologies and Applications. LNCS, vol. 6070, pp. 305–314 (2010)
10. Newman, M.E., Girvan, M.: Finding and evaluating community structure in networks. Phys. Rev. E **69**, 026113 (2004)
11. Hu, J., Wang, B., Tao, Z.: Personalized tag recommendation using social contacts. In: Proceedings of the Workshop SRS 2011, in conjunction with CSCW (2011)
12. Jäschke, R., Hotho, A., Schmitz, C., Ganter, B., Stumme, G.: Discovering shared conceptualizations in folksonomies. Web Semant. **6**, 38–53 (2008)
13. Mezghani, M., et al.: From the influence of user profile enrichment on buzz propagation in social media. Experiments on delicious. J. Sci. Technol. Inf. Série ISI Ingénierie Systèmes d'Information, Lavoisier **21**(4), 67–81 (2016)
14. Ben Hiba, L.: Evaluating virtual teams in social and collaborative platforms based on SNA and BI analaytics. ENSIAS. Mohammed 5 University (2014)
15. Vallet, J.: Where Social Networks, Graph Rewriting and Visualisation Meet: Application to Network Generation and Information Diffusion. Other [cs.OH]. Bordeaux University (2017)
16. Cha, M., Antonio, J., Prez, N., Haddadi, H.: Flash floods and ripples: the spread of media content through the blogosphere. In: Proceedings of the 3rd AAAI International Conference on Weblogs and Social Media, ICWSM 2009 (2009)
17. Furnham, A., Crump, J.: The Myers-Briggs type indicator (MBTI) and promotion at work. Psychology **6**, 1510–1515 (2015). https://doi.org/10.4236/psych.2015.612147
18. Hasan, O., Habegger, B., Brunie, L., Bennani, N., Damiani, E.: A discussion of privacy challenges in user profiling with big data techniques: the EEXCESS use case. In: 2013 IEEE International Congress on Big Data, pp. 25–30. IEEE (2013)
19. Meo, P.D., Ferrara, E., Abel, F., Aroyo, L., Houben, G.-J.: Analyzing user behavior across social sharing environments. ACM Trans. Intell. Syst. Technol. (TIST) **5**(1), 14 (2014)
20. Abel, F., Gao, Q., Houben, G.-J., Tao, K.: Semantic enrichment of twitter posts for user profile construction on the social web. In: Extended Semantic Web Conference, pp. 375–389. Springer, Heidelberg (2011)
21. Benammar, A., Hubert, G., Mothe, J.: Automatic profile reformulation using a local document analysis. In: European Conference on Information Retrieval, pp. 124–134. Springer, Heidelberg (2002)
22. Qassimi, S., Abdelwahed, E.H., Hafidi, M., Lamrani, R.: Towards an emergent semantic of web resources using collaborative tagging. In: Model and Data Engineering, MEDI 2017. LNCS, vol. 10563. Springer, Cham (2017)

The Metabolic Syndrome: Prevalence, Associated Risk Factors and Health Complications in Obese Subjects in Northern Morocco

Nadia Hamjane[1(✉)], Fatiha Benyahya[2], Mohcine Bennani Mechita[1], Naima Ghailani Nourouti[1], and Amina Barakat[1]

[1] Laboratory of Biomedical Genomics and Oncogenetics, Abdelmalek Essaadi University, Tangier, Morocco
hamjanenadia@gmail.com
[2] Institute Pasteur, Tangier, Morocco

Abstract. The metabolic syndrome (MetS) is a major public-health problem; it is associated with increased risk of developing type 2 diabetes and cardiovascular diseases.

This study aimed to estimate the prevalence of MetS and associated risk factors as well as its complications in an obese population of north of Morocco.

This is a cross-sectional study that was undertaken on a population of 485 obese subjects, 339 women and 146 men. A structured questionnaire was used to collect data on demography, lifestyle, medical history and biological parameters.

The mean age of our patients was of 49 ± 11 years, the average of body mass index was of 34.2 ± 7 kg/m^2, and the waist circumference average was of 106.9 ± 15 cm for the women and 104.5 ± 12 cm for the men. Obesity was of class I in 38% of the subjects, class II in 25%, class III in 13%, and 24% of the subjects had an overweight. The prevalence of MetS was 52.4%, higher in females than male subjects (59.24% vs 35.97%). The most commonly associated risk factors of MetS in our population were abdominal obesity plus hyperglycemia plus low HDL cholesterol. The complications found in our population were type2 diabetes and it complications in 42% of the cases and cardiovascular disease in 32%.

Our study showed that MetS was highly prevalent among obese patients. The most prevalent component of MetS in our population was abdominal obesity and hyperglycemia. Targeting obesity and sedentarity is the main solution for the prevention and treatment of the MetS.

Keywords: Metabolic syndrome · Obesity · Complications

M. Ezziyyani (Ed.): AI2SD 2018, AISC 914, pp. 90–99, 2019.
https://doi.org/10.1007/978-3-030-11884-6_8

1 Introduction

Obesity is a major public-health problem; it causes many cardiovascular risk factors such as diabetes, hypertension, dyslipidemia. The association of some of these factors constitutes the metabolic syndrome (MetS) [1]. This MetS represents a major risk of cardiovascular morbidity and mortality [2].

Several definitions of MetS have been proposed by many organizations that have set criteria for the diagnosis of MetS (World Health Organisation (WHO), National Cholesterol Education Program-Adult Treatment Panel III (NCEPATPIII), and International Diabetes Federation (IDF)) [3]. The criteria for all these definitions include abdominal obesity, determined by increased waist circumference, raised triglycerides, reduced HDL, elevated blood pressure, and raised plasma glucose.

The prevalence of MetS is increasing worldwide; it varies substantially between countries [4]. Among Europeans and Americans it varies between 20% and 30% [5, 6]. Among North African populations, the prevalence estimates are 30% in Tunisia and 20% in Algeria [7, 8]. In Morocco, the prevalence of MetS was 35.7% in a recent study (18.56% among men and 40.12% among women) [9].

Studies on metabolic syndrome were conducted in Morocco [9–12], but our study is the first conducted in the North of the country. In addition, our study is the first that studied the MetS and its complications in obese subjects in Morocco.

The main objectives of this study are the description of the epidemiological, clinical and laboratory characteristics of the study population and determination of the prevalence of metabolic syndrome, its associated risk factors and the complications manifested in a population of obese subjects.

2 Materials and Methods

2.1 Study Population

It was a cross-sectional study conducted at the Provincial Specialized Hospital DUC TOVAR, Tangier, Morocco during a period of 12 months (February 2016 to February 2017).

A total of 485 patients with an obesity aged between 18 and 70 years, are from various geographic regions of the north of the country. A structured questionnaire was used to collect data on demography, lifestyle and medical history.

All participants gave written informed consent before including them in this study. The benefit for patients will be the reduction of obesity and its complications.

2.2 Anthropometry, Clinical and Biochemical Measurements

The body weight was measured with an accuracy of 0.1 kg by a battery operated digital balance and the waist circumference was measured by a tape measure.

BMI was calculated using the height and weight of the individual by the following formula:

$$\mathrm{BMI} = \mathrm{Weight}\ (\mathrm{kg})/\mathrm{height}^2(\mathrm{m})^2$$

Systolic and diastolic blood pressures (SBP and DBP) were recorded twice at an interval of three minutes in the sitting position after a 15 min rest, and the mean was then calculated.

The results of the biological analysis were collected from the patient medical record.

2.3 Diagnostic of the MetS

Metabolic syndrome was diagnosed according to the criteria of National Cholesterol Education Program Adult Treatment Panel III according to which an individual with MetS must present any three or more of the following five components: waist circumference ≥ 102 cm for males or ≥ 88 cm for females, raised triglycerides level: ≥ 1.50 g/l; reduced HDL-cholesterol: <0.40 g/l men <0.50 g/l women; raised blood pressure (BP): systolic BP ≥ 130 or diastolic BP ≥ 85 mmHg; raised fasting plasma glucose (FPG): FPG ≥ 1.10 g/l [13].

2.4 Statistical Analysis

Clinical and biochemical data were presented as arithmetic mean standard deviation. Statistical analyses were performed using Epi Info version 3.5.1.

Results are expressed as means ± SD. Statistical comparison of means was performed with the Student's t test; P-values that are less than 0.05 were considered as statistically significant.

3 Results

3.1 Anthropometric and Metabolic Characteristics of the Study Population

The average age of the study population was 49 ± 11 years (51 ± 12.05 years and 48 ± 11.33 years for men and women respectively); female patients were the most represented with a sex ratio of 0.43.

Several anthropometric, biochemical and clinical features showed significant differences between men and women (Table 1). Women were found to have a higher BMI and waist circumference, higher levels of glycemia and higher levels of triglycerides than men. Men showed higher blood pressure levels for systolic blood pressure and diastolic blood pressure, higher level of total cholesterol, higher level of LDL and lower level of HDL than women.

Table 1. Anthropometric and metabolic characteristics of the study population

Parameters	Total population (N = 485) Average ± SD	Men (N = 146) Average ± SD	Women (N = 339) Average ± SD	*P*-value*
Age (years)	49 ± 11	51 ± 12.05	48 ± 11.33	0.8
BMI (kg/m^2)	34.2 ± 7 kg/m^2	32.11 ± 7.99	35.91 ± 8.09	0.52
WC (cm)	105.7 ± 10.24	104.5 ± 12	106.9 ± 15	0.77
Systolic blood pressure (mmHg)	138.60 ± 13.22	137.64 ± 14.79	136.83 ± 13.36	0.51
Diastolic blood pressure (mmHg)	79.27 ± 7.3	78.72 ± 9.46	77.11 ± 9.88	0.87
GLY (g/L)	1.77 ± 0.44	1.69 ± 0.46	1.87 ± 0.43	0.42
TCH (g/L)	2.45 ± 0.52	2.75 ± 0.53	1.98 ± 0.50	0.001
HDL (g/L)	0.41 ± 0.18	0.37 ± 0.20	0.43 ± 0.18	0.13
LDL (g/L)	1.77 ± 0.45	1.99 ± 0.37	1.57 ± 0.44	0.001
TG (g/L)	1.98 ± 0.85	1.60 ± 1.07	2.32 ± 0.711	0.032

**P* is used for comparison between men and women.

Abbreviations: BMI, body mass index; GLY, glycemia; HDL, high-density lipoprotein; LDL, low-density lipoprotein; SD, standard deviation; TCH, total cholesterol; TG, triglyceridemia; WC, waist circumference

3.2 Prevalence of MetS in the Study Population

The prevalence of MetS was 52.4%, higher in females than male participants (59.24% vs 35.97%,) and it increased with age, with the highest prevalence in the age group >50 years ($p < 0.05$) (Fig. 1).

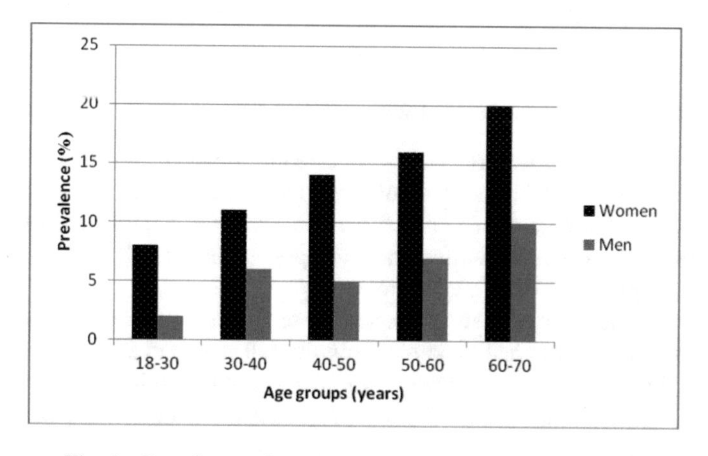

Fig. 1. Prevalence of MetS according to age-groups and sex

The study of the prevalence of MetS according to the classes of obesity showed that the MetS increases with the values of the BMI. Indeed, its prevalence was higher in obese class III (morbid obesity) in both women and men (Table 2).

Table 2. Prevalence of metabolic syndrome and its clinical abnormalities according to the overweight and classes of obesity and sex

	Overweight and classes of obesity	%	MetS (%)	Hight FG (%)	Low HDLc (%)	High Trig %	HBP (%)
All N = 485	Overweight*	24	29.1	50	25	22	16.6
	Class 1*	38	42.9	76.3	55.3	38.6	47.3
	Class 2*	25	72.4	68	68	51.9	44
	Class 3*	13	84.61	76.9	77	79	69.2
	Overall		**52.4**	**68**	**54**	**38.5**	**42**
Men N = 146	Overweight	31.3	18.84	28.75	31.9	30.8	51.1
	Class 1	24.6	36.6	77.23	54.47	35.5	50.8
	Class 2	30	33.3	76.66	60	48.7	60.6
	Class 3	14	78.6	87	71.4	78	78.5
	Overall		**35.97**	**63.3**	**51.42**	**42.1**	**46.7**
Women N = 339	Overweight	20.8	45.1	28.84	48	14.8	43.26
	Class 1	43.7	52.63	80	49.2	41.2	27.45
	Class 2	23	68	78.26	80.43	55.7	47.82
	Class 3	12.5	80	88	80	77.7	64
	Overall		**59.24**	**70**	**60**	**34.5**	**40**

*Overweight: $25 \leq$ BMI < 30 *Class I obesity: $30 \leq$ BMI < 35 *Class II obesity: $35 \leq$ BMI < 40 *Class III obesity: BMI ≥ 40

Abbreviations: FG, fasting glucose; HBP, Height blood pressure; GLY, glycemia; HDLc, high-density lipoprotein cholesterol.

3.3 The Risk Factors Associated with MetS in the Study Population

Abdominal obesity and hyperglycemia were more frequent in our patients with metabolic syndrome. Furthermore, 43.6% of patients had one or two risk factors for developing this syndrome. 28.1% had three and 18.7% expressed four of them. The most common association of risk factors in our population was abdominal obesity plus hyperglycemia plus low HDL-cholesterol.

The distribution of MetS patients according to frequency of NCEPATP III criteria showed that 98% patients had abdominal obesity (all men and 97% women); 68% of them had a hight blood glucose level; 54% had a low HDL-cholesterol level; 38.5% had a hight triglyceride level and 42% were hypertensive. As expected, the frequencies of all abnormalities of MetS increased with the classes of obesity especially hyperglycemia, lowHDLc and hypertriglyceridemia (Table 2).

Furthermore, men had a high proportion of hypertension (46.7%) abdominal obesity (100%) and hypertriglyceridemia (42.1%), whereas women presented more hyperglycemia (70%) and low HDL-cholesterol levels (60%). Low HDL-cholesterol and high triglycerides increase with the classes of obesity in both men and women subjects (Table 2).

3.4 Health Complications of MetS in the Study Population

The most common MetS complications in our obese subjects were: type 2 diabetes (42%) and CVD (32%).

The distribution of diabetic obese patients and obese cardiac patients according to the number of risk factors associated with the MetS showed that the risk of diabetes increased with the existence of a single risk factor, however the risk of cardiovascular disease increases significantly with three or more (Fig. 2).

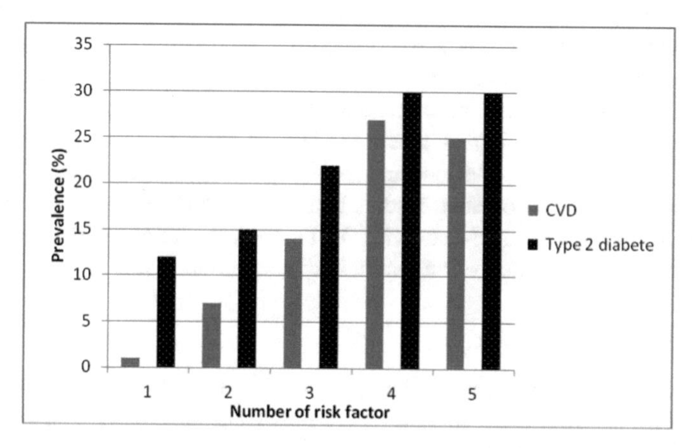

Fig. 2. Prevalence of cardiovascular disease and type 2 diabetes according to the number of risk factors

4 Discussion

4.1 Prevalence of the MetS

We have chosen the definition proposed by the NCEP-ATP III, which is the definition more operational of the syndrome, easy to use in clinical practice [14]. In addition, this definition offer higher waist circumference standards ($\geq$ 102 cm for males or $\geq$ 88 cm for females); which does not lead to an increase in the frequency of the metabolic syndrome since we are working on an obese population.

MetS has become a public health problem, the prevalence of which is increasing worldwide [4]. The prevalence of metabolic syndrome in our study was 52,4%. This result is consistent with results from Spanish study, where the prevalence of MetS was 52% in patients with hypertension [15]. However, it is higher in relation to the national prevalence (35.7%) and to prevalence in the Tunisian population (30%) [7, 9]. This difference is due to the clinical characteristics of our population which is obese.

In addition, this prevalence is lower than an Asian population suffering from sleep apnea (72,3%) and European population with type 2 diabetes (78% and 84% In women and men, respectively) [16, 17]. These differences in the prevalence of MetS can be explained by the difference socio-economic and clinical characteristics between the study population as well as the interaction of genetic and environmental factors, which have long been known to play a key role in the pathophysiology of MetS [18]. In addition, the prevalence of the metabolic syndrome has varied markedly between different studies, most likely due to different criteria used for defining the syndrome [19, 20].

In other hand, our study showed that the prevalence of metabolic syndrome was higher in females than male participants (59.24% vs 35.97%). Similar results have been reported in many studies in other populations [7, 9, 21]. In addition, this MetS increased with age for both men and women, with the highest prevalence in the age group >50 years. This is in agreement with other studies [22]. These results can be explained by the fact that age is associated with evolution in insulin resistance, alteration of other hormones, and increase of abdominal adipose tissue.

Furthermore, we have noticed that the MetS increases with the values of the BMI, indeed, its prevalence was higher in obese class III (morbid obesity) and significant liaison was found between BMI and metabolic syndrome in our study. This result is consistent with the results of other studies that showed that the risk of MetS resulting from being overweight and increases with BMI values, in particular when accompanied by a significant accumulation of abdominal adipose tissue [23, 24].

4.2 Risk Factor of the MetS

The distribution of MetS patients according to frequency of NCEPATP III criteria showed that 98% patients had abdominal obesity. These results are in agreement with those in the literature which have a driving force in the development of the metabolic system with insulin resistance and alteration of adipose tissue lipolysis as a central pathophysiology [25].

The most common association of risk factors in our population was abdominal obesity plus hyperglycemia plus low HDL cholesterol, these components were common in female participants than male participants. Our results are close to those found by a Ghanaian and Turkish study wherein the prominent components of MetS were high BP, low HDL cholesterol and abdominal obesity [26, 27].

Whereas, the sex differences were observed in high blood pressure and high triglycerides levels, which were more elevated in men compared with women, (46.7% vs 40% and 42.1% vs 34.5% respectively). This results is close to another Algerian study [8].

The high level of triglycerides and high blood pressure could be related to smoking, especially in men whose smoking prevalence is higher than women in Arabic population [28].

4.3 Complication of the MetS

Regarding the complications of MetS in the studied population, our results revealed that 42% of MetS patients had type2 diabetes and 32% had a cardiovascular disease. Several studies have shown that the presence of a MetS is a risk factor for developing type 2 diabetes [29, 30]. In addition, systematic review and meta-analysis have demonstrated that presence of MetS is associated with a twofold increase in composite CVD, stroke, myocardial infarction and all-cause mortality [31].

Additionally, the commonest components of MetS in our study, were hyperglycemia and dyslipidemia, these risk factors have been shown to be strong predictors of vascular events [32].

Furthermore, we found that the risk of diabetes increased with the existence of a single risk factor. However, the risk of cardiovascular disease increased significantly with three or more. Another studies showed that the risk of having certain chronic diseases such as diabetes increases with each additional risk marker of MetS [33].

5 Conclusion

From our literature search, this is the first study in northern Morocco that focuses on the estimation of the prevalence of MetS in the obese population by using the NCEP-ATP III definition. In addition, our study is the first studied the complications of MS in Morocco.

The results of this study showed that the prevalence of metabolic syndrome and associated risk factors is high among adults obese in northern Morocco, especially in women, and this syndrome increase with age and with different classes of obesity.

The most prevalent component of metabolic syndrome in our population was abdominal obesity and hyperglycemia. These components play an important role in the development of diabetes mellitus and cardiovascular diseases that impacts their morbidity and mortality.

This observation suggests that early screening and treatment of components MetS may be beneficial in the amelioration of the complications associated with this syndrome.

References

1. Hauhouot-Attoungbre, M.L., Yayo, S.E., Ake-Edjeme, A., Yapi, H.F., Ahibo, H., Monnet, D.: Does metabolic syndrome exist in Ivory Coast? Le syndrome métabolique existe-t-il en Côte d'Ivoire? Immuno-analyse Biologie Spécialisée **23**(6), 375–378 (2008)
2. Scheen, A.J.: Management of the metabolic syndrome. Minerva Endocrinol. **29**, 31–45 (2004)
3. Grundy, S.M.: Diagnosis and management of the metabolic syndrome: an American Heart Association/National Heart, Lung, and Blood Institute Scientific Statement. Circulation **112** (17), 2735–2752 (2005)

4. Kim, M.H., Kim, M.K., Choi, B.Y., Shin, Y.J.: Prevalence of the metabolic syndrome and its association with Cardiovascular Disease in Korea. J. Korean Med. Sci. **19**(2), 195–201 (2004)
5. Qiao, Q.: Comparison of different definitions of the metabolic syndrome in relation to cardiovascular mortality in European men and women. Diabetologia **49**, 2837–2846 (2006)
6. Park, Y.W., Zhu, S., Palaniappan, L., Heshka, S., Carnethon, M.R., Heymsfield, S.B.: The metabolic syndrome: prevalence and associated risk factor findings in the US population from the Third National Health and Nutrition Examination Survey, 1988–1994. Arch. Intern. Med. **163**, 427–436 (2003)
7. Belfki, H., Ben Ali, S., Aounallah-Skhiri, H., et al.: Prevalence and determinants of the metabolic syndrome among Tunisian adults: results of the Transition and Health Impact in North Africa (TAHINA) project. Public Health Nutr. **16**, 582–590 (2013)
8. Houti, L., Hamani-Medjaoui, I., Lardjam-Hetraf, S.A., Ouhaibi-Djellouli, H., Chougrani, S., Goumidi, L., et al.: Prevalence of metabolic syndrome and its related risk factors in the City of Oran, Algeria: the ISOR Study. Ethn. Dis. **26**, 99–106 (2016)
9. El Brini, O., Akhouayri, O., Gamal, A., Mesfioui, A., Benazzouz, B.: Prevalence of metabolic syndrome and its components based on a harmonious definition among adults in Morocco. Diabetes Metab. Syndr. Obes. Targets Ther. **7**, 341–346 (2014)
10. Morjane, I., Kefi, R., Charoute, H., Lakbakbi el Yaagoubi, F., Hechmi, M., Saile, R., et al.: Association study of HNF1A polymorphisms with metabolic syndrome in the Moroccan population. Diabetes Metab. Syndr. Clin. Res. Rev. **11**, S853–S857 (2017)
11. Lakbakbi El Yaagoubi, F., Charoute, H., Morjane, I., Sefri, H., Rouba, H., Ainahi, A., et al.: Association analysis of genetic variants with metabolic syndrome components in the Moroccan population. Curr. Res. Transl. Med. **65**(3), 121–125 (2017)
12. Ajjemami, M., Ouatou, S., Charoute, H., Fakiri, M., Rhaissi, H., Benrahma, H., et al.: Haplotype analysis of the Apolipoprotein A5 gene in Moroccan patients with the metabolic syndrome. J. Diabetes Metab. Disord. **14**, 29 (2015)
13. Expert Panel on Detection, Evaluation, and Treatment of High Blood Cholesterol in Adults: Executive summary of the third report of the National Cholesterol Education Program (NCEP) expert panel on detection, evaluation, and treatment of high blood cholesterol in adults (Adult Treatment Panel III). JAMA **285**, 2486–2497 (2001)
14. Grundy, S.M., Cleeman, J.I., Daniels, S.R., et al.: Diagnosis and management of the metabolic syndrome. An American Heart Association/National Heart, Lung, and Blood Institute Scientific Statement. Circulation **112**(17), 2735–2752 (2005)
15. Barrios, V., Escobar, C., Calderón, A., Llisterri, J.L., Alegría, E., Muñiz, J., et al.: Prevalence of the metabolic syndrome in patients with hypertension treated in general practice in Spain: an assessment of blood pressure and low-density lipoprotein cholesterol control and accuracy of diagnosis. J. Cardiometab. Syndr. **2**(1), 9–15 (2007)
16. Dang Thi Mai, K., Tran Van, N.: Study of the prevalence of metabolic syndrome in patients with sleep apnea syndrome. Fran Viet Pneu **04**(10), 36–42 (2013)
17. Isomaa, B., Almgren, P., Tuomi, T., Forsén, B., et al.: Cardiovascular morbidity and mortality associated with the metabolic syndrome. Diabetes Care **24**, 683–689 (2001)
18. Poulsen, P., Vaag, A., Kyvik, K., Beck-Nielsen, H.: Genetic versus environmental aetiology of the metabolic syndrome among male and female twins. Diabetologia **44**, 537–543 (2001)
19. Nolan, P.B., Carrick-Ranson, G., Stinear, J.W., Reading, S.A., Dalleck, L.C.: Prevalence of metabolic syndrome and metabolic syndrome components in young adults: a pooled analysis. Prev. Med. Rep. **7**, 211–215 (2017)
20. O'Neill, S., O'Driscoll, L.: Metabolic syndrome: a closer look at the growing epidemic and its associated pathologies: metabolic syndrome. Obes. Rev. **16**(1), 1–12 (2015)

21. Prasad, D.S., Kabir, Z., Dash, A.K., Das, B.C.: Prevalence and risk factors for metabolic syndrome in Asian Indians: a community study from urban Eastern India. J. Cardiovasc. Dis. Res. **3**, 204–211 (2012)
22. Shahbazian, H., Latifi, S.M., Jalali, M.T., Shahbazian, H., Amani, R., Nikhoo, A., et al.: Metabolic syndrome and its correlated factors in an urban population in South West of Iran. J. Diabetes Metab. Disord. **12**(1), 11 (2013)
23. Pascot, A., Després, J.P., Lemieux, I., Alméras, N., Bergeron, J., Nadeau, A., et al.: Deterioration of the metabolic risk profile in women. Respective contributions of impaired glucose tolerance and visceral fat accumulation. Diabetes Care **24**(5), 902–908 (2001)
24. Despres, J.-P., Lemieux, I., Bergeron, J., Pibarot, P., Mathieu, P., Larose, E., et al.: Abdominal obesity and the metabolic syndrome: contribution to global cardiometabolic risk. Arterioscler. Thromb. Vasc. Biol. **28**(6), 1039–1049 (2008)
25. Roberts, C.K., Hevener, A.L., Barnard, R.J.: Metabolic syndrome and insulin resistance: underlying causes and modification by exercise training. In: Terjung, R. (ed.) Comprehensive Physiology, vol. 3(1), pp. 1–58 (2013)
26. Soysal, A., Demiral, Y., Soysal, D., Uçku, R., Köseoğlu, M., Aksakoğlu, G.: The prevalence of metabolic syndrome among young adults in Izmir, Turkey. Anadolu Kardiyol Derg. **5**(3), 196–201 (2005)
27. Yeboah, K., Dodam, K.K., Affrim, P.K., Adu-Gyamfi, L., Bado, A.R., Owusu Mensah, R.N. A., et al.: Metabolic syndrome and parental history of cardiovascular disease in young adults in urban Ghana. BMC Public Health **18**(1), 96 (2017)
28. Ben Romdhane, H., Ben Ali, S., Skhiri, H., Traissac, P., Bougatef, S., Maire, B., et al.: Hypertension among Tunisian adults: results of the TAHINA project. Hypertens. Res. **35**(3), 341–347 (2012)
29. Lorenzo, C., Okoloise, M., Williams, K., et al.: The metabolic syndrome as predictor of type 2 diabetes. Diabetes Care **26**, 3153–3159 (2003)
30. Stern, M.P., Williams, K., Gonzalez-Villalpando, C., Hunt, K.J., Haffner, S.M.: Does the metabolic syndrome improve identification of individuals at risk of type 2 diabetes and/or cardiovascular disease? Diabetes Care **27**, 2676–2681 (2004)
31. Mottillo, S., Filion, K.B., Genest, J., Joseph, L., Pilote, L., Poirier, P., Rinfret, S., Schiffrin, E.L., Eisenberg, M.J.: The metabolic syndrome and cardiovascular risk: a systematic review and meta-analysis. J. Am. Coll. Cardiol. **56**(14), 1113–1132 (2010)
32. Dekker, J.M., Girman, C., Rhodes, T., Nijpels, G., Stehouwer, C.D.A., Bouter, L.M., Heine, R.J.: Metabolic syndrome and 10-year cardiovascular disease risk in the Hoorn study. Circulation **112**(5), 666–673 (2005)
33. Ford, E.S.: The metabolic syndrome and mortality from cardiovascular disease and all-causes: findings from the National Health and Nutrition Examination Survey II Mortality Study. Atherosclerosis **173**, 309–314 (2004)

Management of Tensions in Emergency Services

Mouna Berquedich[1(✉)], Oualid Kamach[1], Malek Masmoudi[2], and Laurent Deshayes[3]

[1] Laboratory of Innovative Technologies (LTI), Abdelmalek Saâdi University, Tangier, Morocco
berquedich.mouna@gmail.com
[2] Laboratory of Industrial Engineering, Jean Monnet University, Roanne, France
[3] Polytechnic Mohammed VI University, Ben-Guérir, Morocco

Abstract. The study of emergency services management within hospitals typically requires an effective manipulation and capitalizing of the knowledge. To manipulate and capitalize management strategies, an agile approach of decision making to address massive crowding in emergency department considering constraints such as human resources, costs, patient cases prioritization, capacity and logistics. We inspired from biological immune defense system to design piloting emergency system, basically, the artificial immune system (SIA). The system provides an intelligent assistance to hospital decision-makers to adjust their supplying strategies, and provide relevant traces from previous gathering information assisting hospital staff, facing the massive patient flow, to execute an efficient solution, excellently. In fact, we made a mixture of two related SIA techniques; the negative selection and the clonal selection. The system agility form is gained throughout adopting the approach of components. This paper will focus on the patient overcrowdings dilemmas, raising the reception capacities articulating on coordination networks amid regional hospitals, and simultaneously conserving the safety of the hospitalizing people in every hospital. The main purpose is to decreasing the tension within the emergency department and supplying hospital chiefs working under stress.

Keywords: Hospital environment · AIS · Negative selection · Clonal selection

1 Introduction

At present, there is a tendency towards an emergency service favoring complementarity and coordination of health actors. The vision consists associating an effective production management of care requiring hospital patients' flows control.

Nowadays, the permanent demand of emergency medical care management of hospital emergency services, Emergency Department, (ED) has become increasingly important [1–5]. To anticipate and manage the patient outflow is one of the most important dilemmas within emergency services worldwide. To deal with this patients' fluctuation, EDs require significant human, material resources and a high level of coordination among humans and materials [6]. Unfortunately, these resources are limited.

M. Ezziyyani (Ed.): AI2SD 2018, AISC 914, pp. 100–119, 2019.
https://doi.org/10.1007/978-3-030-11884-6_9

The patients flux generates ED overcrowdings [6]. As a result, ED managers need to monitor patient flow continuously and detect either normal or abnormal patient behavior. Hospital information system plays an important role development hospitals efficiencies. To achieve that, we require a decision-making tool to control these situations.

The manipulation of data and the making of satisfying decisions are major challenges facing the construction of hospital decision support systems [7, 8]. The objective is to realize an excellent control of the patient's flow basing on experience feedback, which often consists a sitting of adverse events knowledge base. This feedback is articulated on a starting loop collected from the ground; retrieving information, analyzing it and finding appropriate solutions. After analyses, it is possible to turn back to it, highlight suitable action to the emergency department, and finally deliver real retroactive loop of continuous updating from data fields.

2 Literature Review

2.1 The Disturbances in the Hospital Environment

In The emergency department is one of the critical infrastructures of a hospital [5]. It often confronts events and/or exceptional situations; the increasing number of patients resulting epidemic episodes (i.e.; natural disasters, terrorist attacks and Accidents, etc.), reduction of resources, and the appearance of complex pathologies requiring considerable time processing.

The consequences of these disturbances on the hospital emergency services can vary from a simple peak of activity to a situation of crisis, passing through situations of tension.

2.2 The Situation of Tension in the Emergency Service

Tension situations can be outlined from different perspectives. It is delimited by different factors. From flow patient paradigm, a tension situation in an emergency department can be defined as an imbalanced load and the care capacity, in which the marginal valuc is cxcccdcd:

1. care load: based on numbers of; patients entering, the outgoing patients, runaways and the number of untreated patients leaving emergencies.
2. capacity of care: represents the emergency department patients' number handled during a given period, taking account of human and material means. This include the number of doctors, nurses, care auxiliaries, number of boxes, beds and medical equipment. It is estimated by emergency department employees.

For the capacity of the care, we will define two types of capacity:

- Capacity required: the gain of the resource working with maximum capacity.
- Available Capacity: the capacity of the resource subtracting from the dysfunction time.

The main factors that can affect balance are:

- factors affecting the number of inflows (patient flows): seasonal epidemics (influenza, colds, gastroenteritis, bronchiolitis, etc.), accidents (works, factories and road accidents).
- Actors influencing faster care and, therefore, the capacity to produce cares:

The nursing staff competences (experience feedback, etc.), internal and external transfer capacity (availability of downstream care services).

2.3 Large Influx of Injured People in Hospital

The hospitality of massive influx victims is taken into account by a recent ministerial circular, called White Plan. This plan displays arranging levels made in every public and private hospitalization facility (with or without emergencies from this facility). The guiding principle of the White Plan is to ensure an optimal reception of victims considering the safety of already hospitalized persons. A crisis unit is the basic structure of the White Plan. Accordingly, deciding planned formalized provisions in reflexing sheets: the establishment of reception points for victims, families, media, access to these points of reception, opportunities to increase the admission capacity of the institution, and the management of the deceased peoples.

2.4 Guiding Principles of the White Plan

The triggering event generates large number of simultaneous victims. It had, for too long, engendered policies of simple transportation to the nearest health facility.

These "wild" made evacuations took place using personal cars or ambulances. They mostly moved the catastrophe from one place to another. Indeed, unwarned and unprepared hospital was too often the cradle of what Professor P. Huguenard described as "an improvisation, a sterile agitation, multiple and contradictory orders, useless good will, unhealthy curiosity" [9].

This wholly unsuitable reception paralyzes the natural operation of the hospital. The basic principle of Emergency Plans is therefore to provide better welcoming to these epidemic victims while disposing security to the already hospitalized patients progressively, and possibly ensuring some usual emergencies functioning. In practice, how to deal with the raising groups of victims?

In this paper, we are particularly interested in increasing the reception capacity via inter-coordination networks linking several regional hospitals, and guaranteeing the safety of the hospitalized persons in each hospital.

2.5 The Increase of Reception Capacity [9]

The White Plan then defines how to increase hospital capacity. Starting from a census as quickly as possible of the existing means (staff, beds, operating rooms, laboratories, etc.) at the time of the alert, several procedures kickoff:

- Keep staff on site especially if an event occurs during a team change.

- Lightening plus deprogramming the activities of operating theaters, radiology departments, and laboratories.
- Move patients whose stable conditions demand less involved services, even towards other institutions.
- Recall staff by:

- A multiplication tested system.
- A graduation according to the projected duration.
- A list of: updating, confidential, and accessible contacts' information.
- A rally to their service or a specific decontamination point.
- An effective functioning of the staff children nursery.

3 Overview of the AIS Techniques

3.1 Basic Concepts

The Artificial Immune System field has been inspired from natural immune system of several species. Ambitiously, to develop systems that operate in environments similar to constraints faced by the natural immune system. De Castro and Timmis defines the AIS as "the adaptive systems, inspired by the theories of the immunology, as well as the functions, the principles and the immune models, in order to be applied to the resolution of problems" [10].

The immunity is subdivided into two distinct systems: innate immune system and adaptive immune system. The adaptive immune system has three principal processes [11]: negative selection, clonal selection and immune network. Whereas, Natural Dendritic Cells are the link between the innate and adaptive immune system.

3.2 Negative Selection

The purpose of negative selection is to provide tolerance for self-cells [12]: The thymus is a gate against the non-self-antigens. The T cells presenting non self antigens are destroyed in this organ. All T cells retiring of the thymus and circulating in the body are said tolerantly towards the self.

3.3 Clonal Selection

The clonal selection algorithm [13] is used by natural immune system to define the basic features of an immune response of an antigenic stimulus. It establishes the idea that only those cells that recognize the antigens are selected to proliferate. The selected cells are subject to an affinity mature process, which improves their affinity to the selective antigens. The readers can read [14] for more details about the main stages of the clonal selection.

3.4 Immune Network

The immune network theory is originally proposed by Jerne [15]. An artificial immune network is a bio-inspired informatics model that uses the ideas/concepts of the immune network theory, mainly, the interaction between B cells and the cloning process. It receives an antigen as entry and sends back an immunized network compound of the B cells that are adjusting in between.

The immune network process is almost the same as clonal selection, except that there exists a mechanism of deletion that destroys the cells having a certain inception of affinity amidst.

3.5 Dendritic Cells (DCs)

The Dendritic Cells Algorithm [16] is a second-generation algorithm based on an abstract model of natural dendritic cells (DCs). It was first introduced in 2005 [17]. Natural DCs are part of the innate immune system. They are responsible for initial pathogen detection, acting as a vital link between the innate and the adaptive system.

Clonal selection algorithms are mostly used as optimizing algorithms. They use fewer classifications. Thus, clonal selection principles first appeared in 1959 [18]. Artificial immune systems algorithms used for classification are considered as classifiers, since they combine the output of many simple classifiers all together.

3.6 Training Methods [19]

The Two types of cells involved to recognize presenting pathogens are; T-cells and B-cells. The population of these present cells in the bloodstream is responsible for recognizing and destructing the pathogens. The population acts collectively. It is capable to identify new pathogens through two training methods: negative selection and clonal selection. Through the process of negative selection, the NIS is able to protect the host organism tissues from being attacked by its own immune system. Some cells generate detectors that recognize proteins, which are present on the surfaces of cells. The detectors are called "antibodies". They are randomly created. Before the cells become fully mature, they are "tested" in the thymus. The thymus, an organ located behind the sternum, is able to destroy any immature cells that identify the tissues of the organism as "non-self" [19]. The process of negative selection maps therefore the negative space of a given class such as given examples of the "self" class. The negative selection algorithm first appeared in 1994 [20]. Using the clonal selection, the NIS is apt to adjust itself to provide the most efficient response against pathogen attacks. Clonal selection happens when a cell detector finds already seen pathogen in the organism, it clones itself then to start the immune response. The cloning process, however, introduces small variations in the pattern that the cell detector recognizes. The number of the clones created by a cell detector is proportional to the new pathogen cell "affinity". It is a measured manner to detect to which extend the cell matches the pathogen. The amount of variation allowed in the clones is negatively proportional to the affinity; the cells with the most affinities are mutated less. The clonal selection algorithms are similar to the natural selection systems. And the clonal selection algorithm is therefore similar to the genetic algorithms based on the natural selection [21]. Nevertheless, clonal selection algorithms have less parameters than genetic algorithms, and potentially, they do not require complex functioning operations. Clonal selection algorithms are mostly used as optimizing algorithms. There have been a few of them used for classification. The clonal selection principle first appeared in 1959 [18]. Artificial immune systems algorithms applied for classifications are considered to being classifiers; they combine the output of many simple classifiers.

4 Analysis of Arrival Patients

Several works stated the management of the sliding flow of the randomly arrivals to hospitals based on different methodologies. In this regard, Tandberg and Qualls used three statistical methods: the moving average and two seasonal decomposition methods. They predict the ED presentations number at any time of the week in the university Hospital of New Mexico [22]. Rotstein and other researchers developed a statistical model of an emergency service in a hospital located in Israel [23].

Abdel-Aal and Mangoud used two univariate time-series analyses to modeling and predicting the monthly volume of patients during eleven-year-period (1986–96) at family and community medicine primary health care clinic of King Faisal University, Al-Khobar, Saudi Arabia [24]. Others scholars adopted Box-Jenkins models to estimate the daily emergent admissions, and the number of emergency often occupied beds at Bromley Hospitals NHS Trust in United Kingdom [24]. Jones, Joy, and Pearson studied ED models at a hospital in Tenerife, Spain. Their analysis was based on time-series of ED presentations number per-hour all along six-year-period (1997–2002). The authors divided the time-series models into linear and non-linear models [25].

Few studies explored the use of knowledge-based-data articulating on the previously achieved solutions, and past scenarios in order to make suitable decisions covering massive flow of patients. Our work will present a proactive approach to solving this problem.

5 Triage of Patients in the Emergency Department

A distinction was made among scales of available patients for triage at the emergency department level. Five classification levels of severity of the arrived patients at ED. Each level assigned weightings according to its severity. We cite the setting tools available as follows:

The Emergency Severity Index (ESI) is a five-point-score indicator developed by American research agency formerly known as the Agency for Healthcare Research and Quality. This validated score borne several modifications making it possible to obtain the current version in 5 points [26, 27]. A score of 1, indicates severe and unstable patient, corresponds to immediate management. A patient with a score of 5 is stable and does not require urgent care.

Another sorting ratio is the Manchester Triage Scale (MTS). It is developed in 1996. The study demonstrates that it can detect severe patients [28]. Subject to good use, including the training of personnel, MTS has good sensitivity. we detect patient levels from MTS1 to MTS5.

Also in Canada, the computerized sorting scale known as the Canadian Emergency Department (CRTC) [29, 30] was introduced in 1998 and widely adopted in the US. It takes into account the speed of implementation of the care and their reassessment time to adopt the consumption of care. It relies on a standardized list of reasons for consultation with the concept of determinant called the first and second order CIMU levels are distinguished from 1 to 5.

It is for this reason that an evaluation of the relevant trace according to three Levels was chosen:

Level one: urgent patients
Level two: moderately urgent
Level three: non-urgent patients.

6 Proposed Filtering Method

Counting the constraints, problems presented in the introduction and on the basis of the AIS techniques (negative selection and clonal selection) adopted, in this section, we will describe our proactive system architecture and our first filtering algorithm.

6.1 System Overview

The main objective of our work is to develop a vital supporting tool for hospital decision-makers to strengthen the quality of their decisions face of the massive flow of patients. The fundamental idea is to detect traces in the database, and to help executives by identifying bad scenarios utilizing AIS techniques, especially negative and clonal selection. The analogy between the principle of the natural immune system and the problem as proposed above (Table 1) has prompted us to develop our system.

Table 1. Analogy between the natural immune system principle and the developed system.

Natural immune system	Artificial immune system applied in our hospital emergency context
Self (antibody)	Relevant trace
Non-self (antigen)	Irrelevant trace
Lymphocyte (B- and T- cell)	Detectors
Detect the antigen	Detect the irrelevant trace
Cloning and memorization	Cloning and update the self-data

6.2 Metrics Distance

A metric distance is a function that measures the similarity in-between two different vectors; xi = [xi1, xi2,..., xiD] and xj = [xj1, xj2,..., xjD]. It yields a non-negative real number, and represents the degree of discrepancy between the two-data points [31].

Although, a large number of distance metrics were proposed in the literature. The widest metric used is still the Euclidean distance. It was established by Euclid past two thousand years ago. Another lengthy applied metric, is the Manhattan one, which is also known as the city-block distance [31].

We will explain the Manhattan distance choice of data based analysis articulating on a comparative study among various methods in terms of efficiency as follows.

6.3 Choice of Manhattan Distance

For Scholars as Noel and Bernardete performed a work that analyze the impact of the distinct distance Metrics in instance-based learning algorithms [32]. Notably, they examined the nearest neighbor algorithm (NN), and the Incremental Hypersphere Classifier (IHC) algorithm, which was proved effective of large-scale problems recognition and e-learning. They provided a detailed empirical assessment on fifteen data sets of several sizes and dimensions. Statistically, they showed that the Euclidean and Manhattan metrics produce significant results in case of wide-range problems. However, grid search methods are often desirable to determine the best matching metric depending on the problem and the algorithm. They concluded that the Manhattan distance is preferred, in particular for large datasets, since it is less computationally demanding. This is what prompted us to adopt this approach.

7 Methodology of Matching with Manhattan Distance

7.1 Definition of the Problem

The problem of supervised learning classification is defined in this section. Giving a sets of data solutions in a knowledge base comprising pairs of inputs and outputs:

$$S = \{(t1, y1), (t2, y2), (t3, y3), \ldots, (ts, yn)\} \quad (1)$$

Where Ti is a vector of parameter values in dimension space (S):

$$t_i \in T \quad (2)$$

A function that maps each vector Ti into Vector space to a class in the set Y, where:

$$T_i \in Y \quad (3)$$

The objective of a learning algorithm [16], is to construct a function F that approaches a function E, where F is the real function which classifies an input vector in T in a Y-category described as follows:

$$F(t) : T \to Y \tag{4}$$

To test our model, we use sets of test data T from an already established knowledge base:

$$Ti = \{t1, t2, t3, \ldots\ldots tn\} \tag{5}$$

$$Tj = \{t1, t2, \ldots\ldots tn\} \tag{6}$$

$$W = \{w1, w2, \ldots\ldots wn\} \tag{7}$$

The W vector is the associated weight vector to T participate in the decision making.

The Manhattan distance is as the following formula indicates [32]:

$$d(Ti, Tj) = \left|\sum((tk(Ti) - tk(Tj))\right| \tag{8}$$

The process of preferences is given as follows:

$$Min\, d(Ti, Tj) = min \frac{\sum((tk(Ti) - tk(Tj)).wi}{\sum wi} \tag{9}$$

7.2 Optimization Framework

In a multi-hospital environment, it is more convenient to transfer the non-emergency patients towards others providing resources hospitals instead of tolerating the not satisfied demands or long-waiting-time within it. As a result, finding the appropriate level of resources, taking into account the patient transfer hypothesis, will considerably reduce overcrowdings in hospitals. In this section, the optimization model considers the component capacity of hospitals. The notations bellow define mathematical model sets of parameters:

i, j: Hospital and demand area indices.
t: Time indices.
l: Patient emergency type indices (1: emergency patients, 2: medium urgent, 3: not urgent).
H: Total number of hospitals.
L: Variants type of the patient.
ci: Cost of increasing a unit of capacity at the hospital i.
di: Overtime cost at the hospital i.
xi: Capacity considered for hospital i.
ni, j: Non-emergency patients number (l = 3) sent from i hospital to j hospital.
di, l, t: Number of l type discharged patients from i hospital at t time.
ki, t: Available capacity in i hospital at t time.
pi, k, t: Number of l type patients admitted to i hospital at t time.

$$Min\sum\nolimits_{i\in H}c_i x_i + \sum\nolimits_{i\in H}\sum\nolimits_{j\in H} z_i, jn_i, j \tag{10}$$

Capacity constraints [R].

All time available capacity equals to the previous capacity changed by accepted and discharged patients.

$$ki, t = ki, t-1 - \sum\nolimits_{l\in L} p_i, l, t-1 + \sum\nolimits_{l\in L} d_i, l, t \tag{11}$$

Total number of accepted patients cannot exceed the available capacity.

$$\sum pi, k, t \leq ki, t \forall i \in H \tag{12}$$

Available capacity should be equal or less than assigned resources to that shift.

$$ki, t \leq xi \forall i \in H \tag{13}$$

Transfer patient constraint should be less than the transfer limit of origin hospital and destination hospital available capacity.

$$ni, j, t \leq kj, t, j \forall i, j \in H \tag{14}$$

In the following section, we present the architecture of our system as well as a description of the algorithms.

8 System Architecture

As indicated by several authors, the traces treatment passes through three main stages: collection, analysis and exploitation. We work on the second and last stage precisely. Indeed, in the second step (i.e. trace analysis), the traces collected in the first step are filtered using the Manhattan distance [32]. In the last step, the objective is to supply hospital decision-makers by suitable traces, and to keep all relevant learning traces in the knowledge base (Fig. 1).

8.1 Collection of Traces

The system brings the actions taken by hospital decision-makers all together. The recorded traces on the Knowledge Base are from the User-system interaction. In addition, other traces may occur from other servers.

8.2 Analysis of Traces

Trace form: A new dataset is created when the traces are reformulated according to the proposed format. The general format of the trace is defined as follows (Fig. 2):

T = {t1, t2, t3, t4, ….}
t: types of cases.

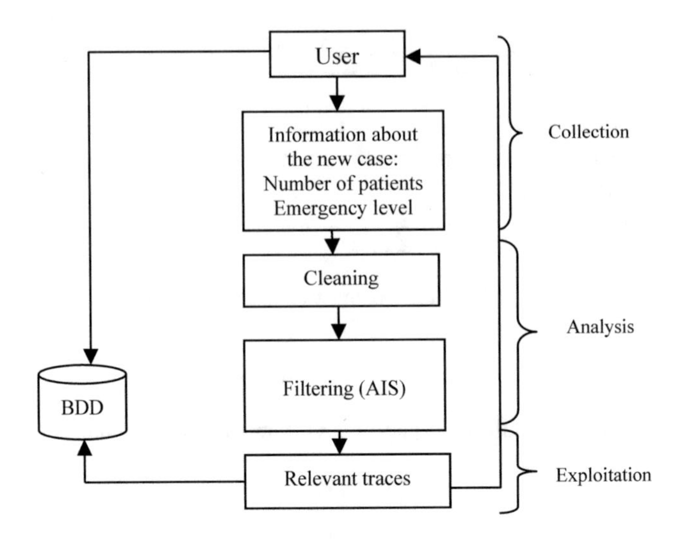

Fig. 1. System architecture

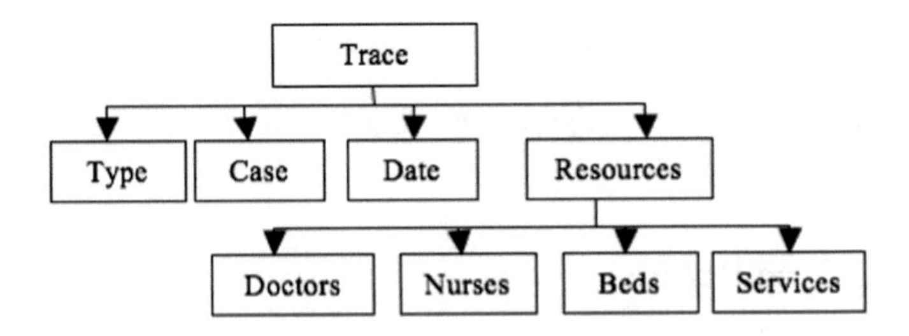

Fig. 2. Trace format

t is characterized by the following 4-tuple:
t = {T, C, D, R}
T: Type.
C: case is the number of patients and their pathology.
D: Date.
R: Resources.
R = {Doc, N, B, S}

Cleaning: to eliminate the noise (the number of patients that did not correspond to the case entered), an algorithm of cleaning of the traces is proposed (see Algorithm 1).

Algorithm1. Cleaning traces

Output:CT=a set of cleaned traces
ND: Nearest distance
NT: set of nearest T
 Begin
For all (trace t ∈ T) then
Ct: case of trace.
D: d(Ct, C)=|C-Ct|
 If (ND is null or D <ND) then
  ND = D
  t ∈ NT
 Else if (d = ND)
  t ∈ NT
End for
End

Filtering: in order to detect automatically the bad scenarios already recorded against the real case entered by the hospital decider, we used an algorithm to filter traces and keep only the relevant elements that will present the relevant traces for the case given by the manager.

9 Computational Results

Global architecture of work entities to guarantee an agility of our system, we applied an approach via work components. We present the global architecture of entities in below:

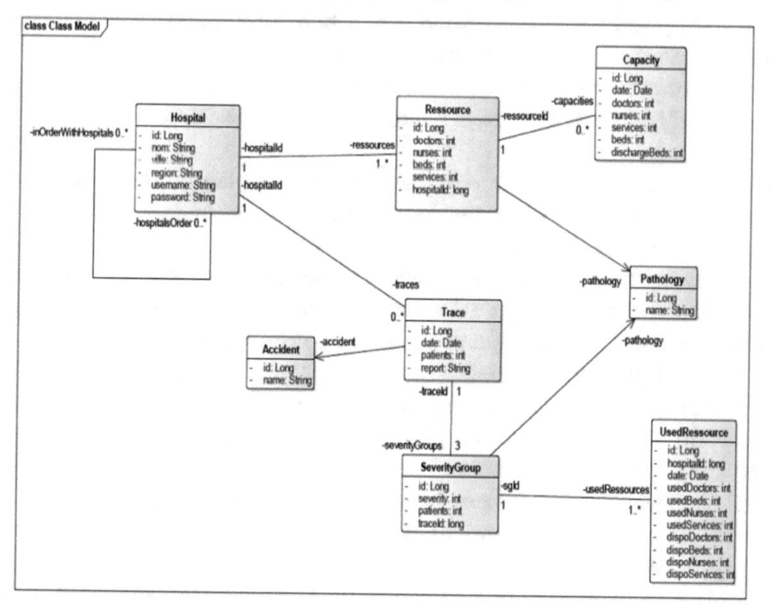

In favor of validating our idea, we have set up a subsystem called Emergency Management (EM). It aims to filter all the traces on the database to display only the relevant traces of the case entered on the interface (Fig. 3).

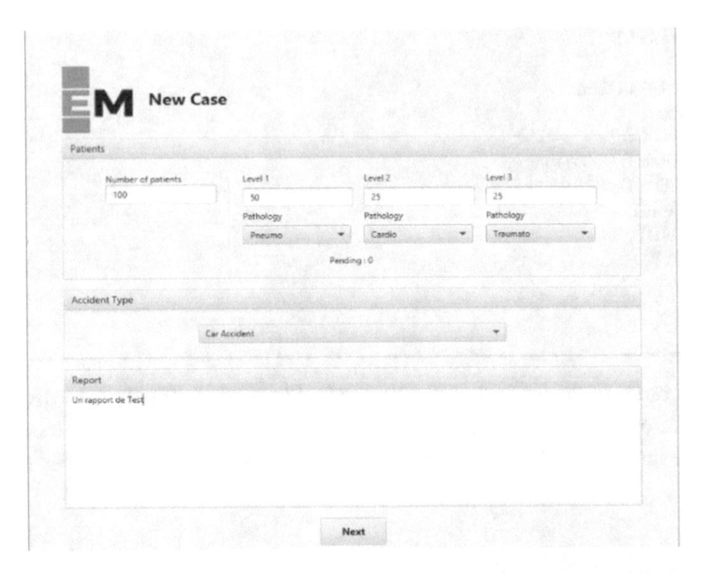

Fig. 3. The results of the proposed algorithm for detecting relevant solutions.

The projected system searches the corresponding case solution on the database according to the available resources, and in collaboration networks with other databases corresponding to the regional hospitals.

The selecting resources process takes into account the host hospital available resources in a real time, and at the same time, it coordinates with other regional hospitals.

The priority selection of the resources of each hospital is given considering the budgetary constraint of patient transfers, the logistical constraints as well as the constraint capacity of each hospital.

The following figures show the results obtained from our system (Fig. 4).

The patients' distribution results are showed according to their urgency level bearing the logistical, capacitive and budgetary constraints (Fig. 5).

We have adapted and applied AIS techniques in a hospital system. The main objective of our work is to provide relevant traces for decision-makers (which go back to the scenarios of the cases already passed by the emergency department), and afford them the most appropriate elements. The objective is to improve real-time scenarios and supply hospital decision-makers with a minimal helpful set of traces. The filtering process integrates AIS techniques in which the negative and clonal selections are associated; the negative selection is applied to detect relevant traces and the clonal selection helps to update the original database. The developed subsystem detects all suited sequences of actions and recommends decision-makers to find the right decision.

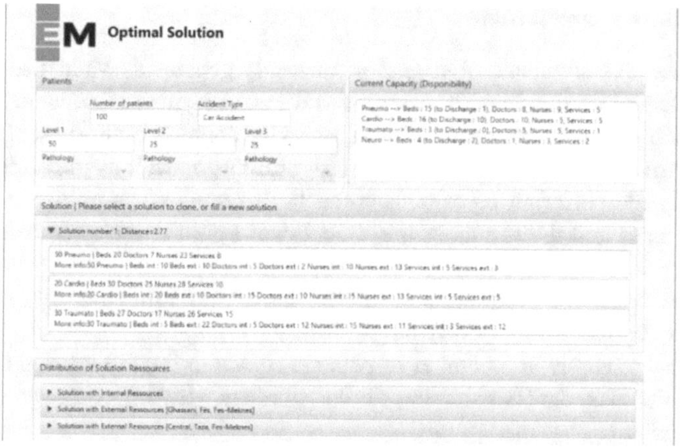

Fig. 4. Displaying optimal solutions.

In this paper, the principles of the white plan have been computerized to bring up real-time responses to the hands of hospital decision makers for distributing patients granting their urgency level. The coordination in-between hospitals admitting of logistical, capacitive and budgetary constraints, and guaranteeing the safety of the already hospitalized patients in the hospital. All talks sum up the objective of this first part.

We are going to fill the white plan boundaries in our system to provide an 'all-risks' strategy in emergencies.

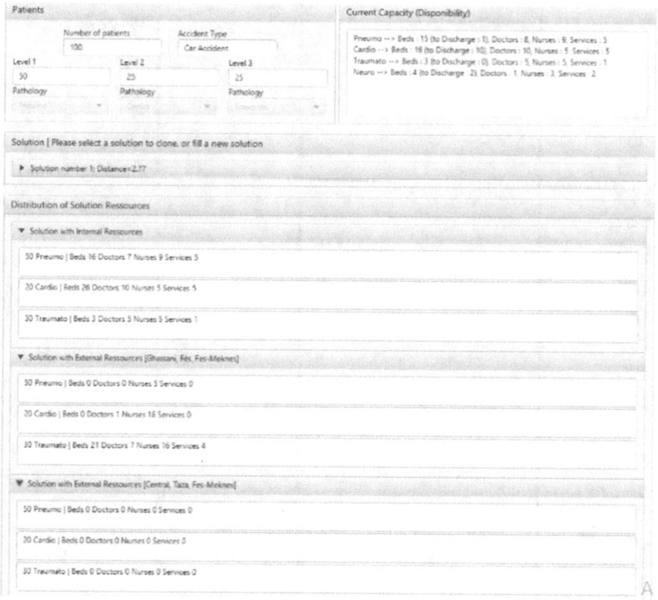

Fig. 5. The distribution of patients between regional hospitals according to their level of urgency

9.1 Database Alimentation

The data base was alimented of scenarios randomly generated, we had selected in the following example a simple of 20 cases. And for each number of patients, there are 50 traces of each single number with different gravity degrees, and different pathologies aiming to prove the results of our filtering algorithms, as well as memorization.

To verify the performance of our approach, this application utilizes a database of 10,000 instances and the results of the executional figure in the table below (Table 2 and 3):

After executing the program, a sample is chosen for validating our approach, we gave the executional time in every single case:

In the first example, the number of patients equals to 90, the looking solution was executed in the local data base among similar numbers with different degrees of gravity and pathologies.

In the second case, the number of patients equals to 60, the searching solution process will due in two different databases presenting multiple similar scenarios of the same number of patients, but with different gravity degrees and pathologies.

Table 2. Sample of study in the database

Hospital	Number of patients by case	Number of traces by patients number	Severity groups number by trace	Utilized resources number by group of severity
1	60 70 80 90 100 110 120 130 140 150 160 170 180 190 200 210 220 230 240 250	Over 50 traces by patients' number with different combinations	3	Min: 1 (internal resources) Max: 3 (1 internal resources + 2 external resources)
Total of a hospital	**Total of cases 20**	**Total of traces more than 1500**	**Total of groups more than 3000**	**With 9000**

Table 3. The results of executional timing during the solution research process over the collaboration among databases

Trace	Maximal hospital participants	Time of execution
Patients = 60 Cardiac (15), Neurotic (15), Nephrotic (30)	1 (Internal only)	Load = 1341 ms Cleaning = 2 ms Filtering = 1 ms Distribution = 1 ms **Total = 1345 ms**
Patients = 70 Orthopedic (20), Neurotic (30), Pneumonic (20)	1 (Internal only)	Load = 1341 ms Cleaning = 2 ms Filtering = 1 ms Distribution = 1 ms **Total = 1345 ms**
Patients = 80 Neurologic (40), Cardiac (10), Pneumonic (30)	1 (Internal only)	Load = 1341 ms Cleaning = 2 ms Filtering = 1 ms Distribution = 1 ms **Total = 1345 ms**
Patients = 90 Cardiac (50), Orthopedic (10), Pneumonic (30)	1 (Internal only)	Load = 1341 ms Cleaning = 2 ms Filtering = 1 ms Distribution = 1 ms **Total = 1345 ms**
Patients = 100 Traumatic (50), Orthopedic (5), Nephrotic (45)	2 (1 Internal + 1external)	Load = 1327 ms Cleaning = 2 ms Filtering = 1 ms Distribution = 8 ms **Total = 1338 ms**
Patients = 110 Cardiac (55), Neurotic (15), Nephrotic (40)	2 (1 Internal + 1external)	Load = 1327 ms Cleaning = 2 ms Filtering = 1 ms Distribution = 8 ms **Total = 1338 ms**
Patients = 120 Orthopedic (90), Traumatic (5), Pneumonic (25)	2 (1 Internal + 1external)	Load = 1327 ms Cleaning = 2 ms Filtering = 1 ms Distribution = 8 ms **Total = 1338 ms**
Patients = 130 Cardiac (85), Neurotic (30), Gastro (15)	2 (1 Internal + 1external)	Load = 1327 ms Cleaning = 2 ms Filtering = 1 ms Distribution = 8 ms **Total = 1338 ms**

(*continued*)

Table 3. (*continued*)

Trace	Maximal hospital participants	Time of execution
Patients = 140 Orthopedic (60), Traumatic (5), Pneumonic (75)	2 (1 Internal + 1external)	Load = 1327 ms Cleaning = 2 ms Filtering = 1 ms Distribution = 8 ms **Total = 1338 ms**
Patients = 150 Gastro (40), Orthopedic (95), Neurotic (15)	2 (1 Internal + 1external)	Load = 1327 ms Cleaning = 2 ms Filtering = 1 ms Distribution = 8 ms **Total = 1338 ms**
Patients = 160 Cardiac (80), Traumatic (10), Pneumonic (70)	2 (1 Internal + 1external)	Load = 1327 ms Cleaning = 2 ms Filtering = 1 ms Distribution = 8 ms **Total = 1338 ms**
Patients = 170 Orthopedic (70), Traumatic (10), Neurotic (90)	3 (1 Internal + 2 externals)	Load = 1462 ms Cleaning = 2 ms Filtering = 1 ms Distribution = 6 ms **Total = 1473 ms**
Patients = 180 Gastro (50), Nephrotic (100), Cardiac (30)	3 (1 Internal + 2 externals)	Load = 1462 ms Cleaning = 2 ms Filtering = 1 ms Distribution = 6 ms **Total = 1473 ms**
Patients = 190 Neurotic (50), Orthopedic (90), Pneumonic (50)	3 (1 Internal + 2 externals)	Load = 1462 ms Cleaning = 2 ms Filtering = 1 ms Distribution = 6 ms **Total = 1473 ms**
Patients = 200 Cardio (50), Traumatic (80), Gastro (70)	3 (1 Internal + 2 externals)	Load = 1462 ms Cleaning = 2 ms Filtering = 1 ms Distribution = 6 ms **Total = 1473 ms**
Patients = 210 Orthopedic (90), Nephrotic (25), Neurotic (95)	3 (1 Internal + 2 externals)	Load = 1462 ms Cleaning = 2 ms Filtering = 1 ms Distribution = 6 ms **Total = 1473 ms**

(*continued*)

Table 3. (*continued*)

Trace	Maximal hospital participants	Time of execution
Patients = 220 Cardiac (110), Traumatic (65), Pneumonic (45)	3 (1 Internal + 2 externals)	Load = 1462 ms Cleaning = 2 ms Filtering = 1 ms Distribution = 6 ms **Total = 1473 ms**
Patients = 230 Orthopedic (70), Traumatic (90), Gastro (70)	3 (1 Internal + 2 externals)	Load = 1462 ms Cleaning = 2 ms Filtering = 1 ms Distribution = 6 ms **Total = 1473 ms**
Patients = 240 Nephrotic (165), Gastro (15), Pneumonic (60)	3 (1 Internal + 2 externals)	Load = 1462 ms Cleaning = 2 ms Filtering = 1 ms Distribution = 6 ms **Total = 1473 ms**
Patients = 250 Cardiac (50), Orthopedic (105), Nephrotic (95)	3 (1 Internal + 2 externals)	Load = 1462 ms Cleaning = 2 ms Filtering = 1 ms Distribution = 6 ms **Total = 1473 ms**

The third case consists of looking for the solution from one internal (Local database) and two external databases (whose representing the 2 external hospitals chosen in this case), likewise, the presence of a couple of similar scenarios, with different gravity degrees and pathologies, however.

Note: (lead-time) signifies the time to load information of the hospital and hospitals contributing in resources distribution. This is performed one time while the application is functioning, and eliminates the frequent demands of information from databases.

10 Conclusion

The anomaly detection is one characteristic of the AIS techniques. We have adapted this feature from our concern, which is filtering and improving the hospital database knowledge. A bad scenario (set of irrelevant traces) is the solution that will not fit the urgent needs of the massive patient flow. We have adapted and applied AIS techniques to supplying hospital decision-makers with a supporting tool. The major ambition of our work is fairly presenting relevant traces to these administrators (which go back to their old solutions) and provide them with the relevant elements in order to satisfy their needs.

References

1. Kellermann, A.: Crisis in the emergency department. N. Engl. J. Med. **355**(13), 1300–1303 (2006)
2. Harrou, F., Kadri, F., Chaabane, S., Tahon, C., Sun, Y.: Improved principal component analysis for anomaly detection: application to an emergency department. Comput. Ind. Eng. **88**, 63–77 (2015)
3. Kadri, F., Pach, C., Chaabane, S., Berger, T., Trentesaux, D., Tahon, C., Sallez, Y.: Modelling and management of strain situations in hospital systems using an orca approach. In: Proceedings of 2013 International Conference on Industrial Engineering and Systems Management, IESM, pp. 1–9. IEEE (2013)
4. Kadri, F., Harrou, F., Chaabane, S., Tahon, C.: Time series modelling and forecasting of emergency department overcrowding. J. Med. Syst. **38**(9), 1–20 (2014)
5. Harrou, F., Sun, Y., Kadri, F., Chaabane, S., Tahon, C.: Early detection of abnormal patient arrivals at hospital emergency department. In: 6th IESM Conference, Seville, Spain (2015)
6. Kadri, F., Chaabane, S., Tahon, C.: A simulation-based decision support system to prevent and predict strain situations in emergency department systems. Journal **42**, 32–52 (2014)
7. Carey, P., Cuthbert, G., Dang, R., Greystoke, B., McGregor, A., Oakes, R., Wallis, J.: A more devolved and inclusive approach to integrated reporting facilited by an IT system (Haemosys) networked to local information management systems (LIMS) in all participating regional hospitals. Br. J. Haematol. **173**(1), 43 (2016)
8. Carvalho, D., Joao, V., Rocha, A., Vasconcelos, J.: Towards an encompassing maturity model for the management of hospital information systems. J. Med. Syst. **39**(9), 99 (2015)
9. Virenque, C.: Large influx of injured people in hospital. Hôpital Purpan, TSA 40031, 31059 Toulouse cedex 09 (2016). Journal, 712–715
10. De Castro, L.N., Timmis, J.: Artificial immune systems: a novel paradigm to pattern recognition. In: Corchado, J.M., Alonso, L., Fyfe, C. (eds.) Artificial Neural Networks in Pattern Recognition, pp. 67–84. Springer, Berlin (2002)
11. Timmis, J., Hone, A., Stibor, T., Clark, E.: Theoretical advances in artificial immune systems. Theor. Comput. Sci. Rev. **403**(1), 11–32 (2008)
12. Aickelin, U., Dasgupta, D.: Artificial immune systems. In: Burke, E.K., Kendall, G. (eds.) Research Methodologies, pp. 375–399. Springer, New York (2005)
13. De Castro, L.N., Von Zuben, F.J.: The clonal selection algorithm with engineering applications. Paper presented at The Workshop on Artificial Immune Systems and Their Applications, Las Vegas, USA (2000)
14. De Castro, L.N., Von Zuben, F.J.: Learning and optimization using the clonal selection principle. IEEE Trans. Evol. Comput. **6**(3), 239–251 (2002)
15. Jerne, N.K.: Towards a network theory of the immune system. Ann. Immunol. **125**, 373–389 (1974)
16. Greensmith, J., Aickelin, U., Tedesco, G.: Information fusion for anomaly detection with the dendritic cell algorithm. Inf. Fusion J. **11**(1), 21–34 (2010)
17. Greensmith, J., Aickelin, U., Cayzer, S.: Introducing dendritic cells as a novel immune-inspired algorithm for anomaly detection. In: Jacob, C., Pilat, M.L., Bentley, P.J., Timmis, J. I. (eds.) Proceedings of the 4th International Conference on Artificial Immune Systems, pp. 153–167. Springer, Heidelberg (2005)
18. Burnet, M.: The Clonal Selection Theory of Acquired Immunity (1959)
19. Schmidt, B., Ala, A., Ajay, G., Dionysios, K.: Optimizing an artificial immune system algorithm in support of flow-Based internet traffic classification (2017)

20. Forrest, S., Perelson, A., Allen, L., Cherukuri, R.: Self-nonself discrimination in a computer. In: Proceedings of the 1994 IEEE Computer Society Symposium on Research in Security and Privacy, pp. 202–212. IEEE (1994)
21. De Castro, L.N., Von Zuben, F.J.: Learning and optimization using the clonal selection principle. IEEE Trans. Evol. Comput. **6**(3), 239–251 (2000)
22. Tandberg, D., Qualls, C.: Time series forecasts of emergency department patient volume, length of stay, and acuity. Ann. Emerg. Med. **23**(2), 299–306 (1994)
23. Rotstein, Z., Wilf-Miron, R., Lavi, B., Shahar, A., Gabbay, U., Noy, S.: The dynamics of patient visits to a public hospital: a statistical model. Am. J. Emerg. Med. **15**(6), 596–599 (1997)
24. Abdel-Aal, R., Mangoud, A.: Modeling and forecasting monthly patient volume at a primary health care clinic using univariate time-series analysis. Comput. Methods Programs Biomed. **56**(3), 235–247 (1998)
25. Jones, S., Joy, M., Pearson, J.: Forecasting demand of emergency care. Health Care Manag. Sci. **5**(4), 297–305 (2002)
26. Eitel, D., Travers, D., Rosenau, A., Gilboy, N., Wuerz, R.: The emergency severity index triage algorithm version 2 is reliable and valid. Acad. Emerg. Med. **10**(10), 1070–1080 (2003)
27. Tanabe, P., Gimbel, R., Yarnold, P., Adams, J.: The emergency severity index (version 3) 5-level triage system scores predict ED resource consumption. J. Emerg. Nurs. **30**(1), 22–29 (2004)
28. Cooke, M., Jinks, S.: Does the Manchester triage system detect the critically ill? J. Accid. Emerg. Med. **16**(3), 179–181 (1999)
29. Jimenez, J., Murray, M., Beveridge, R., Pons, J., Cortes, E., Garrigos, J., et al.: Implementation of the Canadian Emergency Department Triage and Acuity Scale (CTAS) in the Principality of Andorra: can triage parameters serve as emergency department quality indicators? CJEM **5**(5), 315–322 (2007)
30. Bullard, M., Unger, B., Spence, J., Grafstein, E.: Group CNW. Revisions to the Canadian Emergency Department Triage and Acuity Scale (CTAS) adult guidelines. CJEM **10**(2), 136–151 (2008)
31. Duda, R.O., Hart, P.E., Stork, D.G.: Pattern Classification. Wiley, New York (2001)
32. Noel, L., Bernardete, R.: On the impact of distance metrics in instance-based learning algorithms. UDI, Polytechnic of Guarda, Portugal (2017)

Decision System for the Selection of the Best Therapeutic Protocol for Breast Cancer Based on Advanced Data-Mining: A Survey

Sarah Khrouch[1(✉)], Mostafa Ezziyyani[1], and Mohammed Ezziyyani[2]

[1] Faculty of Sciences and Techniques, Abdelmalek Essaâdi University, Tangier, Morocco
rhksara@gmail.com, ezziyyani@gmail.com
[2] Polydisciplinary Faculty, Abdelmalek Essaâdi University, Larache, Morocco
mohammed.ezziyyani@gmail.com

Abstract. Sometimes the experience of Doctors is not enough sufficient to guide patients perfectly and predict exactly the best treatments to follow and give results with high accuracy. For this reason, it is very important to get a predictive model, resulting in effective and accurate decision making. Our main goal is to make a significant contribution toward improving the quality of healthcare. This work strives to create a dynamic graph of treatments which is able to predict the suitable therapeutic protocol. The objective of this graph is to help doctors classify breast cancer patients depending on the type of breast cancer and the appropriate therapeutic protocol and the optimal dose. In this article we focus on the use of the patient's personal data and medical history for each patient, input features and the medical tests that patient already have done. The predictive machine learning model based on Neural Network, as well as on different input features and using other advanced Data mining algorithms.

Keywords: Breast cancer · Machine learning · Neural network · Therapeutic protocol · Data mining · Predictive model

1 Introduction

No one can deny that cancer is one of the major health problems worldwide. The statistics have shown that 8.8 million people worldwide died from cancer in 2015, that is nearly 1 in 6 of all global deaths (WHO) [1].

The World Health Organization WHO has estimated that cancer causes more deaths than all cardiovascular diseases [1].

Cancer is an excessively complex disease and can become a real danger to the survival of the living being. Besides, cancer is a disease caused by a change that arises in genes or by a lesion to genes what's called a genetic mutation, this disease characterized by the division of abnormal cells that form lumps or growing mass of cancer cells, called a tumor which may invade other normal body tissue.

A single tumor can have more than 100 billion cells and each cell can acquire individual mutations.

M. Ezziyyani (Ed.): AI2SD 2018, AISC 914, pp. 120–128, 2019.
https://doi.org/10.1007/978-3-030-11884-6_10

In Morocco, it is estimated that cancer is a major health problem requiring a global policy of care and it is the second leading cause of mortality after cardiovascular diseases with 10.7% of all deaths [2].

Cancer genes may be changed by several mechanisms presenting a complex evolution. To understand the basic of cancer development and progression, it is therefore necessary to analyze and interpret thousands of genetic compositions of the tumor. However, it becomes a complex and difficult task for clinicians and scientists.

This review will give a brief description of breast cancer in Morocco, the use of machine learning applications in cancer diagnosis, breast cancer and presents the results of many researches works which are applied to data mining. The next step will be to create a predictive model which can help to improve the quality of clinical decisions.

The rest of this paper is organized as follows Sect. 2 represents a breast cancer in brief. Section 3 an overview of the machine learning that employed for modeling breast cancer diagnosis and studies which are related to data mining application in breast cancer diagnosis. Section 4 is about predictive model. Section 5 concludes the paper and presents future works.

2 Breast Cancer

2.1 A Brief Description

The breast cancer is very frequent, and is at the top of the list for the cancers that still kill too many women worldwide.

In Morocco, breast cancer is the most common cancer disease among women and it is a major public health problem.

Several Moroccan researchers still search to learn more about breast cancer in order to find the best medicines which help to fight against this disease. It is in this context that work took place; it involved the setting up of an intelligent system based on the advanced data mining algorithms. With the objective to enhance patient's safety and quality of care in the healthcare field.

In [4] Elidrissi Errahhali, Elidrissi Errahhali, Ouarzane, Boulouiz and Bellaou among their study they registered the distribution of the 7,872 incident cases by cancer type in October 2005–December 2012, as it's shown in Fig. 1 beneath.

According to the Fig. 1 above, breast cancer came first, and overtaken the other cancers, with 30.75% of all cancer [3].

Breast cancer can affect men too, but it is less common in men than women.

There are two types of breast cancers are:

Benign breast lump or non-cancerous: the size of tumor and its texture is understandable during the roughly examination.

Malignant breast lump or cancerous: clinical diagnosis requires for predicting this type of cancer two types of M cancer are

Non-invasive

Invasive.

Type of cancer	Female N.	Male N.	Total N.	%
All incident cases	5220	2652	7872	100
Breast	2368	53	2421	30.75
Cervix uteri	716	-	716	9.1
Colon-rectum	333	309	642	8.16
Lung	90	503	593	7.53
Nasopharynx	153	243	396	5.03
Stomach	164	185	349	4.43
Skin	109	145	254	3.23
Prostate	-	220	220	2.79
Ovary	197	-	197	2.5
Brain	77	94	171	2.17
Bladder and urinary tract	33	126	159	2.02
Bone	62	70	132	1.68
Thyroid	99	23	122	1.55
Esophagus	42	52	94	1.19
Pancreas	48	43	91	1.16
larynx	12	78	90	1.14
Gallbladder	67	12	79	1
Oral cavity and oropharynx	39	37	76	0.97
Corpus uteri	75	-	75	0.95
Soft parts	32	42	74	0.94
Liver	35	24	59	0.75
Kidney	19	24	43	0.55
Peritoneum	28	11	39	0.5
Vulva	32	-	32	0.41
Salivary gland	11	19	30	0.38
Eye	10	13	23	0.29
Testicles	-	20	20	0.25
Pharynx (unspecified)	8	9	17	0.22
Small intestine	10	4	14	0.18
Vagina	10	-	10	0.13
Tonsil	0	5	5	0.06
Mediastinum	1	3	4	0.05
Pleura	2	1	3	0.04
Trunk	1	-	1	0.01
Penis	-	1	1	0.01
Other	337	283	620	7.88

Fig. 1. The distribution of the cancer by type.

2.2 Grade or Stage of Breast Cancer

Breast cancer grade or the extent of cancer refers to

- The size and the shape of the cancer tumor.
- whether the cancer has spread from where it first started and where cancer has spread.

There are five grades, grade 0 followed by grades I, II, III, and IV. Stage 0 stage IV.

According to Rabat cancer registry (in 2005) was found about half of the cases are diagnosed at stages I and II and less than 15% are diagnosed at the stage IV means that cancer has spread to other body in Fig. 2 below [4].

3 State of the Art

Making the right decision in the field of medical must be made effectively and with accuracy. In recent years data mining has played a very important role in the healthcare industry and are becoming very important in medical decision making. In Data mining is an essential step of knowledge discovery. Besides data mining techniques are very useful in the field of healthcare. In addition, data mining has the potential to predict breast cancer and better effective therapeutic protocol, which can help to significantly improve the quality of clinical decision.

Data mining is the process of extracting and analyzing the huge volume of raw or multi-dimensional data.

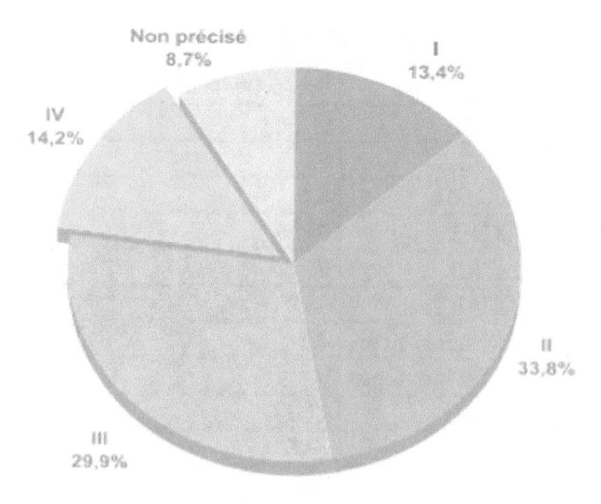

Fig. 2. Distribution of breast cancer in women by stage.

There are various data mining techniques like classification regression, etc.

3.1 Classification

Classification is one of the most important data mining technique and it is a supervised learning, that assigns classes or categories to a collection of data in order to aid in more accurate predictions and analysis.

Besides, classification is one of several methods intended to make the analysis of a very huge dataset effective. It is a supervised learning having known class category.

Following are the various classification algorithms used in the healthcare sector:

3.2 Decision Tree (DT)

A decision tree is one of a predictive model that have been widely applied for classification based on a branching series of Boolean tests that use specific facts to make more generalized conclusion.

Using decision tree, decision makers can choose best alternative and traversal from root to leaf indicates unique class separation based on maximum information gain [6].

Decision tree is widely used by many researchers in healthcare field.

In [7] Decision tree are a reliable and effective decision making that provide high classification accuracy with a simple representation of gathered knowledge.

Several advantages of decision tree as follows: decision trees are self-explanatory and when compacted they are also easy to follow.

The Table 1 below represents the usage frequency of various decision tree algorithms [8].

3.3 Support Vector Machine (SVM)

SVMs are a set of supervised learning methods used for classification, regression and outliers detection. However, it is mostly used in classification problems. In this

Table 1. Frequency usage of decision tree algorithms.

Algorithm	Usage frequency (%)
CLS	9
IDE	68
IDE3+	4.5
C4.5	54.55
C5.0	9
CART	40.9
Random tree	4.5
Random forest	9
SLIQ	27.27
PUBLIC	13.6
OCI	4.5
CLOUDS	4.5
SPRINT	31.84

algorithm, we plot each data item as a point in n-dimensional space (where n is number of features you have) with the value of each feature being the value of particular coordinate. Then, we perform classification by finding the hyper-plane that differentiate the two classes very well [].

In Fig. 3 below shows how an SVM work for classifying tumors (benign and malignant) by their size and patients age the circles presented the misclassified tumors.

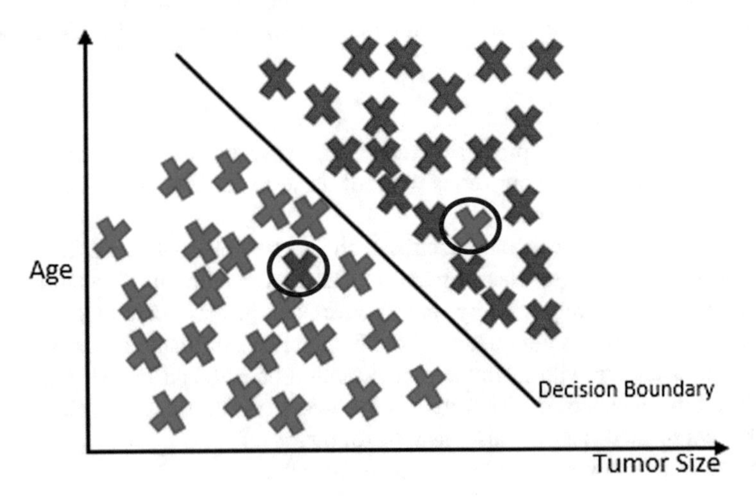

Fig. 3. Example of a linear SVM classification.

3.4 Neural Network

Neural networks those systems modeled based on the human brain working. As the human brain consists of millions of neurons that are interconnected by synapses, a neural network is a set of connected input/output units in which each connection has a weight associated with it [9].

Before the introduction of decision trees and the Support Vector Machine (SVM) it was regarded as the best classification algorithm [5]. This was one of the reasons which encouraged NN as the most widely used classification algorithm in various biomedicine and healthcare fields [5] (Fig. 4).

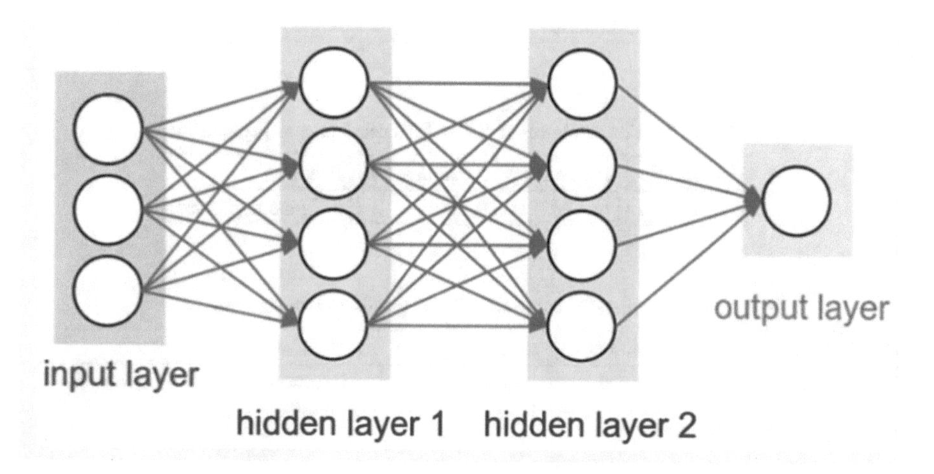

Fig. 4. Example of the neural network structure.

3.5 Naïve Bayes

Naïve Bayes has been one of the popular machines learning methods for many years and is a quick method for creation of statistical predictive models. NB is based on the Bayesian theorem with an assumption of independence among predictors. This technique analyses the relationship between each attribute and the class for each instance to derive a conditional probability for the relationships between the attribute values and the class.

3.6 Diagnosis

Clinical diagnosis of breast cancer helps in predicting the malignant cases. For this reason, many researchers attempt to create intelligent systems for diagnosing breast cancer earlier.

Various common methods for breast cancer diagnosis are Mammography, Positron Emission Tomography, Biopsy and Magnetic Resonance Imaging. Based on the results obtained from these methods are used to recognize the patterns which are aiming to help the doctors to classify the malignant and benign cases. There are various data mining techniques, statistical methods and machine learning that are applied for this purpose. We will see the review of different technical and review articles of data mining techniques applied in breast cancer diagnosis.

Chaurasia et al. [10] applied three algorithms for predicting breast cancer survivals Table 2 (Tables 3, 4 and 5).

Table 2. Performance of algorithms for breast cancer prediction

Publication	Classifiers	Accuracy (%)	Features
Chaurasia et al. [10]	RepTree	71.32%	Tumour size, patient' age, menopause, degree of malignancy and etc.
	RBF network	73.77%	
	Simple logistic	74.47%	

Table 3. Performance of SVM for breast cancer prediction

Publication	Classifiers	Accuracy (%)	Features
Xu et al. [11]	SVM	97%	50-gene signature

Table 4. Performance of DT for predicting breast cancer

Publication	Classifiers	Accuracy (%)	Features
Delen et al. [12]	DT	93%	Tumour size, age, histological, number of nodes

Table 5. Performance of the classifier

Publication	Classifiers	Accuracy (%)	Data
Asri et al. [13]	C4.5	95.13%	The Wisconsin Breast cancer dataset
	SVM	97.13%	
	BN	95.99%	
	K-NN	95.27%	

Shrivastava et al. [14] compare the performance between different neural network techniques (MLP, RBF, Self-Organizing Map) and Probabilistic Neural Network (PNN) for diagnosis of breast cancer, the experimental result shows that PNN is more accurate than other techniques.

4 Proposed Predictive Model

We propose this study to identify a predictive model which help prevents, diagnose, treat, follow the evolution of the disease on patients and propose effective recommendations.

It is therefore important to build a knowledge base contains all information of each patients including their medical history, results and impact of various treatment and etc.

Based on this medical knowledge we can select and decide the best treatment.

Figure 5 shows our model predictive.

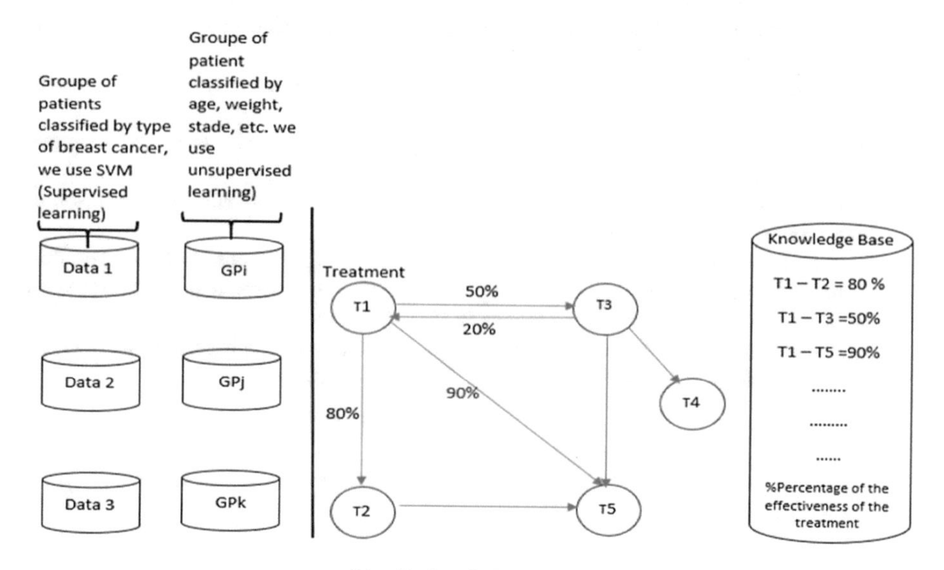

Fig. 5. Predictive model.

5 Conclusion and Perspectives

In this work we see a brief description of breast cancer, provides a study of various technical, we summarizing different algorithms of data mining and we present the research review in the use of data mining. Proposed a structure of our predictive model and the Machine learning applied for.

In our future work, a predictive model will be more developed and further enhanced with the objective to be more reliable and effective.

References

1. WHO: World Health Organization
2. Lalla Salma Foundation - Cancer Prevention and Treatment
3. Elidrissi Errahhali, M., Elidrissi Errahhali, M., Ouarzane, M., Boulouiz, R., Bellaou, M.: Cancer incidence in eastern Morocco: cancer patterns and incidence trends. BMC Cancer **17**, 587 (2017). https://doi.org/10.1186/s12885-017-3597-6. (2005–2012)
4. Rabat cancer registry (2005)
5. Parvez, A., Qamar, S., Rizvi, S.Q.A.: Techniques of data mining in healthcare: a review. Int. J. Comput. Appl. (0975 – 8887) **120**(15), 38–50 (2015)

6. Apte, C., Weiss, S.M.: Data mining with decision trees and decision rules. T.J. Watson Research Center
7. Podgorelec, V., Kokol, P., Stiglic, B., Rozman, I.: Decision trees: an overview and their use in medicine. J. Med. Syst. **26**(5), 445–463 (2002)
8. Sujatha, G., Usha Rani, K.: Evaluation of decision tree classifiers on tumor datasets. Int. J. Emerg. Trends Technol. Comput. Sci. (IJETTCS) (2013)
9. Gupta, S., Kumar, D., Sharma, A.: Data mining classification techniques applied for breast cancer diagnosis and prognosis (2011)
10. Chaurasia, V., Pal, S.: Data mining techniques: to predict and resolve breast cancer survivability. Int. J. Comput. Sci. Mob. Comput. **3**(1), 10–22 (2014)
11. Xu, X., Zhang, Y., Zou, L., Wang, M., Li, A.: A gene signature for breast cancer prognosis using support vector machine. IEEE, 16–18 October 2012
12. Delen, D., Walker, G., Kadam, A.: Predicting breast cancer survivability: a comparison of three data mining methods. Artif. Intell. Med. (2004)
13. Asri, H., Mousannif, H., Al Moatassime, H., Noel, T.: Using machine learning algorithms for breast cancer risk prediction and diagnosis. In: The 6th International Symposium on Frontiers in Ambient and Mobile Systems (FAMS 2016) (2016)
14. Shrivastava, S.S., Sant, A., Aharwal, R.P.: An overview on data mining approach on breast cancer data. Int. J. Adv. Comput. Res. **3**(4), 256–262 (2013)

Obtaining an X-Ray of the Zubal Phantom by Monte Carlo Simulation

Hassane El Bekkouri(✉), Ahmed Dadouch, Abdessamad Didi, and Abdelmajid Maghnouj

Laboratory of Integration System and Technology Advanced (LISTA), Department of Physics, Faculty of Science, University of Sidi Mohamed Ben Abdellah, Fez, Morocco
{hassane.elbekkouri,Abdessamad.didil}@usmba.ac.ma, ahmeddadouch@gmail.com, maghnouj2002@yahoo.fr

Abstract. Radiation transport in matter has attracted great interest since the beginning of the 20th century. High-energy photons, electrons, and positrons penetrate the matter undergoing multiple interactions where his energy is transferred to the atoms and molecules of the material, and secondary particles are produced. By multiple interactions a high energy particle produces a cascade of particles that is usually referred to as a shower. In each interaction, the energy of the particle is reduced and particles can be generated so that the evolution of the shower represents a degradation of the energy. The purpose of this work is to obtain x-ray images of the human body using the Zubal phantom. The transport of the radiation, crossing the phantom and arriving on the detector, is realized using the code MCNP (Monte-Carlo N-Particle transport). The images obtained are comparable to those obtained by a real radiological imaging system.

Keywords: Monte Carlo code · Simulation · Computed Tomography · X-ray · Numerical phantom

1 Introduction

Medical imaging has led to improvements in the diagnosis and treatment of numerous medical conditions in children and adults. There are many modalities of medical imaging procedures, each of which uses different technologies and techniques. Computed tomography (CT), fluoroscopy and radiography use ionizing radiation to generate images of the body. Ionizing radiation is a form of radiation that has enough energy to potentially cause damage to DNA and may elevate a person's lifetime risk of developing cancer. CT, radiography, and fluoroscopy all work on the same basic principle: an X-ray beam is passed through the body where a portion of the X-rays are either absorbed or scattered by the internal structures, and the remaining X-ray pattern is transmitted to a detector for recording or further processing by a computer. These exams differ in their purpose: – Radiography: a single image is recorded for later evaluation. Mammography is a special type of radiography to image the internal structures of breasts. – Fluoroscopy: a continuous X-ray image is displayed on a monitor, allowing for real-time monitoring of a procedure or passage of a contrast agent

M. Ezziyyani (Ed.): AI2SD 2018, AISC 914, pp. 129–139, 2019.
https://doi.org/10.1007/978-3-030-11884-6_11

through the body. Fluoroscopy can result in relatively high radiation doses, especially for complex interventional procedures which require fluoroscopy be administered for a long period of time. – CT: many X-ray images are recorded as the detector moves around the patient's body. A computer reconstructs all the individual images into cross-sectional images or "slices" of internal organs and tissues.

Computed tomography is one of the diagnostic procedures that can cause relatively high radiation exposure to the patient. Over the last two decades, the increasing use of CT in clinical practice and the relatively high dose delivered to the patient during such examinations have made CT a significant contributor to the total collective dose from all medical X-ray examinations. With the introduction of multi-slice CT (MSCT) scanners, the number of clinical applications of CT procedures has continued to increase due to the greater volume coverage and faster rotation times that have provided significantly higher performance. According to recent surveys [1–4], CT was estimated to contribute around 67% of the total collective dose in the USA and about 40% in the UK and Germany, although CT examinations represent only about 11% in the USA and 4% in the UK and Germany, of all radiology examinations. Therefore, there is interest in assessing and optimizing CT radiation doses to patients. The motivation to develop tools to quantitatively assess 3D dose distributions and to derive organ dose values for CT examinations is accordingly very high. Although Monte Carlo (MC) techniques for dose calculation purposes in diagnostic radiology are not new, only lately have they become extensively used in this field mainly due to the increasing computational power of present day personal computers with performances approaching or even exceeding the performances of the supercomputers of a decade ago. Generally, MC simulations are used when physical experiments yielding the same data are impossible, too laborious or too expensive to perform [5]. Several MC tools are available within the scientific community, for example Geant4 [6], MCNP [7] or EGS4 [8].

In Computed Tomography (CT), an X-ray source and an arc of detectors rotate around a body that is positioned in the center of rotation to record X-ray projections from different directions. The measured X-ray projections are then translated into sectional images using reconstruction algorithms [9]. The resulting CT images are used as a quantitative measure of tissue properties for radiotherapy treatment planning. Computed tomography has emerged as one of the most important medical imaging modalities. In fact, the number of CT examinations is still increasing, a significant disadvantage of CT, however, is the exposure to ionizing radiation inherent in the technique [10]. Therefore, it is common to keep the radiation dose as low as reasonably achievable (ALARA). Unfortunately, lowering the dose gives a lower signal-noise and thus poor image quality that may hinder further diagnosis. Optimizing the trade-off between dose and quality is a far from trivial problem, as subjects cannot simply be exposed to a range of radiation doses for ethical reasons. In general, measurements on anthropomorphic phantom may not capture the great variability of structures that can be encountered in real life. The interest of the simulation makes it possible to optimize the quality of the image, to know the importance of the physical properties, the influence of the geometry of the detector and to estimate in a precise way the absorbed doses during radiotherapy or for radiation protection measures. The reconstruction of a radiological or dosimetry image for radiotherapy or radiation protection requires the use of a phantom associated with a Monte Carlo code in order to simulate the patient and his environment. The first anthropomorphic numerical models during the 70's made it possible to represent the organs using mathematical equations. These are the phantom of MIRD (Medical Internal Radiation Dose) committee. The phantom was to approach the main characteristics of the organs using equations that are easy to solve in order to minimize the calculation time. But this mathematical description remained very approximate. The purpose of our work is to obtain X-ray images of the human body using the Zubal anthropomorphic phantom.

2 Methods and Materials

2.1 The Monte Carlo Method

The physical laws and mathematical formalisms that govern the elemental interactions of particles with matter are well known. But the number of high, successive interactions and their stochastic nature makes the task difficult, hence the use of Monte Carlo techniques. Monte Carlo methods are based on microscopic modeling resulting in a 3-dimensional simulation. Particle interactions are simulated individually from a series of random numbers and cross-sections charged to reproduce the actual physical phenomenon. MCNP is a general-purpose Monte Carlo N-Particle code that can be used for neutron, photon, electron, or coupled neutron/photon/electron transport. Specific areas of application include, but are not limited to, radiation protection and dosimetry, radiation shielding, radiography, medical physics, nuclear criticality safety, detector design and analysis, accelerator target design, fission and fusion reactor design, decontamination and decommissioning [11].

The Monte Carlo method is a statistical sampling technique that involves the use of random numbers and probability distributions to solve complex mathematical problems [12]. The emergence of the Monte Carlo method is historically attributed to Stanislaw Ulam. This mathematician worked with John von Neumann on the Manhattan project on research into the manufacture of the atomic bomb during the Second World War. This work consisted of modeling the trajectories of neutrons and gamma rays produced by a nuclear explosion. In 1946, Ulam proposed the Monte Carlo method. He took advantage of the appearance of the computer and his collaboration with Von Neuman and Nicholas Metropolis, to develop implementable Monte Carlo algorithms, the execution of which makes it possible to make non-random problems in stochastic forms which can thus be easily treated by statistical sampling [13]. It was Metropolis who gave the name Monte Carlo to these methods by analogy with the random character of the roulette of the famous Casino of Monte-Carlo.

In 1976, Raeside [14] was the author of the first retrospective on the Monte Carlo method and its applications in medical physics. In his book he breaks down the principle of the Monte Carlo method into three essential parts: random number generation, sampling methods, and variance reduction. The drawing of random numbers is essential for sampling probability functions; sampling methods are the basis for equalities of dispersion functions (cumulative probability density functions) for integral calculation. Finally, variance reduction techniques are essential for effective calculations Monte

Carlo. Early applications of Monte Carlo simulation in medical physics have focused on determining camera detection efficiency for gamma rays and on the calculation of absorption fractions useful for dose calculation absorbed by a patient undergoing a diagnostic nuclear medicine examination.

A classic and amusing exercise that can be used to introduce the Monte Carlo method is the problem of the Count of Buffon's needle. This is one of the first famous historical experiments of stochastic calculus in 1777, making it possible to determine an approximate value of the number π by means of repeated experiments [15]. See Fig. 1.

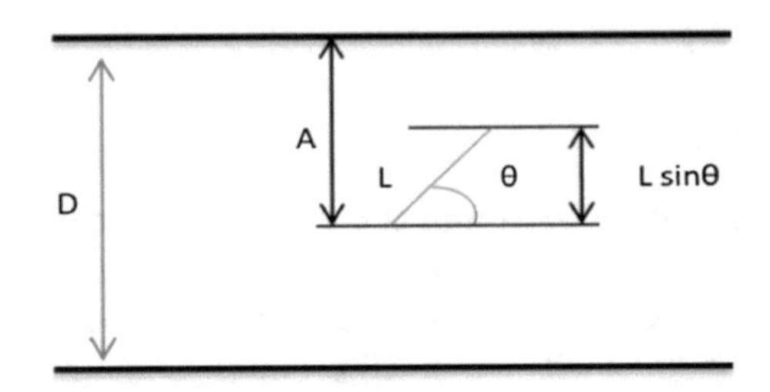

Fig. 1. Schematic representation of Buffon's problem

The problem is as follows: if a needle of length L is thrown randomly into a plane in which two parallel lines separated by a distance D > L. If we throw the needle n times and cut one of the lines m times, the estimated value of π is as follows:

$$\pi \approx \frac{n}{m} \times \frac{2L}{D}$$

2.2 The MCNPX Simulator

This paragraph is intended to briefly introduce the Monte Carlo simulation code we have chosen to use: MCNPX. In what follows we will recall the origin of MCNPX and the statement of its main characteristics. But before dealing with these points, a first question can be asked: why did you choose MCNPX rather than another code? The EGS (Electron Gamma Shower) code [16] is the most widely used code in the field of radiation transport. The PENELOPE code [17] deals in detail with the efficient sections for low energy photon transport and has a flexible geometry allowing simple modeling of linear accelerators. The GEANT4 code [18] was developed for particle physics applications. It is used for radiation simulation in radiotherapy [19] and forms the core of the GATE interface [20] for simulating imaging systems in nuclear medicine. Despite their differences, they all use the Monte Carlo method and the calculated value of a deposit of energy is essentially the same regardless of the code used. We chose MCNPX for the following reasons: Its efficiency in photon and electron transport; the ability to calculate virtual dose grids.

2.3 General Information

MCNPX is a universal radiation transport code that includes 3D geometry, continuous energy particle transport, various source descriptions, flow calculations, dose calculations, etc., and a graphical interface. It is necessary to imagine a delimited geometrical universe, of known atomic composition, in which particles, coming from a radiation source or created by interaction, will be transported. This universe may itself contain other universes of various geometries and atomic compositions. The particles, along their trajectory, will undergo interactions at the origin of energy transfers and/or particle creation, which in turn will be transported. The MCNPX code will generate the random paths of all particles of the problem and throughout the defined universe. In practice, the user builds geometry and fixes the atomic elements that constitute the life universe of particles. It determines the nature of the particles that will be transported; it defines the source of radiation (type of particles, energy, etc.), and chooses its calculation (particle flux, dose deposition, etc.), specifying its location in geometry. The user codifies this information by writing a file, called input file, which will be subject to the code.

2.4 Physical Transport of Particles

Monte Carlo particle transport algorithms implemented in MCNPX use different theories depending on whether the particle is charged or not. In the case of neutral particles, such as photons, algorithms calculate the distance between the particle and the nearest geometric edge, and compare it to the distance from the next collision. If the minimum distance corresponds to a collision, sampling techniques are called for drawing the interaction type and calculating post-collision parameters such as energy and trajectory of primary and secondary particles. On the other hand, if the minimum distance corresponds to a geometric border, the code updates the position of the particle in the new cell. In the case of charged particles, such as electrons, there are several so-called condensed story theories introduced by Berger [21] that simplify their transport.

MCNPX uses a sequence of pseudo-random numbers to sample probability distributions. This sequence is generated by an algorithm based on the congruently form of Lehmer [22]. The period of this algorithm is 2 exponent 46.

A particle is transported if it is activated in simulated physical processes. There is a map entitled mode which allows fixing one or several types of particles that the code will have to carry. In our situation, only photon transport will be active over a default energy range of 1 keV to 100 GeV. For understand photon transport modeling, it is necessary to introduce the notions of trace and weight:

The Trace
The emission of a source particle initiates a story. The trace reflects the trajectory of the source particle during its history. The source particle can interact and provide a secondary particle that will have its own trace. Several traces may belong to the same story. A story ends when the trajectories of the source particle and the secondary particles leave the geometric limits of the observed universe or when their kinetic

energy reaches the minimum (default = 1 keV or the one specified by the user). The trace has a great importance in the calculation of the physical quantities requested by the user. Indeed, the passage of a trace through a surface, as well as its length inside a volume makes it possible to calculate particle flows and energy deposits in the volume.

The Weight
Ideally, each real particle of a physical problem should be simulated by a fictitious MCNPX particle. In reality, to limit the duration of simulations and improve computation efficiency, an MCNPX particle does not exactly simulate a physical particle but rather represents a number w of physical particles. The number w is the initial weight of the source MCNPX particle. This weight remains constant throughout the history of the particle. If in the course of its history, the particle gives birth by interaction to two other particles, the latter will have an identical weight equal to w/2, and so on. The sum of the weights thus remains constant throughout the history of the source particle. The physical particles w all have a distinct random path while the single particle MCNPX, representing these physical particles w, will follow a single random path. Finally, this is not an exact simulation however; the true number of physical particles is preserved by statistical averages within the limit of a large number of MCNPX source particles. Each result from an MCNPX particle is multiplied by its weight so that the expected results for physical w particles are counted in the final result. This principle allows the user to normalize his result according to the weight he has chosen. By default, the normalization is 1, which means that the result obtained is normalized by source particles. A second normalization with respect to the number of Monte Carlo stories is made in the final results so that their average is independent of the number of source particles actually initiated in the calculation. In other words, if twice as many source particles are used, the expected result will not be twice as large but more accurate. Apart from saving time and standardization facilities, the weight of a particle has a great importance on the calculation of physical quantities. Indeed, the contribution of a particle passing through a volume of interest is given by its weight. The weight represents the relative contribution of the particle to the expected result. As a result, the weight can be used for certain bias techniques whose goal is to increase the convergence speed of the calculation while maintaining accuracy. Indeed, when a volume is little visited by particles when it corresponds to the location of the requested calculation, the weight of particles reaching this volume can be increased in order to improve the statistics while respecting the proportionality with respect to its probability of presence. To illustrate the traces and weights, we propose to follow three source particles whose stories are schematized by the following Fig. 2. Stories are dealt with one after the other. Tracks are the paths between two Collisions (tracks 3, 5, 6 and 11) or between a collision and a surface (tracks 2, 4, 9, 10, 12, 14 and 15) or between two surfaces (track 8). The particle is followed until it stops by collision or by interception of the surface of the universe. After a collision, the created particles share the weight of the particle that has just interacted.

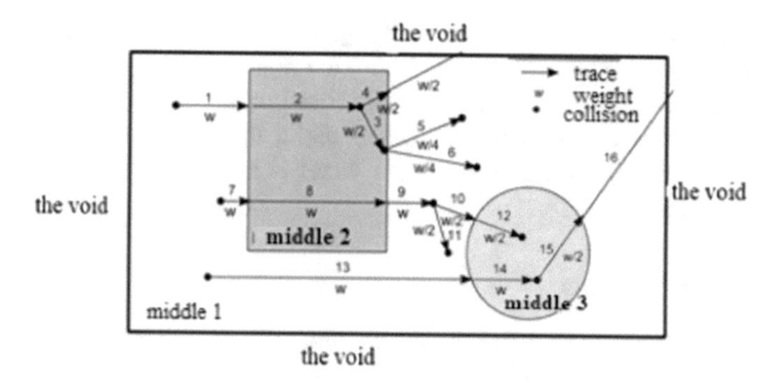

Fig. 2. Monte Carlo problem of three backgrounds with three stories

2.5 Phantom

There are currently two types of models used in ionizing radiation dosimetry: mathematical models, simple to use but representing the human body in a rather unrealistic way, and voxelized models, more complex but representing a much more precise the human body.

Thanks to advances in medical imaging such as computed tomography or magnetic resonance imaging, new anthropomorphic phantoms called voxelized phantom have been developed. In this model, the human body is represented as a matrix of small cubes called voxel. The best known of these are the Zubal phantom illustrated in Fig. 3 which can be freely used from (http://noodle.med.yale.edu/zubal/). This phantom, without arms or legs, consists of a voxelized volume of $128 \times 128 \times 293$ pixels and each voxel has a volume of $0.4 \times 0.4 \times 0.4$ mm^3 and contains a given material or

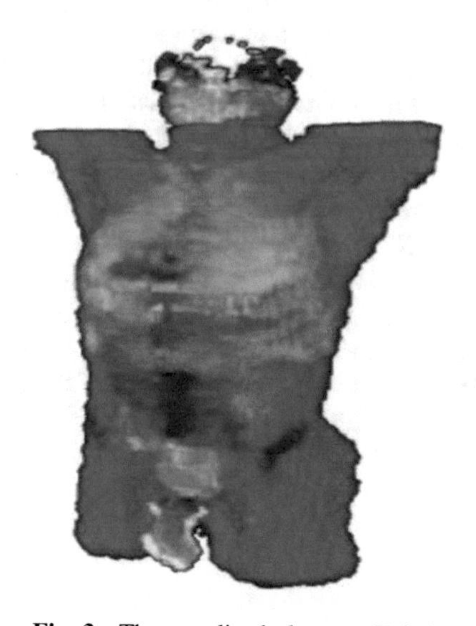

Fig. 3. The voxelized phantom Zubal

tissue of fifteen: air, muscles, soft tissues or organs, cortical bone, cartilage, fat, blood, skin, the lungs, the glandular tissue, the brain, the marrow, the liver, the stomach and finally the water. The voxelized phantom Zubal used in this work consist of 128 pixels along the anteroposterior (x) axis, 128 pixels along the transverse axis (y) and 243 pixels along the longitudinal axis (z). Each voxel is a cube of 0.4 mm of side containing a given tissue.

2.6 Simulation Methods

We placed our x-ray source 1.5 m from the phantom centered in the frontal plane (xoz), which is the projection plane of the image. The X-ray beam is isotropic and conical in shape, with a half-angle equal to 18°. The energy of the X photons is constant and equal to 50 keV. The detector is a thin layer of cesium iodide (CsI), 100×120 cm^2 in size and 0.06 cm thick, placed 0.8 cm behind the phantom. The resolution of the detector is 600×600 pixels. We simulated 10 to the power 9 events. We first counted the energy deposited in each pixel by the primary photons only, that is to say the non-diffused photons. Then, in a second step, the energy deposited by the primary and diffused photons. Figures 2 and 3 illustrate the images obtained. A larger number of events would reduce noise and achieve sharper images. My available computing power limits the increase in the number of events. Another point demonstrated by the simulation is the interest of using an anti-diffusion grid in reality to eliminate the scattered photons which generate a blur on the image.

3 Results and Discussion

After the simulation, we first obtained an X-ray of the Zubal phantom represented in Fig. 4 with the energy deposited on each pixel by all the scattered or primary photons, and in a second step: an X-ray of the same phantom with the energy deposited on each pixel by the primary photons and simulating the use of anti-diffusion grids (Fig. 5).

Our work consisted of Monte Carlo simulations of an X-ray of a digital phantom representing a geometric modeling of anatomical structures and their physical properties. We used for this the code MCNP6 which describes using Monte Carlo techniques the transport of electrons, positrons and photons in matter. The X-ray source had an isotropic emission of X photons of energy equal to 50 keV. The voxelized anthropomorphic phantom Zubal has been used to describe the human body. The images obtained are comparable to those obtained by a real radiographic imaging system but with limits that are those of the phantom and the detector model used. The interest of the anti-diffusion grid in the improvement of the quality of the image was illustrated by the images obtained by the simulation.

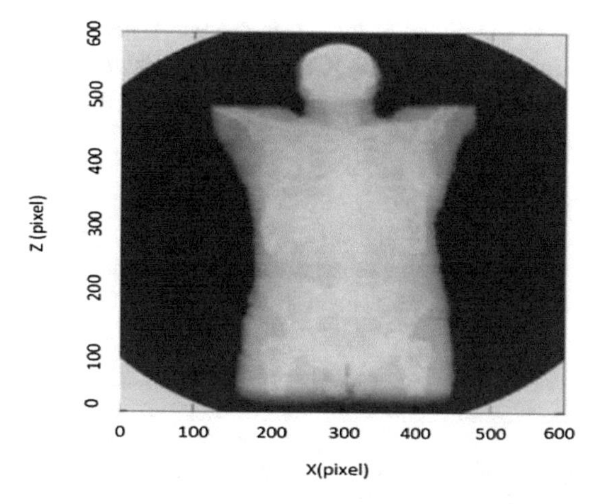

Fig. 4. X-ray of the Zubal phantom obtained by Monte Carlo simulation. The energy deposited on each pixel by all the diffused or primary photons (eV/cm^2 photons).

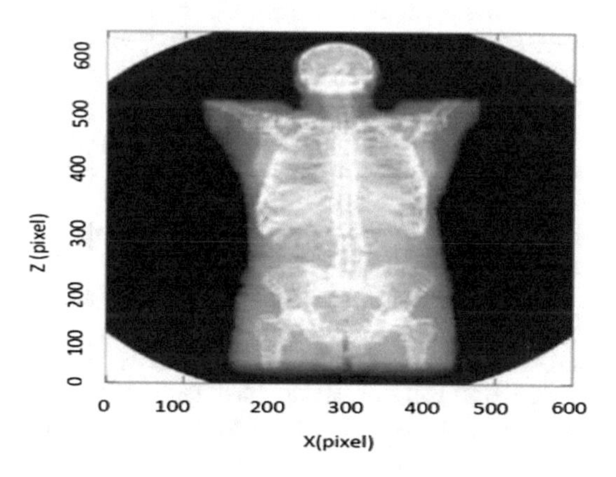

Fig. 5. X-ray of the Zubal phantom obtained by Monte Carlo simulation. The energy deposited on each pixel by the primary photons and simulating the use of anti-diffusion grids.

4 Conclusion

Our work consisted in carrying out by Monte Carlo simulations an X-ray of a digital phantom representing a geometrical modeling of the anatomical structures and their physical properties. The voxelized anthropomorphic phantom Zubal was used to describe the human body. The images obtained are comparable to those obtained by a real radiographic imaging system but with limits that are those of the ghost and the model of detector used. The interest of the anti-diffusion grid in the improvement of the image quality was illustrated by the images obtained by the simulation.

As a perspective to this work, it is possible to use a poly-energetic X-ray source closer to the spectrum emitted by an X-ray tube. Digital phantom having a higher resolution with a more detailed description of the Zubal anatomy allow obtaining images of better qualities. Finally, the dosimetry calculation, measuring the energy deposited in each voxel, makes it possible to address the aspects radiotherapy and radioprotection which becomes easily accessible. It is possible to use, for example, high energy electrons, between 6 and 20 meV, products by particle accelerators or a Cobalt 60 radioactive source using gamma photons of 1.17 and 1.33 meV and visualize the distribution of the absorbed dose for a given geometry.

References

1. Mettler, F.A., Wiest, P.W., Locken, J.A., Kelsey, C.A.: CT scanning: patterns of use and dose. J. Radiol. Prot. **20**, 353–359 (2000)
2. Shrimpton, P.C., Edyvean, S.: CT scanner dosimetry. Br. J. Radiol. **71**, 1–3 (1998)
3. BfS: Jahresbericht 2003. Annual rep., Bundesamt für Strahlenschutz, Salzgitter (2003)
4. Brix, G., Nagel, H.D., Stamm, G., Veit, R., Lechel, U., Griebel, J., Galanski, M.: Radiation exposure in multi-slice versus single-slice spiral CT: results of a nationwide survey. Eur. Radiol. **13**, 1979–1991 (2003). https://doi.org/10.1007/s00330-003-1883-y
5. Andreo, P.: Monte Carlo techniques in medical radiation physics. Phys. Med. Biol. **36**(861), 920 (1991)
6. Geant4 Collaboration: Introduction to Geant4 (2007). http://geant4.web.cern.ch/geant4
7. Team XBMC: MCNP-general Monte Carlo N-particle transport code, version 5. LA-UR-03-1987 RSICC, Los Alamos, USA (2003)
8. Nelson, W.R., Hirayama, H., Rogers, D.O.W.: The EGS4 code system. Stanford Linear Accelerator Center, Stanford University, USA (1985)
9. Kalender, W.A.: Computed Tomography: Fundamentals, System Technology, Image Quality, Applications. Wiley, New York (2000)
10. Zubal, I.G., Harrell, C.R., Smith, E.O., Rattner, Z., Gindi, G., Hoffer, P.B.: Computerized three-dimensional segmented human anatomy. Med. Phys. **21**(2), 299–302 (1994)
11. X-6 Monte Carlo Team. a. MCNP, A General Monte Carlo N-Particle Transport Code, Version 1.0: Initial MCNP-6 Release Overview -MCNP6 (2014)
12. Charlie Ma, C.-M.: Calcul Monte Carlo de la dose en radiothérapies. Focus on Radiosurgery, Newsletter No. 1 (2008)
13. Ulam, S.M., von Neumann, J.: On combination of stochastic and deterministic processes. Bull. Am. Math. Soc. **53**, 1120 (1947)
14. Raeside, D.E.: Monte Carlo principles and applications. Phys. Med. Biol. **21**, 181–197 (1976)
15. Buffon, G.: Essai d'arithmétique Supplément à la naturelle (1777)
16. Bielajew, A.F., Hirayama, H., Nelson, W.R., Rogers, D.W.O.: History, overview and recent improvements of egs4. Technical Report, PIRS-0436 (1994)
17. Baro, J., Sempau, J., Fernandez-Varea, J.M., Salvat, F.: Penelope: an algorithm for Monte Carlo simulation of the penetration and energy loss of electrons and positrons in matter. Nucl. Instrum. Methods B **100**, 31–46 (1995)
18. Agostinelli, S.: Geant4-a simulation toolkit. Nucl. Instrum. Methods A **506**, 250–303 (2003)
19. Carrier, J.F., Archambault, L., Beaulieu, L., Roy, R.: Validation of geant4, an objectoriented Monte Carlo toolkit, for simulations in medical physics. Med. Phys. **31**, 484–492 (2004)

20. Jan, S.: Gate: a simulation toolkit for pet and spect. Phys. Med. Biol. **49**, 4543–4561 (2004)
21. Berger, L.: Utilisation d'un système d'imagerie portale électronique avec détecteur au slicium amorphe pour vérifier la dose reçue par les patients en radiothérapie. These (2006)
22. Zubal, I.G., Harrell, C.R., Smith, E.O., Smith, A.L., Krischlunas, P.: Two dedicated software, voxel-based, anthropomorphic (torso and head) phantoms. In: Proceedings of the International Workshop, vol. 6, no. 7. National Radiological Protection Board, Chilton, UK, July 1995

Genetic K-Means Clustering Algorithm for Achieving Security in Medical Image Processing over Cloud

Mbarek Marwan(✉), Ali Kartit, and Hassan Ouahmane

LTI Laboratory, ENSA, Chouaïb Doukkali University,
Avenue Jabran Khalil Jabran, BP 299, El Jadida, Morocco
marwan.mbarek@gmail.com, alikartit@gmail.com,
hassan.ouahmane@yahoo.fr

Abstract. In healthcare domain, there is persistent pressure to improve clinical outcomes while lowering costs. In this respect, healthcare organizations can leverage cloud computing resources to avoid building an expensive in-house data center. More specifically, this new trend offers the opportunity to rent the use of imaging tools in order to process medical records. Additionally, cloud billing is based on a pay-per-use model to achieve cost savings. However, security and privacy concerns are the main disadvantages of cloud-based applications, especially when it comes to managing patients' data. The commonly used techniques for protecting data are homomorphic algorithms, Service-Oriented Architecture (SOA) and Secret Share Scheme (SSS). These traditional approaches have some limitations that provide a boundary to its use in practice. Precisely, the implementation of these security measures in cloud environment does not have the ability to maintain a good balance between security and efficiency. From this perspective, we propose a hybrid method combining a genetic algorithm (GA) and K-Means clustering technique to meet privacy and performance requirements. This approach relies on distributed data processing (DDP) to process health records over multiple systems. Consequently, the proposal is designed to help protect clients' data against accidental disclosure as well as accelerating the computations.

Keywords: Image processing · Cloud · K-Means · Security · Genetic algorithm

1 Introduction

Cloud computing has demonstrated effectiveness for improving the quality of care through innovative technologies. In fact, this model has the potential to overcome challenges associated with the management of local data centers. The main objective behind this new paradigm is to achieve cost savings and flexibility by using shared resources and pay-per-use model. More importantly, health IT applications can be quickly provisioned and released with minimal management effort [1]. These advantages represent the main reasons for cloud adoption in healthcare domain. Nowadays, this new paradigm is being utilized by medical professionals to rapidly process large

M. Ezziyyani (Ed.): AI2SD 2018, AISC 914, pp. 140–145, 2019.
https://doi.org/10.1007/978-3-030-11884-6_12

volumes of medical data. Hence, cloud computing has emerged as an important strategy to improve clinical quality and reduce costs. The goal of this model is to eliminate the need to purchase and maintain in-house built applications. First and foremost, this technology was designed to overcome the burden of traditional systems by providing ubiquitous and on-demand computational resources. In addition to this, clients are charged according to usage of these resources. In simple terms, cloud-based applications are an easy and effective method to process health records, as illustrated in Fig. 1.

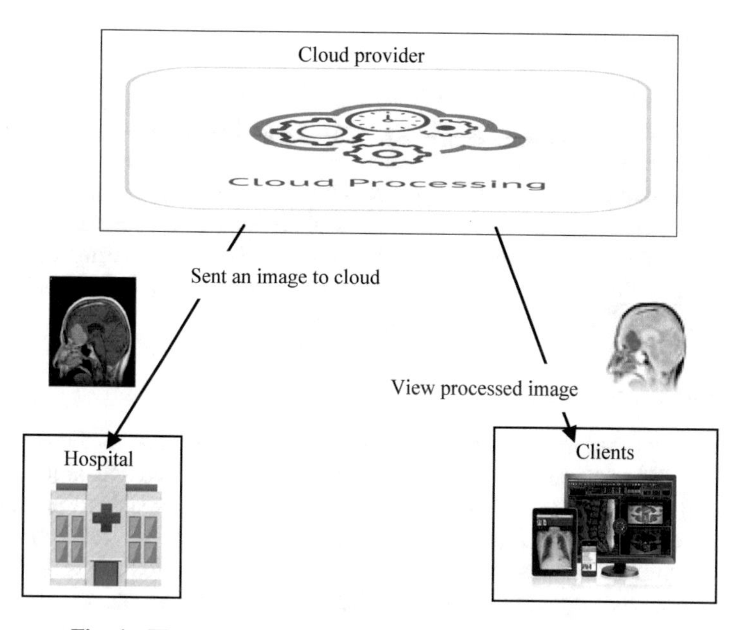

Fig. 1. The principle of medical image processing-as-a-service

Despite the great utility of cloud services, the implementation of a cloud-based system brings a number of privacy and security concerns [2–5]. Broadly speaking, there are various solutions to keep medical records safe when using cloud-based image processing tools. In this context, Homomorphic Encryption (HE) [6, 7], Secret Share Scheme (SSS) [8, 9] and Service-Oriented Architecture (SOA) [10, 11] are among the most commonly techniques used in cloud environment to address security risks. Although these techniques have the potential to maintain confidentiality of medical data, they have a negative impact on the running time, especially for homomorphic encryption and Secret Sharing Scheme. In the same line, SOA does not protect data from unauthorized access, regardless of its utility to achieve interoperability. In light of these facts, we propose a method based on K-Means technique and Genetic Algorithm (GA) to preserve the privacy of the data when using cloud services. Compared to traditional solutions, this method splits an image into many segments to maintain a secure environment for data processing and improve system running performance as well.

The rest of this paper is structured as follows. Section 2 presents the proposed method to address security problems and provide overview of the differences used techniques to comply with data protection requirements. In Sect. 3, we end this study by concluding remarks and recommendations for future work.

2 Proposed Solution

The utilization of cloud services in healthcare domain has many potential benefits. Although classical encryption techniques have the ability to preserve the privacy of sensitive data, they usually involve a set of complex mathematical operations. As a result, these techniques can have a negative impact on system performance. In light of this fact, this section presents a secure way of processing data over cloud computing. The proposed solution is basically a combination of K-Means clustering technique and a genetic algorithm. Essentially, this approach aims primarily at achieving an acceptable trade-off between performance and security.

2.1 Proposed Approach

In general, segmentation is an effective tool to partition an image into many parts. In this context, the clustering method is one of the widely used techniques for data processing. In this study, we intend to use segmentation approach to address security and privacy issues in cloud environments. To this aim, we rely on K-Means algorithm to group pixels into homogeneous regions according to their features such as intensity, color and texture. In order to reach the highest levels of accuracy, we introduce a genetic algorithm (GA) to find optimal or near-optimal solutions [12, 13]. Simply put, K-means aims at minimizing the distances between data and the corresponding cluster centroid a in such a way that similar pixels are in one cluster [14, 15]. Meanwhile, we use the GA algorithm to search for the appropriate cluster centers that minimize the clustering metric. In this respect, we evaluate the individual fitnesses of each chromosome. Thus, we rely on crossover and mutation operations to generate high-quality solutions [16–18]. Consequently, the proposed method GA-Kmeans consists of six steps, as summarized in Algorithm 1 [19–21].

Algorithm 1. pseudo-code of GA-KMeans

Inputs: I (x×y), k, where I is an image and k is the number of regions
Outputs: < M_s>, where M_s segmented image
Step 1: Set parametres
Clusters Set C={c_1, c_2,..., c_k} of k cluster centers)
Step 2: Choose encode method
Convert input image into data Set X = {x_1, x_2,..., x_n} of n object
Step 3: Intilize_population ();
Step 4: Optimize the individuals of initial population
Selection ();
Crossover ();
Mutation ();
Fitness ();
Step 5: Repeat Step until the fitness of the population no longer improves;
Step 6: Return < M_s>

2.2 Proposed Framework

Upon successful completion of segmentation process, the secret image is divided into multiple parts. Since, the exact number of regions is known a priori, each region is sent to a distinct cloud computing. In this case, cloud provider process only a single part of the secret data, so that sensitive data disclosure might seem more difficult. Finally, we need to combine all processed regions to obtain desired results, as illustrated in Fig. 2.

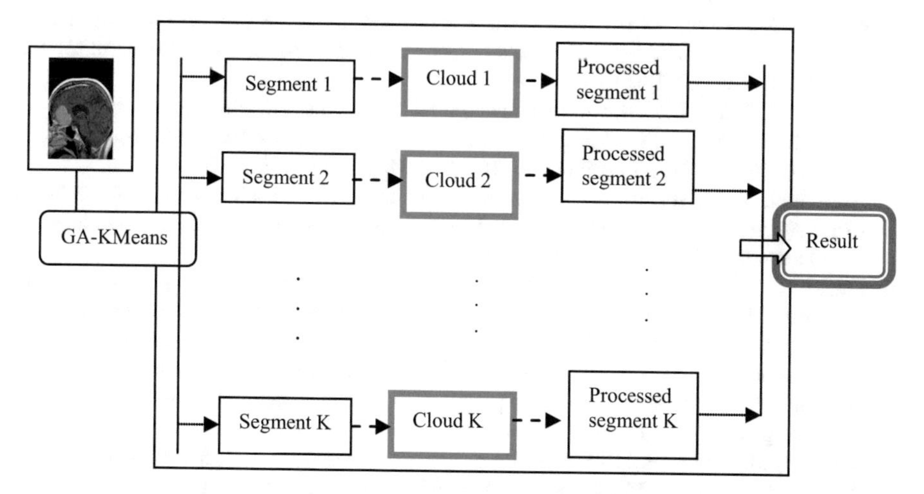

Fig. 2. An overview of the proposed approach

In light of this, the proposed approach uses GA-KMeans as a way to produce small portions in order to prevent unauthorized access, use, or disclosure of medical data.

3 Conclusion

The purpose of cloud-based services is to reduce costs and facilitate access to advanced imaging tools. However, despite its many benefits, a malicious cloud provider or unauthorized users might access sensible medical data in a cloud computing. To address these security threats and challenges, there are many techniques available for the security of image processing over cloud computing. More specifically, Homomorphic Encryption (HE), Service-Oriented Architecture (SOA) and Secret Share Scheme (SSS) are the main solution to keep medical data secure. Nevertheless, these traditional techniques have certain inherent drawbacks that limit the utility of these solutions, especially in terms of the quality of service (QoS). In light of this fact, we propose a method that ensures both security and performance. To this aim, we use Genetic K-means algorithm to split the input image into many segments. The key concept behind this new method is to reduce security risks and improve performance. Precisely, this method ensures that only authorized users can view, use medical data when using cloud services. For future work, we intend to implement this method and perform complex image processing tasks. In addition, we plan to compare the proposed solution with others approaches, especially in terms of computational complexity.

References

1. Mell, P., Grance, T.: The NIST definition of cloud computing. Technical report, National Institute of Standards and Technology, vol. 15, pp. 1–3 (2009)
2. Marwan, M., Kartit, A., Ouahmane, H.: Cloud-based medical image issues. Int. J. Appl. Eng. Res. **11**, 3713–3719 (2016)
3. Marwan, M., Kartit, A., Ouahmane, H.: A framework to secure medical image storage in cloud computing environment. J. Electron. Commer. Organ. **16**(1), 1–16 (2018). https://doi.org/10.4018/JECO.2018010101
4. Abbas, A., Khan, S.U.: e-Health cloud: privacy concerns and mitigation strategies. In: Gkoulalas-Divanis, A., Loukides, G. (eds.) Medical Data Privacy Handbook, pp. 389–421. Springer, Cham (2015). https://doi.org/10.1007/978-3-319-23633-9_15
5. Al Nuaimi, N., Al Shamsi, A., Mohamed, N., Al-Jaroodi. J.: e-health cloud implementation issues and efforts. In: Proceedings of the International Conference on industrial Engineering and Operations Management (IEOM), pp. 1–10 (2015)
6. Challa, R.K., Kakinada, J., Vijaya Kumari, G., Sunny, B.: Secure image processing using LWE based homomorphic encryption. In: Proceedings of the IEEE International Conference on Electrical, Computer and Communication Technologies (ICECCT), pp. 1–6 (2015)
7. Gomathisankaran, M., Yuan, X., Kamongi, P.: Ensure privacy and security in the process of medical image analysis. In: Proceedings of the IEEE International Conference on Granular Computing (GrC), pp. 120–125 (2013)
8. Mohanty, M., Atrey, P.K., Ooi, W.-T.: Secure cloud-based medical data visualization. In: Proceedings of the ACM Conference on Multimedia (ACMMM 2012), Japan, pp. 1105–1108 (2012)

9. Lathey, A., Atrey, P.K.: Image enhancement in encrypted domain over cloud. ACM Trans. Multimedia Comput. Commun. **11**(3), 38 (2015). https://doi.org/10.1145/2656205
10. Todica, V., Vaida, M.F.: SOA-based medical image processing platform. In: Proceedings of the of IEEE International Conference on Automation, Quality and Testing, Robotics (AQTR), pp. 398–403 (2008). https://doi.org/10.1109/aqtr.2008.4588775
11. Chiang, W., Lin, H., Wu, T., Chen, C.: Building a cloud service for medical image processing based on service-orient architecture. In: Proceedings of the 4th International Conference on Biomedical Engineering and Informatics (BMEI), pp. 1459–1465 (2011). https://doi.org/10.1109/bmei.2011.6098638
12. Lim, Y.W., Lee, S.U.: On the color image segmentation algorithm based on the thresholding and the fuzzy c-means techniques. Pattern Recogn. **23**, 1935–1952 (1990)
13. Nascimento, S., Moura-Pires, F.: A genetic approach to fuzzy clustering with a validity measure fitness function. Lectures Notes in Computer Science, vol. 1280, pp. 325–335 (1997)
14. Gan, G., Ma, C., Wu, J.: Data Clustering: Theory, Algorithms and Applications. Society for Industrial and Applied Mathematics. SIAM, Philadelphia (2007)
15. Ravichandran, K.S., Ananthi, B.: Color skin segmentation using K-Means cluster. Int. J. Comput. Appl. Math. **4**(2), 153–157 (2009)
16. Di Gesù, V., Bosco, G.L.: Image segmentation based on genetic algorithms combination. In: Roli, F., Vitulano, S. (eds.) Image Analysis and Processing, ICIAP 2005, Lecture Notes in Computer Science, vol. 3617, pp. 352–359. Springer, Heidelberg (2005). https://doi.org/10.1007/11553595_43
17. Holland, J.H.: Adaptation in Natural and Artificial Systems. University of Michigan Press, Ann Arbor (1975)
18. Goldberg, D.E.: Genetic Algorithms in Search, Optimization, and Machine Learning. Addison-Wesley, New York (1989)
19. Lo Bosco, G.: A genetic algorithm for image segmentation. In: Proceedings of ICIAP 2001, Palermo, Italy, pp. 262–266. IEEE Computer Society Press, Los Alamitos (2001)
20. Chehouri, A., Younes, R., Khoder, J., Perron, J., Ilinca, A.: A selection process for genetic algorithm using clustering analysis. Algorithms **10**(4), 123 (2017). https://doi.org/10.3390/a10040123
21. Lamine, B., Nadia, B.: Image segmentation using clustering methods. In: Bi, Y., Kapoor, S., Bhatia, R. (eds.) Proceedings of SAI Intelligent Systems Conference IntelliSys 2016. Lecture Notes in Networks and Systems, vol. 16, pp. 129–141. Springer, Cham (2018). https://doi.org/10.1007/978-3-319-56991-8_11

E-Health or the Human 2.0!

Moulay Hicham El Amrani(✉)

Territorial Governance, Human Security and Sustainability Research Laboratory, Ibn Zohr University, Agadir, Morocco
elamrani@mondeannuaires.com

Abstract. In the few last years, the revolution of big data in the industry is a new field of research and source of riches to many businessmen. The healthcare gets benefits of the massive amounts information of the big data that it never had access to before. It let to have access to billion of samples, that can do any experience on it, then, gets more efficient results. The new technologies lead to create more health apps and personal fitness tools, which permit to have more sources of downloadable patient's data. That has surely a double face, the first one, the data is going to help to find more medicines for several diseases, in the other hand, the question that will be hold is the data's security, and what is going to be the future of the human being in this case.

Keywords: Human 2.0 · E-Health · Human's future

1 Introduction

In the few last years, the revolution of big data in the industry is a new field of research and source of riches to many businessmen. The healthcare gets benefits of the massive amounts' information of the big data that it never had access to before. It let to have access to billion of samples, that can do any experience on it, then, gets more efficient results.

The new technologies are going to create more health apps and personal fitness tools, which will permit to get, easily, more information about patients. That has double challenge, the first one, the data is going to help to find more medicines for several diseases, in the other hand, the question that will be hold is the data's security, and what is going to be the future of the human being in this case.

The second dimension of the new technologies that it provides an easy access to the whole information of the patients, from anywhere and at any time.

The use of the new technologies would help, indeed, to increase the human's life expectancy. By analysing the last three centuries life expectancy, we can note that it increased from 40 years old at the beginning of the 19th to 85 years in the 21st century (2012).

This evolution is thanks to the development of medicines and the medical's technology, which we use massively nowadays to preserve the human's life and guaranty his longevity, which is a project of some of the most developed companies in the world, like Google, Facebook, Amazon… those companies are actually investing,

M. Ezziyyani (Ed.): AI2SD 2018, AISC 914, pp. 146–153, 2019.
https://doi.org/10.1007/978-3-030-11884-6_13

massively, in the NBIC technologies to reach this goal in the next few years (2030 as it fixed by the Google company).

The human's body is very difficult to understand and complicated to analyse, to decrypt, but the new technologies, such as, robotics, would let scientists to understand, repair, modeling our organs, even to a small-scale, and more than that, it leads creating artificial organs, from the biggest one to the nano organs. All these things are available now, thanks to powerful computers. The Moore's Law is the basis of this technological revolution. Today, the computer is able to do 1018() (Exaflop) operation by second, what means, that it will be able to analyse the DNA cell in some hours, thing which let the scientists and doctors to develop the new nano tools to work, to discover how to manipulate the cell, and in consequence to increase the life expectancy of the human being.

This situation will raise some ethical and economic questions beside the regulation dimension.

So, in this paper, we propose to analyse this subject by adopting the two following points:

- The ethic dimension of the new waves of medical technology
- The economic challenges by using the new technologies in the medical field.

2 The Ethic Dimension of the New Waves of Medical Technology

This following figure (Fig. 1) represents the evolution of life expectancy during the last 200 years, which was multiplied by three.

Today, and according to this graph, our life expectancy grows with three months per year. So, how much the life expectancy would be able to go?

To answer this question, four scenarios are possible:

- Life expectancy will be abbreviate, because of the pollution, climate changes, quality and composition of nutrition, which, unfortunately, accelerate by an unreasonable behavior of human, and the excessive consumption over his real needs;
- The limit of the technology, when it will reach a certain level, it will surely limited and will not be able to get more than it reaches;
- The pursuit of development and increasing of the human longevity to be 150 and 200 years, by controlling the negative effects and developing more efficient and safer solutions;
- The technological explosion, which will help to reach, the stage of 2 or 3 centuries, maybe more, of life, which is an idealistic and unbelievable goal.

The human body is very complicated, our cells, organs, tissues… are very difficult to understand and analyse, for the last years, but now, with technological tools, we are able to understand, manipulate and modify, even, the most complicated element of the human body.

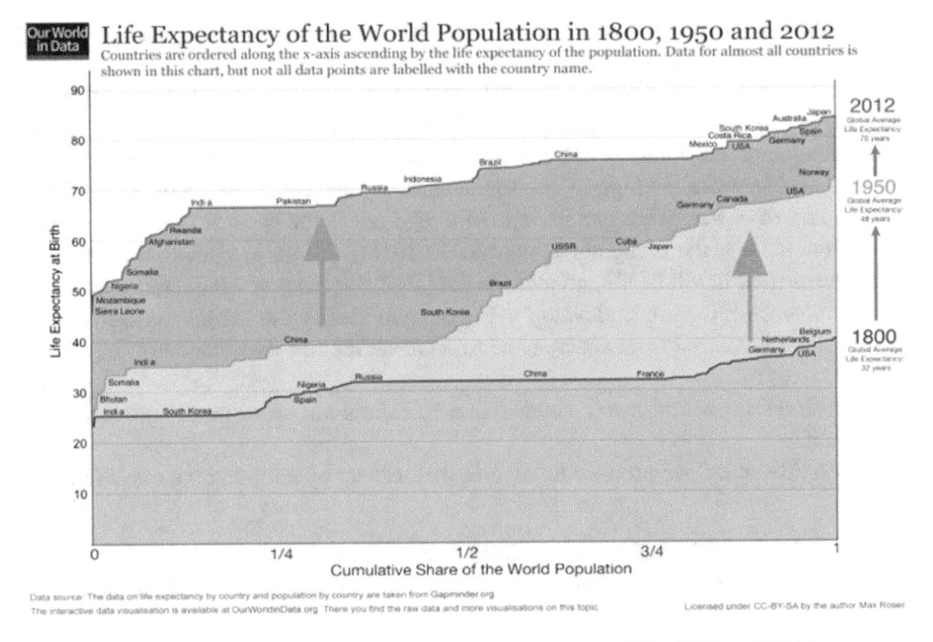

Fig. 1. Life expectancy of the world population in 1800, 1950 and 2012

Today, we are able to change cell's chromosomes, - a technique - known as gene editing- which means that we are able to change the human's body configuration; for instance, the first experiences have begun about 2 years ago. Indeed, a Londoner team (The Francis-Crick Institute) had got, On 1st February 2016, the authorization to begin the manipulations on human embryo, with a new gene engineering technics called Crispr-Case9.

The following figure (Fig. 2) shows the possibility of preventing or repairing a faulty gene, by changing the cell's faulty DNA:

The Chinese worked, also, on the same project, and they have done some scientific experiences on non-viable human embryos, in order to jam a genetic blood's disease called beta thalassemia.

This new revolution research had raised lots of ethical questions. Because, in the case, these experiences have success, which means that we will be able to create genetically modified babies by editing the germ cell, in the absence of ethical rules, which will modify the human's being future and its balance.

The United Kingdom had authorized, since 2009 researches on human embryos, and it has not agreed on the Oviedo convention, which is signed by the most European countries. On December, 15th, 2015, an international meeting was held in Washington and composed by three members: England, Americans and Chinese in order to discuss the ethical DNA and embryos manipulations; the final result was that "it will be irresponsible to pursuit the clinical usage and modifying the germ cells", in this meeting some scientists were for this idea and others were against.

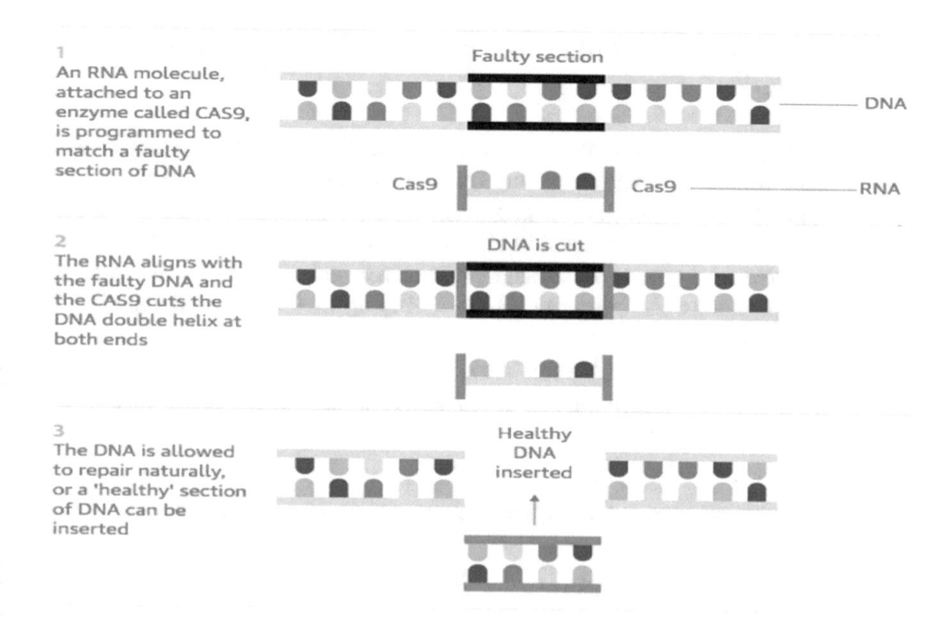

Fig. 2. Repairing a faulty gene

In reality, the ethics could easily be changed, for instance, the use of the pill in the 50th was not accepted by most societies in the world, but today it's a normal act to do in order to prevent having babes.

Else, what would be the reality if we will have biological differences?

Nowadays, we try to struggle, to fight against gender and financial inequality. With the biological manipulations, we will be faced to fight also for the biological equality. Because, people will get smarter, healthier and faster… only by being able to afford these possibilities, what means, that it will be available just for the wealthy person; thing which was expressed by Dr. David King: "It is critical that we avoid a eugenic future in which the rich can buy themselves a baby with built-in genetic advantages", he also adds "Human gene editing will lead to greater social inequality and more designer babies".

In the future, maybe, tiny nano-robots in our bloodstream could be able to detect diseases and might even eradicate the word symptom in as much as no one would have them any longer. In the future, these microscopic robots, maybe, will be able to alert us or our doctors, before, even, a disease could be developed in our body, and prevent to get ill. If it becomes reality, and micro-robots swimming in bodily fluids, how can we prevent terrorists from trying to hack these devices by controlling not only our health but also our lives?

This is also a big question, which we are unable to find answers right now.

3 The Economic Challenges by Using the New Technologies in the Medical Field

Any healthcare performance in the world depends on the economy, especially nowadays, because, we are strongly depending on technologies to do all the analyses and medical exams. So we should invest massively in the technologies industry. So, the future of the humanity is to invest in artificial intelligence to help the health care system to be competitive and give more efficient results for patients. Indeed, the artificial intelligence applications can create an annual saving up to 150 billion dollars for the U.S.A healthcare economy by 2026.

The Artificial Intelligence (AI) market is getting bigger and bigger, for instance, this market will reach 6.6 billion dollars by 2021, what will represent 40% of the annual growth rate (Fig. 3).

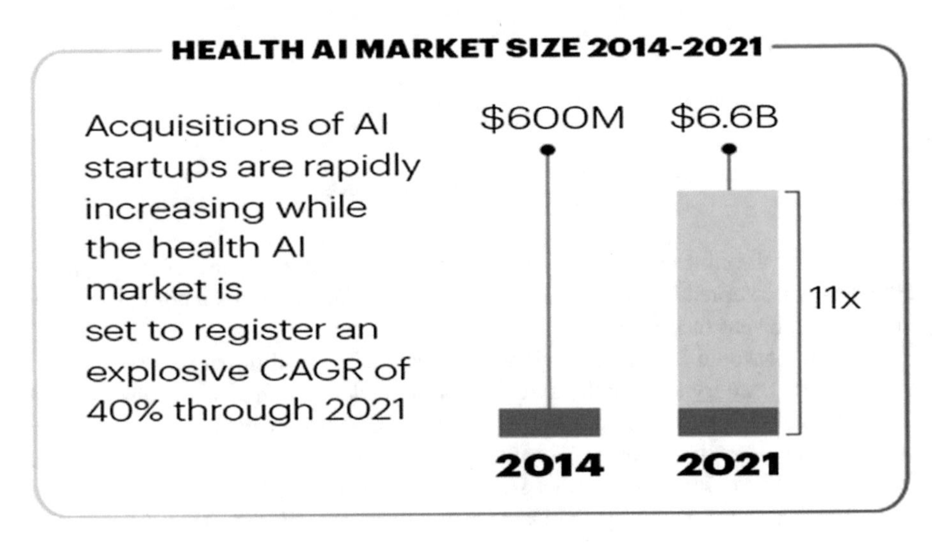

Fig. 3. Health AI Market size 2014–2021

This market is dominated by the big companies in the world, which developed medical applications like (Table 1):

Table 1. Applications Market size

Application	Value
Robot-assisted surgery	40 B dollar
Virtual nursing assistants	20 B dollar
Administrative workflow assistance	18 B dollar
Dosage error reduction	16 B dollar

This size will be increased in the next few years, because of the entrance of new companies, and the explosion of data, which lead to smarter systems, and by consequence, the Artificial Intelligence will get stronger than ever, especially with the deep learning, that makes the machine able to learn by itself. So, robot-assisted surgery, for instance, would be able to integrate information from medical records in real-time and enhance the physician's instrument precision. Which lead to earn lots of time and more efficiency to do surgical operations. This will let clinics and hospitals to save money and invest more in Artificial Intelligence.

For instance, the AI is used largely in hospitals in China, especially to read CT scans and x-rays and help to detect suspicious lesions and nodules in the case of cancers. In another way, it lets a lot of time to doctors to work and provide their patient with earlier treatment in order to avoid heavy patient, in case the disease will diagnosis lately (Fig. 4).

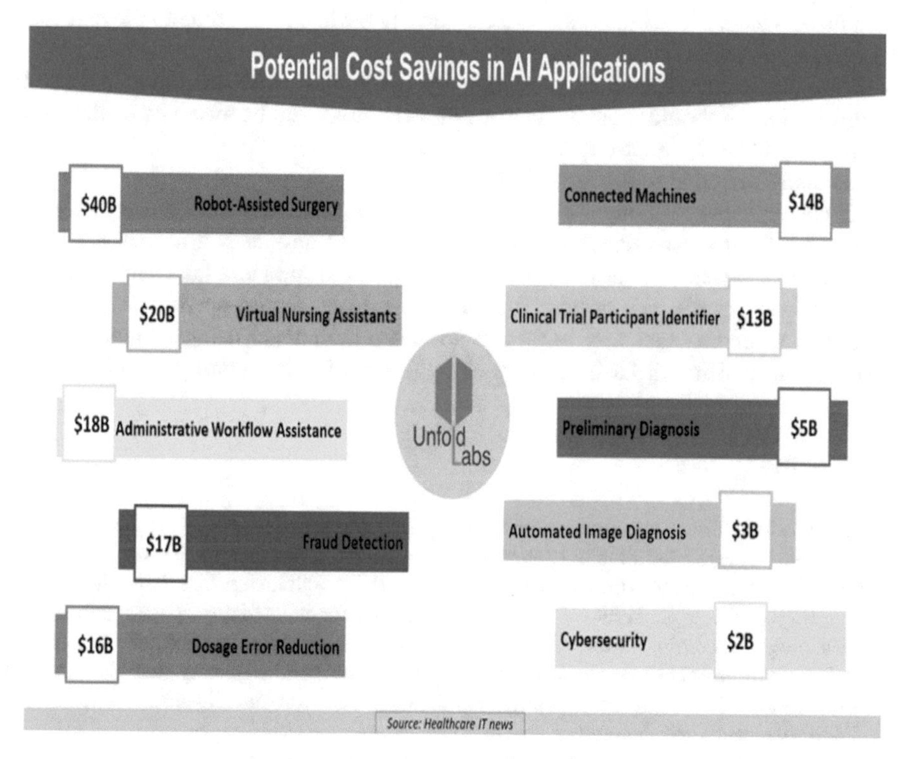

Fig. 4. The potential cost savings in AI applications, in the healthcare system

But the dark side of this revolution is the unemployment will get higher and higher and will cause social drams for the society, that should find solutions, and we should think to these scenarios from now. Because, the AI will take the place of human, and will destruct the job position. For instance, virtual nursing assistants would reduce waste of money by reducing the unnecessary visits to the hospital, because the AI solution remotely assesses a patient's symptoms and deliver alerts to clinicians when patient care is needed.

4 Conclusion

The artificial intelligence represents a real threat for the humanity, if it is not regulated.

Some AI researchers recognise that there are valid concerns about its impact on health care, jobs and the privacy of the human.

But, what is the best way?

Is it to slow the development, stop it or let it go so fast, but to put some rules to regulate it?

In reality, we will be able, in the few next years, to know, at the beginning of the pregnant, the whole genome of the babe, by a simple blood test, thanks to power computers. That means simply, that we can modify the cell at any time to prevent some diseases, or abort it if there is a potential one.

Sure, the science should help to improve the human's life condition, but not to change it. So, we should regulate the uses of technology and be aware of its danger to be able to prevent it, in case it will be an exceeding.

Is simply the ethic will be enough?

Of course, it is not enough, because it can be changed at any time; for instance, the in vitro fertilization was unacceptable in the 1930, but now, it is a normal act and it does not raise any ethical question now. We accept more and more the contravention to avoid suffering or die. So, besides the ethical field, we should open an international discussion to find a legal way to protect and keep the human being without a major modification, which will have negative consequences for the future generations.

References

1. Our World in Data. https://ourworldindata.org/life-expectancy. Accessed 21 Apr 2018
2. Nanotechnology, Biotechnology, Information technology, Cognitive science (NBIC): The Nanotechnology is referring to act in the billionth of millimeter; The Biotechnology is referring to the exploitation of biological processes for industrial purposes; Information technology is referring to the use of computers to store, retrieve, transmit, and manipulate data, or information; Cognitive science is referring to the interdisciplinary study of mind and intelligence, embracing philosophy, psychology, artificial intelligence, neuroscience, linguistics, and anthropology
3. Moore's Law is the observation made in 1965 by Gordon Moore, co-founder of Intel, that the number of transistors per square inch on integrated circuits had doubled every year since the integrated circuit was invented. Moore predicted that this trend would continue for the foreseeable future. In subsequent years, the pace slowed down a bit, but data density has doubled approximately every 18 months, and this is the current definition of Moore's Law
4. Exaflop is the equal of 1.000.000.000.000.000.000
5. Deoxyribo Nucleic Acid
6. The actual DNA sequencer is able to analyse the whole component of the cell in only 4 hours, and that is thanks to powerful computer available now

7. The Francis-Crick Institute. For more information about the institute https://www.crick.ac.uk/. Accessed 24 Apr 2018
8. The authorization had been given by Human Fertilisation and Embryology Authority
9. Morin, H.: Des manipulations génétiques d'embryons humains autorisées au Royaume-Uni, LE MONDE SCIENCE ET TECHNO, Science, Biologie, 01 January 2016. LE MONDE.FR .http://www.lemonde.fr/biologie/article/2016/02/01/des-manipulations-genetiques-d-embryons-humains-autorisees-en-grande-bretagne_4857389_1650740.html. Accessed 04 May 2018
10. The Guardian. https://www.theguardian.com/science/2016/feb/01/human-embryo-genetic-modify-regulator-green-light-research. Accessed 10 May 2018
11. The Convention for the Protection of Human Rights and Dignity of the Human Being with regard to the Application of Biology and Medicine: Convention on Human Rights and Biomedicine (ETS No 164) was opened for signature on 4 April 1997 in Oviedo (Spain). This Convention is the only international legally binding instrument on the protection of human rights in the biomedical field
12. Agence Universitaire de la francophonie, lettre de la ciruisef Sciences et Francophonie, Conférence Internationale des Responsables des Universités et Institutions Scientifiques d'Expression Française, p. 2
13. Dr. David King is a former molecular biologist and founder of Human Genetics Alert, an independent secular watchdog group that supports abortion rights. The Guardian. https://www.theguardian.com/profile/dr-david-king. Accessed 17 May 2018
14. Telgraph. https://www.telegraph.co.uk/news/science/11558305/China-shocks-world-by-genetically-engineering-human-embryos.html. Accessed 18 May 2018
15. The Guardian. https://www.theguardian.com/profile/dr-david-king. Accessed 18 May 2018
16. Accenture, Artificial intelligence: Healthcare's new nervous system, p. 8 (2017)
17. Accenture, Artificial intelligence: Healthcare's new nervous system, p. 2 (2017)
18. Medium. https://medium.com/@Unfoldlabs/the-impact-of-artificial-intelligence-in-health-care-4bc657f129f5. Accessed 23 May 2018

3D MRI Classification Using KNN and Deep Neural Network for Alzheimer's Disease Diagnosis

El Mehdi Benyoussef[1(✉)], Abdeltif Elbyed[1], and Hind El Hadiri[2]

[1] LIMSAD, Faculty of Science, Hassan II University, Casablanca, Morocco
elmehdibenyoussef@gmail.com, a.elbyed@fsac.ac.ma
[2] Geriatric Service, Emile Roux Hospital, Paris, France
hind.elhadiri@aphp.fr

Abstract. Alzheimer's disease (AD) is known as one of the most common neurodegenerative diseases which causes permanent damage to the brain cells related to memory and thinking skills. Research in this field aims to identify the most specific structures directly related to the changes in AD. MRI is one of the main imaging modalities which plays a huge role in AD diagnosis. Images produced in MRI helps us get information on anatomical structures in the brain and can also be used for clinical diagnosis of AD stages. In the recent years, deep learning has gained huge fame in solving complex problems from lots of fields, medical image analysis is one of them. This work proposes a K-Nearest Neighbor and a Deep Neural Network combined model for the early diagnosis of Alzheimer's disease and its stages using 3D magnetic resonance imaging (MRI) scans.

Keywords: Magnetic resonance imaging · Machine learning · Brain · Data modeling · Alzheimer's disease · Image classification · Neural networks

1 Introduction and Related Works

Alzheimer's disease (AD), known as the common cause of dementia, is a neurodegenerative disorder that leads to neuronal losses and brain's volume reduction. Definitive diagnosis can only be made with histopathological confirmation of amyloid plaques and neurofibrillary tangles, usually at a postmortem stage i.e. autopsy. Early detection of AD is important allowing the treatment to be introduced at an early stage, making it efficient.

Related to the Moroccan context where there is a lack of medical facilities especially in rural areas, there are currently no accurate figures regarding Alzheimer's patients and insufficient diagnosis equipment. Following these facts, Moroccan health institutes require an efficient and accurate automated system for earlier AD diagnosis.

M. Ezziyyani (Ed.): AI2SD 2018, AISC 914, pp. 154–158, 2019.
https://doi.org/10.1007/978-3-030-11884-6_14

Historically, brain imaging, especially MRI, has largely been used to help define causes of dementia [4]. More recently, there has been a realization that MRI has been shown to be a surrogate for early diagnosis of AD and may add a high positive predictive value to early Alzheimer's disease diagnosis [3]. Several studies demonstrate that using MRI to evaluate atrophy of temporal lobe structures can contribute to diagnosis accuracy [1]. Even if there is a high trend in AD researches, these findings have not been yet applied to daily clinical practices.

Computer-aided diagnostics (CAD) and Machine Learning (ML) have been of growing interest in the field of medical imaging. Generally speaking, a supervised machine learning algorithm is "trained" to produce a desired output from a set of input data known as training set. As such, the trained algorithm may be treated as a "black box" encapsulating knowledge acquired from the training data whose inputs are useful for producing the expected outcome. The supervised machine learning algorithms used in this paper are K-Nearest Neighbor (KNN) and Deep Neural Network (DNN).

Support vector machines (SVM), K-nearest neighbor (KNN), artificial neural networks (ANN) [6], and convolutional neural network (CNN) [5], are some of the most known Machine Learning algorithms used for classification tasks in medical settings [6].

In our previous work [2], we proposed a combination of three Data Mining algorithms for Alzheimer's Disease classification based just on clinical data.

The aim of the paper is to optimize and train an automated model based on a combination of KNN and DNN for AD subjects' classification based on OASIS library of MRI scans from 416 clinically diagnosed subjects.

The remainder of this paper is organized as follows. In the following section we describe our motivating context then our methodology whilst we present extensive experiments and discussion in Sect. 3 and we conclude in Sect. 4.

2 Context and Methodology

The diagnosis process in the medical field can be considered as a decision-making process in which the diagnosis of a new case is made by medical practitioner - a geriatrician in the case of AD - from the information extracted from available data. To make this decision-making process easy for specialists, faster, efficient and accurate, the clinical data processing can be automated.

The Moroccan context is in a real need for automated solutions to early diagnose Alzheimer's disease subjects.

As it's shown in Fig. 1, our solution's Architecture contains an MRI dataset from Open Access Series of Imaging Studies (OASIS). This data was first prepared to obtain the gray matter (GM) and the white matter (WM) from the brain's MRI. Then we performed a dimensionality reduction technique to extract important features. Our two models, KNN and DNN, are fed with prepared data to train on performing classification and prediction tasks.

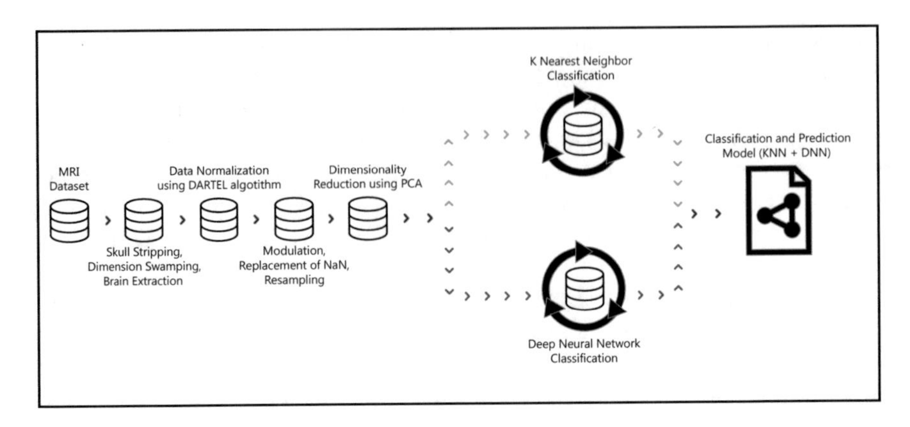

Fig. 1. The model's definition.

2.1 Dataset

MRI scans come from Open Access Series of Imaging Studies (OASIS) database, which provides datasets freely for the aim of research and data analysis. The dataset of 416 subjects are provided with a known diagnosis result as a target for our classification purposes.

2.2 Data Preparation

MRI scans provided from OASIS are in the form of 3D Analyze 7.5 volumes. First, we performed brain extraction by skull stripping to remove skull and other non-brain tissues from the MRIs because their presence is considered as an obstacle for automatic brain image analysis. Then gray matter (GM) and white matter (WM) segmentation is carried out using Statistical Parametric Mapping SPM8. Then normalization using DARTEL algorithm then replacement of NaN values with 0 in gray/white matter density maps then resampling to reduce shape and make it correspond to the shape of the non-DARTEL data and replacement of values less than "1e-4" with zeros to reduce the file size. We obtain then separate GM and WM 3D Niftii volumes for each subject.

2.3 K-Nearest Neighbor

K-nearest neighbors (KNN) is a simple algorithm that stores all available cases and classifies new cases based on a similarity measure. KNN is by definition an instance-based learning, sometimes called a lazy learner because of its tend to give a null answer in cases where it gets no similarity. We used a 1 Nearest Neighbor to help Deep Neural Network discriminate strongly diagnosable subjects from weakly diagnosable ones.

2.4 Deep Neural Network

Deep neural network (DNN), as its name indicates is a stacked representation of the single layer Neural Network which is the key to non-linearly separable problems because almost all of the complex problems are non-linearly separable. Our proposed model is based on a network configuration starting with the number of relevant features coming as outputs from PCA, and then two layers of 100 neurons for each one and at the end an output layer of 3 neurons which are the three classes (or stages) of Alzheimer's disease.

Table 1. The model's prediction results

Patient.ID	Real CDR	1NN predicted CDR	DNN predicted CDR	Predicted score
390	0.5	-	0.5	1
399	1	1	1	1
401	0	0	1	1
404	0	0	0.5	1
405	1	-	1	1
422	0	-	0	1
425	1	-	1	1
428	0	-	0	1
430	1	-	1	1
438	0	-	0	1
441	0.5	-	1	0
443	0	-	0.5	0
445	0	0	1	1
446	0	0	1	1
454	0.5	0.5	0.5	1
	Accuracy		—	13/15

3 Results and Discussion

Table 1 summarizes our results. Starting from the left, P.ID corresponds to the patient ID in OASIS dataset. CDR is known as Clinical Dementia Rating which describes the real subjects' stages of AD. KNN Predicted CDR is the K-Nearest Neighbor's output of Clinical Dementia Rating and it corresponds to one of the three AD classes, respectively Non-Demented (ND), Mild Cognitive Impairment (MCI) and suffering patients (AD), so the choice of the class where belongs a subject is based on the output of KNN's similarity measure between them. [1, 0, 0], [0, 1, 0] and [0, 0, 1] are respectively referring to ND, MCI and AD. Our KNN's output can be one of the three values or sometimes "-" referring to

[0, 0, 0] which means that a subject is not similar to any other one from a class. This is where combination can be useful. On the other side Deep Neural Network produces prediction probabilities like [0.25, 0.22, 0.32] which can be seen as 25% ND, 22% MCI and 32% AD. Combining the two models results in increasing a single probability if KNN gives a class or keeping the same probabilities if KNN gives a "-" (no class answer).

Deep Neural Network proved its classification power but can't converge to a generalization with a small number of samples so it's combination with K-Nearest Neighbor proved usefulness. The K-Nearest Neighbor helped Deep Neural Network because of its less data quantity sensitive.

4 Conclusion

In this paper, we presented a Machine Learning approach for Alzheimer's disease classification using a combination of K-Nearest Neighbor and Deep Neural Network. We introduced a probability combination which gave us a representative accuracy. Following our principal purposes which are to give Moroccan health institutes a new way of diagnosing Alzheimer's disease in an easy, faster, efficient and accurate way, we believe that our proposed model is still on iterations but can be leveraged to become performant in few years.

References

1. Barnes, J., Scahill, R.I., Boyes, R.G., Frost, C., Lewis, E.B., Rossor, C.L., Rossor, M.N., Fox, N.C.: Differentiating ad from aging using semiautomated measurement of hippocampal atrophy rates. Neuroimage **23**(2), 574–581 (2004)
2. Benyoussef, E.M., Elbyed, A., El Hadiri, H.: Data mining approaches for alzheimer's disease diagnosis. In: International Symposium on Ubiquitous Networking, pp. 619–631. Springer (2017)
3. Fox, N.C., Schott, J.M.: Imaging cerebral atrophy: normal ageing to Alzheimer's disease. The Lancet **363**(9406), 392–394 (2004)
4. Marcus, D.S., Wang, T.H., Parker, J., Csernansky, J.G., Morris, J.C., Buckner, R.L.: Open access series of imaging studies (OASIS): cross-sectional mri data in young, middle aged, nondemented, and demented older adults. J. Cogn. Neurosci. **19**(9), 1498–1507 (2007)
5. Payan, A., Montana, G.: Predicting Alzheimer's disease: a neuroimaging study with 3D convolutional neural networks. arXiv preprint arXiv:1502.02506 (2015)
6. Tufail, A.B., Abidi, A., Siddiqui, A.M., Younis, M.S.: Automatic classification of initial categories of Alzheimer's disease from structural MRI phase images: a comparison of PSVM, KNN and ANN methods. In: Proceedings of World Academy of Science, Engineering and Technology, p. 1731. World Academy of Science, Engineering and Technology (WASET) (2012)

Task-Specific Surgical Skill Assessment with Neural Networks

Malik Benmansour(✉), Wahida Handouzi, and Abed Malti

AutoMed (LAT), Tlemcen University, Tlemcen, Algeria
benmansour1994@gmail.com, wahida.handouzi@gmail.com, abed.malti@gmail.com

Abstract. Many studies on surgical skill analysis have reported results on classification of different skills. However, regardless of the classification problem, only few of them have addressed the problem of task evaluation. In this paper, we propose a simple and computationally lightweight neural network to provide evaluation scores on a given surgery task. The used neural network has three hidden layers and one output node. The output is trained so that it fits average scores of performance on a single known surgery task. Three levels of performance are used: expert, intermediate and novice. We evaluate the performance of the proposed approach on three different surgical gestures: knot-tying, needle passing and suturing. To each surgery gesture, we associate one instantiation of the designed network, which is trained with the corresponding data. We show that this method gives evaluation scores that are more plausible than a single network, which is requested to provide evaluation scores for different tasks.

Keywords: Skill assessment · Deep learning

1 Introduction

The minimally invasive surgery approach was widely used these last years. Such a surgery requires particular skill set since the manipulability of the surgery tools is reduced and the surgeon has only a tight range of moving tools in a critical environment. The required skill set is even more critical when using tele-operated robots like the DaVinci.

To acquire surgery expertise, trainees have to continuously practice and thus be continuously evaluated. This practice can be either on animal, surgical simulator [1] or real patients in a controlled context. In either case, conventional methods requires medical experts to fill out an evaluation checklist for global and task specific performance of surgery gestures. These gestures can be either basic or complex. The same medical expert has to evaluate same tasks for many students. This evaluation has to be cross-validated with other evaluation from other medical experts. The subjective and manual character of such a procedure make it non scalable for continuous evaluation of multiple trainees. An objective and automatic evaluation will obviously solve this issue and provide the trainees with reliable feedback to improve their surgical skills.

M. Ezziyyani (Ed.): AI2SD 2018, AISC 914, pp. 159–167, 2019.
https://doi.org/10.1007/978-3-030-11884-6_15

To achieve this non-subjective and automatic goals, many methods from machine learning [2, 3], like support vector machine, K-nearest neighbors, deep neural networks for which new architectures are currently being developed to improve results.

In this paper, we consider only the evaluation problem where we provide scores for three given surgery tasks: suturing, knot tying and needle passing. We draw our evaluator on a light weight neural network inspired from [5]. The author used a simple yet efficient architecture of three layers and 20 nodes per layer to classify five digits. We adapt the number of input to handle a fixed number of inputs. We extend the original input to an appropriate size to be used with kinematic data (position, velocity and acceleration) with a fixed sequence length. We experimentally prove that we can distinguish surgical skills by using specifically one neural network per given task. The simple and efficient neural network gives good, average and bad scores according to whether the subject is an expert, an intermediate or a novice. Studying other configurations will be the object of our future works. This paper is organized as follows. First, we present some researches on the used of some machine learning to recognize and evaluate surgery skill. Second, we present the proposed neural network architecture and the training setup. After that, results and discussions are presented. We conclude with a synthesis of our contribution and future work.

2 Related Work

In 2016, a research group studied fine-grained actions recognition on two datasets: 50 Salads which represents fine-grained action in the cooking domain [6], JIGSAWS [7]. They used a Spatiotemporal Convolutional Neural Network (ST-CNN). The obtained results shown that ST-CNN takes less time to compute features improved dense trajectories (IDT) and so highlight the effectiveness of ST-CNN on cooking and surgical action datasets [8].

The first work proposing the using of crowdsourcing and deep neural networks to track instruments and assess the surgeons technical skill level was done by Law et al. [9].

Also, recently, Jin et al. [10] studied tool detection and operative skill assessment in surgical videos. The used method was region-based convolutional neural networks and running in real time. JIGSAWS dataset [7, 11] and three other videos datasets containing daily living tasks were used in the studied of Doughty et al. [12]. The goal was proposing a solution for the pairwise and overall ranking using supervised deep ranking. The results were about 76% of correctly ordered pairs for the four used datasets.

Development and validation of an objective method of assessing surgical skill was performed by Poddar et al. [13]. The used features were three (feature 1: Stroke Curvature Consistency (SCC), feature 2: Stroke Duration Consistency (SDC), feature 3: Coverage Rate (CR)). HMM model and SVM classification yielded good accuracy. Zapella et al. [14] studied surgical gesture classification from video and kinematic data. Three methods were tested to classify video clip. The first one was linear dynamical system (LDS) and metrics in the space of LDSs. The second one, spatio-temporal features extracted from video clip a bag-of-features (BoF). And the final one, was multiple kernel learning (MKL) to combine the LDS and BoF approaches. For kinematic data LDS approach was used. To combine video and kinematic data, MKL was used. Results shown that the visual features could be more discriminative than kinematic data if they are selected from meaningful locations.

Surgical activities from kinematics data using recurrent neural networks were proposed by Dipetro et al. [15]. Using a single model and a single set of hyper parameters, the RNN shown good performance for recognizing gestures and maneuvers in terms of both accuracy and edit distance. The ability of trainees was evaluated using three machine learning methods: linear discriminant analysis, support vector machines, and artificial neural network classifiers. The comparison between the three methods results shown that ANN achieved best performances [16].

In real surgery applications, several deep network frameworks have been proposed. Twinanda et al. [17] used CNN for surgery phase recognition from cholecystectomy videos. The approach carried out both phase recognition and tool presence detection. A similar method was recently used for cataract surgery [18]. Rafii-Tari et al. [19] used catheter-tissue interaction and motion patterns across different skill levels to deliver an automated and objective assessment of performance.

To contribute in the advance of state-of-the-art performance, we propose in this work a simple and computationally light weight neural network to provide evaluation scores on three given surgery task. The used neural network has three hidden layers and one output node. The output is trained so that it fits average scores of performance on a single known surgery task. Three levels of performance are used: expert, intermediate and novice.

3 Methodology

We established three independent models to evaluate performance of the trainees on three basic tasks in surgery. These models are artificial neural networks. Each model is responsible to learn gestures (that are interpreted by kinematic data) of one task only.

Here is a figure representing the general model of the utilized neural network. We will talk about the number of the hidden layers and the number of nodes later in the paper (Fig. 1).

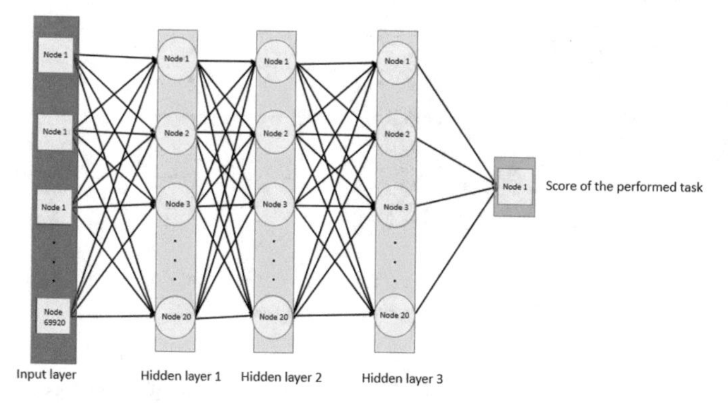

Fig. 1. Architecture of a single network for specific task evaluation

Inputs: The inputs are kinematic data from the JIGSAWS dataset [11]. Each kinematic represents in rows the numbers of frames i.e. the duration of the task completed by the surgeon and in columns, 76 kinematic data of the DaVinci robot tools (positions and velocity of the different tools…etc.). For more information about the DaVinci surgical robot and its components, please refer to [7].

Outputs: The output of each neural network is a scalar rating between 0 and 1 of the performance of a surgeon who completed one of the three tasks.

Layers: Each neural network contains h hidden layers with n nodes per hidden layer. The activation function used on the hidden layers and the output layer is a Sigmoid function. The training method is described in the following sections.

We can find, in the JIGSAWS dataset [7, 11], kinematic data of the DaVinci robot tools that give us information about the performed gesture by many surgeons. These surgeons have more or less time experience in the robotic surgical domain: novice subjects have less than 10 h experience, intermediate subjects have between 10 and 100 h practice in the domain while expert subjects have more than 100 h experience. Each surgeon performed five trials on each task.

1st model: Its goal is to evaluate performances in the Knot-Tying task only. It receives as inputs kinematic data of the Knot-Tying task of three trials done by all expert, intermediate and novice subjects for the learning phase. Some of the remaining trials of novice and intermediate subjects are used to test the network after training it. We named this model by "Knot-Tying Neural Network" which we abbreviate by "KTNN". The following figure shows on left, a sample frame from the Knot-Tying task and shows on right the curves of the spatial positions of one Patient Side Tool (which is a component of the DaVinci robot that can be seen in the sample frame) during the time the surgeon completes the task.

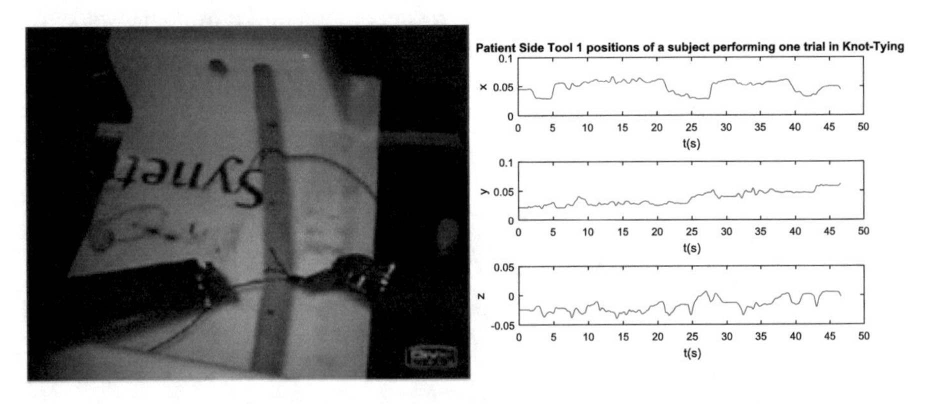

Fig. 2. On left: sample frame of the Knot-Tying task. On right: evolution of the spatial positions of one Patient Side Tool while the task is performed by a surgeon.

2nd model: this model is responsible in assessment of the Needle-Passing task performance. It receives as inputs kinematic data of the Needle-Passing task. As in the first model, only three trials are picked for all the subjects and the test is done with some of the remaining trials performed by novice and intermediate subjects. The model is named "Needle-Passing Neural Network" abbreviated by "NPNN" (Fig. 3).

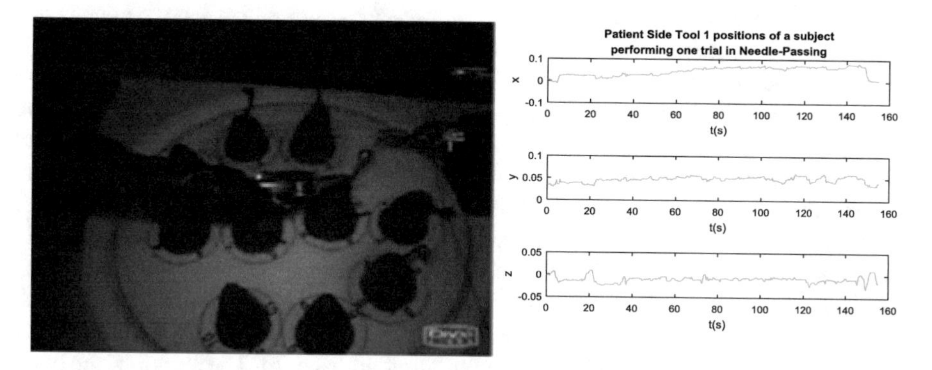

Fig. 3. On left: sample frame of the Needle-Passing task. On right: evolution of the spatial positions of one Patient Side Tool while the task is performed by a surgeon.

3rd model: this third and last model evaluates the Suturing task performances. It follows the same procedure of the two previous models for the training and the test. We named it by "Suturing Neural Network" abbreviated by "STNN" (Fig. 4).

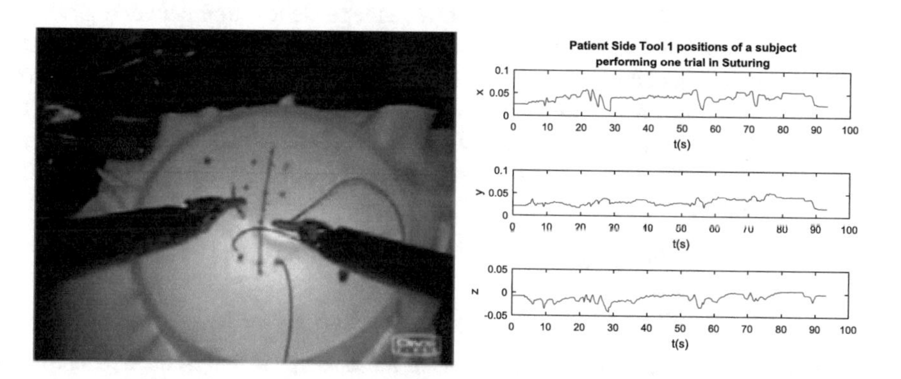

Fig. 4. On left: sample frame of the Suturing task. On right: evolution of the spatial positions of one Patient Side Tool while the task is performed by a surgeon.

4 Experimental Results

In the following section, we will present two experimental setups we have used and compared to get a performance evaluation of all surgical trainees mentioned in the JIGSAWS paper [7] after performing the three tasks. The first setup is the presented approach. The second setup is a single global network that evaluates the three tasks at once.

4.1 Experimental Setups

1st setup: we designed three independent fully connected neural networks and each one is intended to learn kinematic data of one task only. As depicted in Fig. 2, each of the three networks is a fully connected neural network composed of three hidden layers each of which contains 20 nodes. The input layer contains 69920 nodes because it is the size of each kinematic data used for the training and the test. In order to train these networks, we used the backpropagation algorithm. To compute the training error, we have chosen the cross-entropy loss function. The desired output depend on the subject who is operating. Therefore, we give the output score 1 if the kinematic data of an expert subject is given as input, 0.7 for kinematic data of an intermediate subject and 0.4 for kinematic data of a novice subject. We have chosen these ratings according to the number of hours in practicing of each subject (more than 100 h for the experts, between 10 h and 100 h for the intermediate subjects and less than 10 h for the novices). Concerning the choice of the number of hidden layers and the number of nodes in each hidden layer, we took this configuration from [5]. The author of the book used this network for a classification problem: classifying five digits of dimension 5×5 into five categories, which are numbers from 1 to 5.

This network yielded great results and thus, we decided to try it to apply our approach. We did not use other configurations because the purpose of this paper is to prove that we can assess surgical skills by using specifically one neural network to assess performance of trainees on one task.

2nd setup: we used a single fully connected neural network that has the same number of hidden layers and nodes as each of the three independent neural networks of the 1st setup. The Sigmoid activation function and the Softmax activation function are used respectively in the hidden layers and the output layer. For the training step, the network receives as inputs the data of all trials but of the expert subjects only performing the three tasks. The learning phase is completed using the Backpropagation algorithm and the training cost is computed with the cross-entropy loss function. The desired output is encoded as follows:

[1 0 0] for the Knot-Tying task.
[0 1 0] for the Needle-Passing task.
[0 0 1] for the Suturing task.

The main difference between the models in these setups is that in the 2nd setup, the neural network is designed to evaluate performance of novice and intermediate trainees after learning kinematics of expert subjects only. In addition, we did not give ratings according to subjects as desired outputs as in the 1st setup but instead, we gave binary codes as desired outputs. Each binary code represents one task. We have decided to employ this approach in order to have an assessment of one task from a network that have learned kinematic of this task and was not disrupted by data of the other tasks. On the contrary, in the setup that consists of one global artificial neural network, we may get different results from those of the 1st setup, results that we will discuss in the following subsection.

4.2 Surgical Skill Evaluation and Discussion

We run the evaluation procedure on the test data. It contains two intermediates and four novices. The intermediate subjects are labeled with the letters C and F and the novice subjects are labeled with the letters B, G, H and I. For the first setup, we give for each network, as test data, one trial of each subject performing the task the network is responsible to assess. For the model of the second setup, the test data contains one trial of each intermediate and novice subject performing each task.

The following table shows the scores of each novice and intermediate subject after performing the three tasks. For more convenience, we abbreviate the names of the tasks Knot-Tying, Needle-Passing and Suturing respectively as KT, NP and ST. We labeled any task performed by any subject by the abbreviation of the task concatenated with the label representing the subject followed by the number of the trial. For example, KTB4 stands for "novice subject B performing Knot-Tying task, trial 4". In the "Rate" rows, the green colored cells show the test results of the model of the 2nd setup while the yellow colored cells show the test results of the three independent models of the 1st setup.

Subject and task	KTB4		KTG4		KTH4	
Rate	60.8%	39.0%	98.6%	36.5%	58.2%	39.9%
Subject and task	KTI5		KTC4		KTF4	
Rate	0.8%	50.8%	98.9%	87.7%	85.2%	50.9%
Subject and task	NPB4		NPG4		NPH4	
Rate	99.7%	43.5%	32.9%	50.0%	99.9%	31.1%
Subject and task	NPI4		NPC4		NPF4	
Rate	99.8%	33.7%	32.5%	100%	60.3%	64.4%
Subject and task	STB4		STG4		STH4	
Rate	0.05%	26.9%	0.01%	46.8%	0.00%	27.3%
Subject and task	STI4		STC4		STF4	
Rate	3.8%	34.5%	0.02%	78.2%	27.3%	45.2%

As it can be seen, the three independent models yielded globally better test results than those of the single model. We can also see that particularly, the two intermediate subjects C and F got better ratings than all the novice subjects B, G, H and I with the three neural networks than with the single neural network; which seems logical since intermediate subjects have more time experience in the domain than the novice subjects. The reason the 1st setup yielded better results is because each model focuses only on assessing performance of the desired task that the model learned from the given kinematic data unlike the model of the 2nd setup which objectively assesses performance of the subjects on all tasks at once. Another reason why the model of 1st setup gave better results is because the single network must assess performance of subjects on the three tasks simultaneously. Thus, we can say that at the same time that the network was learning data of one task, it was disrupted by data of the two remaining tasks. We do not find this issue in the second setup since we have three independent models. Speaking about the time required for training the networks of both setups; the training loop of each of the three networks is performed on 1000 epochs. Consequently, the training of the three networks is completed after 3000 epochs against 1000 epochs for the single neural network. However, the single neural network takes the data of the three tasks for the training step while each of the three independent networks takes only data of the concerned task. Consequently, the amounts of time required to train networks of both setups are practically the same. We precise that the three independent networks weren't trained in parallel.

5 Conclusion

In this paper, we presented an approach with the purpose of surgical skills evaluation. This method consists on assigning three independent fully connected neural networks that were trained on all subjects performing three corresponding gestures. The training scores for assessment were assigned according to the subject experience. Thus, each network is responsible on rating the performance of one task. We compared this approach with a basic fully connected neural network that was trained with all subject database performing the three tasks and it was intended to evaluate the three tasks simultaneously through the kinematic data given as test. We have experimentally shown that the proposed approach yields better assessment results since specifying to each network a given task allows us to put more focus on the evaluation of the concerned task and therefore, we avoid any disruption during the learning step. As future work, we intend to design a task specific recurrent neural network that will be able to learn from sequences of images that show the gestures composing each task.

References

1. Dubin, A.K., Julian, D., Tanaka, A., Mattingly, P., Smith, R.: A model for predicting the GEARS score from virtual reality surgical simulator metrics. Surg. Endosc. **32**, 3576 (2018)
2. Vapnik, V.N.: An overview of statistical learning theory. IEEE Trans. Neural Netw. **10**(5), 988–999 (1999)
3. Hastie, T., Tibshirani, R., Friedman, J.: The Elements of Statistical Learning: Data Mining, Inference, and Prediction, 2nd ed. Springer, New York (2009)
4. LeCun, Y., Bengio, Y., Hinton, G.: Deep learning. Nature **521**(7553), 436–444 (2015)
5. Kim, P.: MatLab Deep Learning: with Machine Learning, Neural Networks and Artificial Intelligence. Apress (2017)
6. Stein, S., McKenna, S.J.: Combining embedded accelerometers with computer vision for recognizing food preparation activities. In: Proceedings of the 2013 ACM International Joint Conference on Pervasive and Ubiquitous Computing - UbiComp 2013 (2013). http://eprints.gla.ac.uk/134991/. Accessed 07 Apr 2018

7. Gao, Y., Vedula, S.S., Reiley, C.E., Ahmidi, N.: JIGSAWS: The JHU-ISI Gesture and Skill Assessment Working Set. CIRL, 04 September 2014. https://cirl.lcsr.jhu.edu/research/hmm/datasets/jigsaws_release/
8. Lea, C., Reiter, A., Vidal, R., Hager, G.D.: Segmental spatiotemporal CNNs for fine-grained action segmentation. ArXiv160202995 Cs, February 2016
9. Law, H., Ghani, K., Deng, J.: Surgeon technical skill assessment using computer vision based analysis. In: Machine Learning for Healthcare Conference, pp. 88–99 (2017)
10. Jin, A., et al.: Tool detection and operative skill assessment in surgical videos using region-based convolutional neural networks. ArXiv180208774 Cs, February 2018
11. Ahmidi, N., et al.: A dataset and benchmarks for segmentation and recognition of gestures in robotic surgery. IEEE Trans. Biomed. Eng. **64**(9), 2025–2041 (2017)
12. Doughty, H., Damen, D., Mayol-Cuevas, W.: Who's better? Who's best? Pairwise deep ranking for skill determination. ArXiv170309913 Cs, March 2017
13. Ahmidi, N., et al.: Automated objective surgical skill assessment in the operating room from unstructured tool motion in septoplasty. Int. J. Comput. Assist. Radiol. Surg. **10**(6), 981–991 (2015)
14. Zappella, L., Béjar, B., Hager, G., Vidal, R.: Surgical gesture classification from video and kinematic data. Med. Image Anal. **17**(7), 732–745 (2013)
15. DiPietro, R., et al.: Recognizing surgical activities with recurrent neural networks. In: Medical Image Computing and Computer-Assisted Intervention – MICCAI 2016, pp. 551–558 (2016)
16. Sbernini, L., Quitadamo, L.R., Riillo, F., Lorenzo, N.D., Gaspari, A.L., Saggio, G.: Sensory-glove-based open surgery skill evaluation. IEEE Trans. Hum. Mach. Syst. **48**(2), 213–218 (2018)
17. Twinanda, A.P., Shehata, S., Mutter, D., Marescaux, J., Mathelin, M., Padoy, N.: EndoNet: a deep architecture for recognition tasks on laparoscopic videos. IEEE Trans. Med. Imaging **36**(1), 86–97 (2017)
18. Charrière, K., Quellec, G., Lamard, M., Martiano, D., Cazuguel, G., Coatrix, G., Cochener, B.: Real-time analysis of cataract surgery videos using statistical models. Multimed. Tools Appl. **76**(21), 22473–22491 (2017)
19. Rafii-Tari, H., Payne, C.J., Liu, J., Riga, C., Bicknell, C., Yang, G.-Z.: Towards automated surgical skill evaluation of endovascular catheterization tasks based on force and motion signatures. In: IEEE International Conference of Robotics and Automation – ICRA 2015, pp. 1789–1794 (2015)

Development of a New Diagnostic Tool in the Field of Endoscopy and Telemedicine Applications

Yassine Baskoun[1(✉)], Salah D. Qanadli[2], Moha Arouch[1], Mohamed Taouzari[3], Mustafa Elalami[1], and Aziz Hraiba[1]

[1] Laboratory of Engineering, Mechanics, Industrial Management and Innovation, Faculty of Science and Technology, University Hassan 1st, Settat, Morocco
y.baskoun@uhp.ac.ma

[2] Cardio-Thoracic and Vascular Unit, Department of Radiology, University Hospital of Lausanne, Bugnon 46, 1011 Lausanne, Switzerland

[3] Laboratory LISA, Superior School of Technology Berrchid, University Hassan 1st, Settat, Morocco

Abstract. The use of smartphone in healthcare field is increasing, in particular within the field of endoscopy that usually involves expensive and often cumbersome equipment. The objective is to offer a novel adapter connected to the smartphone with modern endoscopes, exploiting the camera for viewing and recording. The design and operation are described in this article. The adapter demonstrated feasibility of coupling endoscopes to a smartphone. It makes endoscopy easier and unrelated to location and time.

Keywords: Smartphone · Endoscopy · Telemedicine · Adapter

1 Introduction

Since their inception in the mid-twentieth century, the use of endoscopes has revolutionized the practice of otolaryngology, urology and gastroenterology. Harold Hopkins was first researcher who is clarified the optics of the flexible fibrocable and invented the rod lens system in 1959. With the addition of fiber-optic light transmission by Karl Storz the following year, the modern endoscope was realized [1]. Actually, the endoscopic images obtained can be viewed directly through a monocular lens or on a portable stacking system linked via a compatible camera. This latter usually involves expensive, often cumbersome equipment and always electricity needed.

The use of mobile phone technology in health-related fields is increasing [2]. A smartphone is accessible around the world. There are 2.53 billion smartphones in use in the world, and that number is expected to grow [3]. Researchers are now realizing the great potential of using mobile health technology, such as smartphones, for electronic health services. Mobile health can also support the daily practice of health care workers via the dissemination of clinical updates, learning materials, and reminders particularly in underserved rural locations, as well as in low-income and middle-income countries.

M. Ezziyyani (Ed.): AI2SD 2018, AISC 914, pp. 168–173, 2019.
https://doi.org/10.1007/978-3-030-11884-6_16

With the development of smartphone technology, mobile health can support daily practice in the field of telemedicine [4, 5].

The purpose of this work is based on the drawbacks of the materials recently existing which are mentioned above. Thus, the new mobile technology offers the good advantages including high quality photos, manual control of focus, exposure, ISO, zoom, and color temperature. While, we record the video, photos can be captured and extracted in order to share them. An adapter combining endoscopes with smartphone innovated as viewing systems for endoscopy is ideal idea for the best useful. This concept is facilitated by the fact that all of the endoscopes used come with a 32-mm eyepiece as standard regardless of manufacturer. As the smartphone cameras are equipped with autofocus and autoaperture capabilities, the resulting image is digitally reconstructed and viewed in high definition on screen. The use of the latter has the advantage that the image can be shared with the patient, facilitating their understanding of their condition. Displayed images can also be used to educate trainees and students.

There are a few alternative devices on the market which also offer smartphone adapted endoscopic viewing systems. Endoscope-i [6, 7]: designed for use with iphone's smartphones. Endockscope [8, 9]: offers an adaptor to couple an endoscope to an iPhone to produce a mobile endoscopic viewing system. Karl Storz smart scope [10]: For use with some iPhone and Samsung models. But we should change the holder of mobile.

The structure of this work is as follow: The first section focuses on the working principle, designing and discussion. The second section is about a 3d design prototype. The last section gives the comparison with alternative devices. Finally, a conclusion is given.

2 Description of the Adapter Design and Operation

The different elements of the proposed adapter are illustrated in the Fig. 1 and given in details in [11].

The use the proposed adapter is working as follow, we firstly connect the horizontal and vertical sliding bracket on the smartphone. Secondly, the Endoscope and its fixation support connected to sliding bracket support is adjust with camera in order to capture the photos which will be displayed on smartphone screen.

3 3D Design Prototype

The 3D concept of the proposed system is presented in the two parts illustrated in Fig. 2, which describes the movement of endoscope to focus with camera.

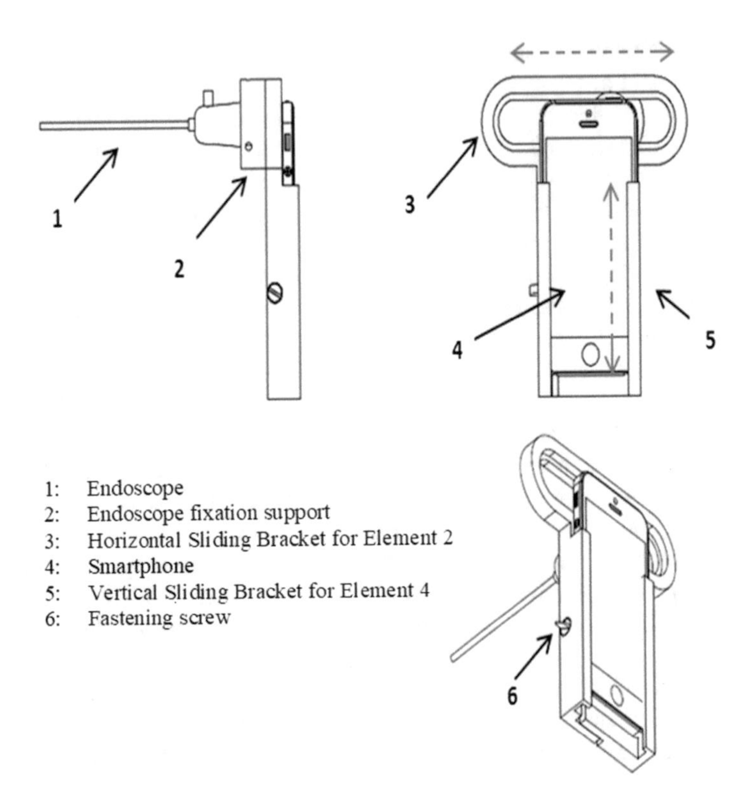

Fig. 1. Original prototype for the adapter and its components

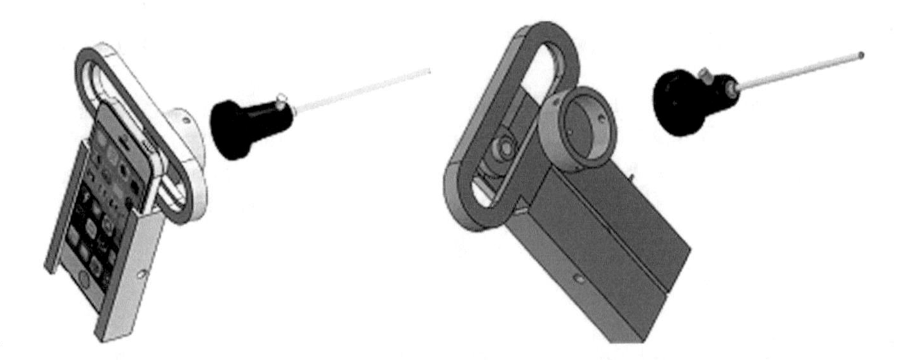

Fig. 2. 3D concept of the system

4 Comparison with Alternatives Devices

The different existing adapters (endoscope-i, Smart Scope and endosckscope) are listed in Table 1 and Fig. 3, they are limited in terms of smartphone compatibility such as the size and camera position. For the proposed system, it offers the good reliable connection with all types of the smartphone.

Table 1. Comparison with alternatives devices

Device	Smartphone compatibility
Endoscope-i [6, 7]	iPhone 4s/5/5s/6/6s and 6/6s Plus, and 7/7 Plus, iPod Touch (6th gen)
Endockscope [8, 9]	iPhone 4/4s and 5/5s
Karl Storz smart scope [10]	Adapter for each smartphone
Proposed adapter	All smartphone's brand and size

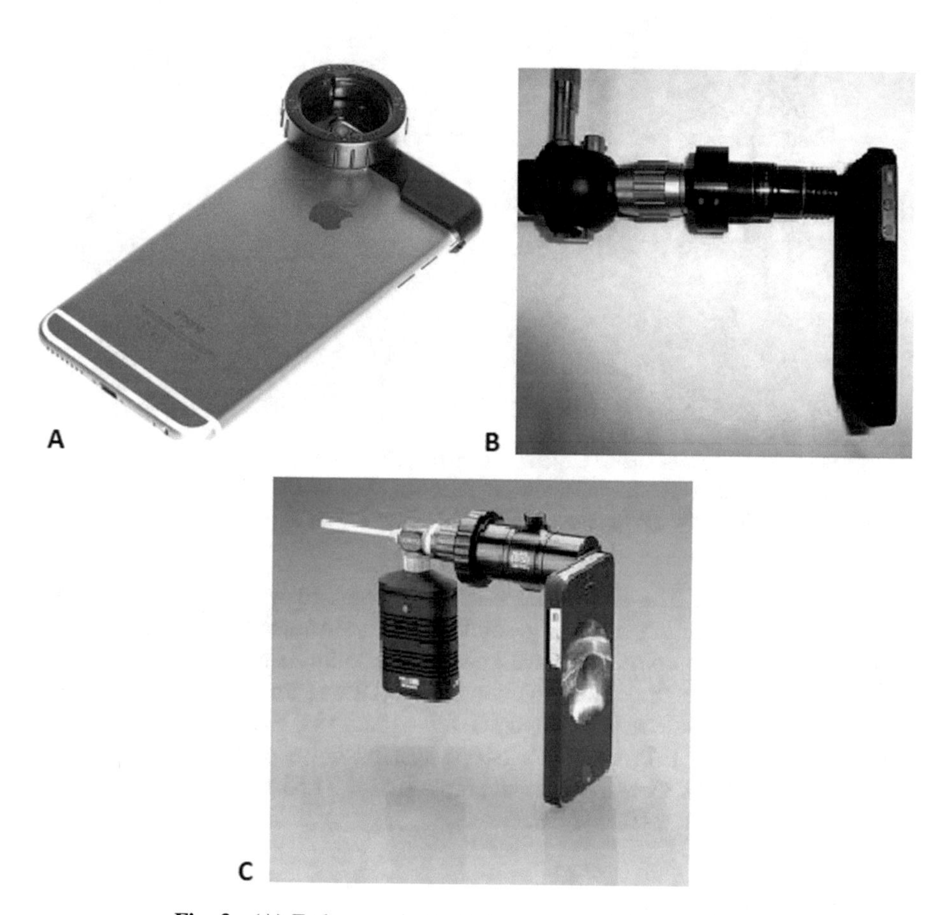

Fig. 3. (A) Endoscope-i, (B) Endosckscope, (C) Smart Scope

5 Comparison Between Traditional and Mobile Phone Based Endoscopy

As shown in Fig. 4, images captured by Endockscope+iPhone 4S and Storz HD [8].

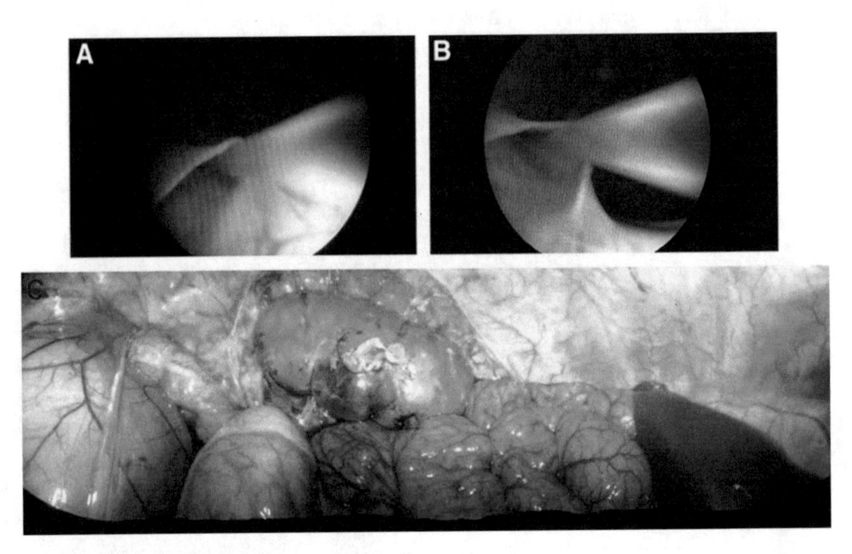

Fig. 4. Flexible cystoscope image of porcine ureteral orifice with nitinol guidewire in place with Endockscope (A) and Storz high definition (B). Panoramic image of the entire abdominal porcine cavity using the Endockscope system coupled to a laparoscope (C).

Image resolution: The Endockscope system compared with a Storz HD system revealed no difference in the image resolution (line pairs/mm) (4.49 vs 4.49 lp/mm). Color resolution: The color difference between the color samples and the reference (DE) demonstrated that the color resolution for red (DE = 9.26 vs 9.69) was similar for the two systems. There was better orange (DE = 18.13 vs 8.54) and yellow resolution (DE = 24.47 vs 20.51) for the Endockscope system; however, green (DE = 7.76 vs 10.95), blue (DE = 12.35 vs 14.66), and purple (DE = 11.55 vs 29.1) color resolution were better for the Storz HD system.

6 Conclusion

The use of smartphone technology has a significant impact in underserved areas and developing countries, where the health care infrastructure is limited. The proposed system is portable, easy to use, it makes the exams, simpler and quicker. This adapter will be beneficial in telemedicine that uses a variety of telecommunication devices including smartphones and mobile wireless devices to deliver health care. Benefits include increasing access to health care, reducing costs, and the provision of a more convenient and economic service.

References

1. Linder, T.E., Simmen, D., Stool, S.E.: Revolutionary inventions in the 20th century. The history of endoscopy. Arch. Otolaryngol. Head Neck Surg. **123**, 1161–1163 (1997)
2. Clemmensen, P., Loumann-Nielsen, S., Sejersten, M.: Telemedicine fighting acute coronary syndromes. J. Electrocardiol. **43**, 615–618 (2010)
3. The statistics portal, June 2016. https://www.statista.com/statistics/330695/number-of-smartphone-usersworldwide
4. Matusitz, J., Breen, G.M.: Telemedicine: its effects on health communication. Health Commun. **21**(1), 73–83 (2007)
5. Dorsey, E.R., Topol, E.J.: State of telehealth. N. Engl. J. Med. **375**, 154–161 (2016)
6. Mistry, N., Kulasegarah, J., George, A., Coulson, C.: Endoscope-i: transforming endoscopic technology and the delivery of patient care in ENT. J. Laryngol. Otol. **130**(S3), S206 (2016)
7. Endoscope-i. http://endoscope-i.com. Last Accessed 09 Aug 2018
8. Sohn, W., Shreim, S., Yoon, R.: Endockscope: using mobile technology to create global point of service endoscopy. J. Endourol. **27**, 1154–1160 (2013)
9. Endockscope. http://endockscope.weebly.com. Last Accessed 09 Aug 2018
10. karl-storz-smart-scope. https://www.karlstorz.com/fj/en/karl-storz-smart-scope.htm. Last Accessed 09 Aug 2018
11. Taouzari, M., Arouch, M., Baskoun, Y., Mouhsen, A., Hraiba, A., Fassi, H.F.: Patent: Adaptateur ajustables entre les endoscopes et les smartphones, OMPIC, MA 37682 (2016)

Smart Emergency Alert System Using Internet of Things and Linked Open Data for Chronic Disease Patients

Hajar Khallouki[1(✉)], Mohamed Bahaj[1], and Philippe Roose[2]

[1] Mathematics and Computer Science Department, Faculty of Sciences and Techniques, Hassan I University, Settat, Morocco
Hajar.khallouki@gmail.com

[2] LIUPPA – T2I, 2 Allée du Parc Montaury, 64600 Anglet, France

Abstract. Nowadays, the widespread deployment of more powerful devices (sensors, smartphones, tablets, etc.) has provided us with great number sources of sensing data that are exploited in several domains namely the healthcare domain. Chronic diseases are the most common causes of death and disability worldwide. These types of diseases require more and more studies to help patients and notify cases of crises that lead to death. Representing knowledge through building an ontology for emergency alert system is important to achieve semantic interoperability among health information, predict the patient real-time context and to better execute decision notification. Linked Open Data services are used in our paper in order to provide with the semantic description of collected data from different sources (wearable sensors, environmental sensors, etc.).

Keywords: Devices · Sensing data · Chronic diseases · Ontology · Emergency alert · Real-time context · Linked Open Data

1 Introduction

Since the last decade, the amount of data, the one on the Web as well as the one provided by Sensor Networks, is increasingly growing. Sensor Networks are the main parts of the Internet of Things (IoT). The term "Internet of things" was initially proposed by Kevin Ashton [1] in 1999 to describe things which are equipped with radio frequency identification chips (RFID chips). However, the concept has been developed during the last years and generalized towards an approach connecting a very large number of things to the internet, enabling them to provide services and collect context information independently.

The context awareness is a key element for creating smart applications. The collected contextual data is generally raw information from different distributed sources, which needs to be interpreted. Based on ontologies, it is possible to build semantic models which will be fed by this raw data and thus not only to increase their level of semantic representation but especially of being able to use them to make automatic decisions of adaptation of applications based on the context to the runtime.

M. Ezziyyani (Ed.): AI2SD 2018, AISC 914, pp. 174–184, 2019.
https://doi.org/10.1007/978-3-030-11884-6_17

The idea is to profit from the context-awareness functions to enable the chronically ill to live a normal life and to benefit from flexible and automated medical surveillance. In fact, several cases appear among which we can mention the patients with chronic kidney disease who suffer from an irreversible decrease in glomerular filtration rate, the best indicator of renal function.

The objectives of our work include:

- To model a smart system that enables predicting the patient's real-time context, detecting their critical situation and send an emergency alert when needed.
- A real-time data modeling and knowledge representation through ontology with examples of inference rules.
- A mechanism for collecting raw data from different sources.
- A smart emergency mechanism that locates the patient in emergency conditions along with the closest hospital then sends an emergency notification.

In the rest of this paper, we first introduce some related work on smart healthcare paradigm and existing approaches. Next, we present our proposed system architecture and its components. Finally, we conclude our paper.

2 Related Work

Over the last decade, interest in well-being has increased among the population. Several approaches have been proposed in order to improve the healthcare systems. Solanas et al. [1] introduced the new concept of smart health, which is the context-aware complement of mobile health within smart cities. They provided an overview of the main fields of knowledge that are involved in the process of building this new concept. Moreover, they presented the main challenges and opportunities that s-Health would imply and provide a common ground for further research.

In [2] Liu et al. proposed the concept of IoT-enabled intelligent assembly system for mechanical products (IIASMP). They described the IIASMP framework, which is based on advanced techniques such as information and communication technology, sensor network, and radio-frequency identification.

Venkatesh et al. [3] proposed an approach which integrates smart health applications with the connectivity of the Internet of Things (IoT), facilitating the use of machine learning and improving the complexity of context-aware designs. Their proposed approach allows designing more complex health applications with limited resources, using sensors both on the user and in the surrounding spaces.

In their work [4] Zamanifar et al. introduced a novel hierarchical scalable network scheme, DSHMP-IOT, for mobility management of IP-based sensors, which get the benefit of predicting the movement direction of mobile nodes in health-care applications to reduce the hand-off cost. Venkatraman et al. [5] developed user ontology for a Smart Health Information Portal (SHIP) to provide collaborative health terms in holistic medicine. The proposed approach integrates conventional medical terms related to cardiac conditions along with Homeopathy and Ayurvedic terms towards providing meaningful complementary heart health information within an existing SHIP.

In [6] Azimi et al. started with studying the state-of-the-art IoT-based elderly monitoring approaches to investigate their advantages and shortcomings from a different viewpoint by considering the elderly requirements at the center of attention. Thus, they presented a modernized classification and proposed a hierarchical model for elderly-centered monitoring to investigate the current approaches, objectives and challenges in a top-down fashion.

Muhammad et al. proposed in [7] a solution for voice pathology monitoring of people using IoT–cloud. More specifically, a voice pathology detection system was proposed inside the monitoring framework using a local binary pattern on a Mel-spectrum representation of the voice signal, and an extreme learning machine classifier to detect the pathology. The proposed monitoring framework can achieve high accuracy of detection.

An ontology model is a framework for describing domain knowledge, considering relevant concepts and their connections [8]. Kim et al. presented in [9] an ontology-driven interactive healthcare (OdIH_WS) to apply real-time information acquired from wearable sensors to services.

In [10] Ko et al. proposed context modeling and context reasoning in a context-aware framework which is executed on an embedded wearable system in a ubiquitous computing environment for U-Healthcare.

3 Proposed System Architecture

Our main objective is to design an innovative architecture able of predicting the patient's real-time context, detecting their critical health situation and send an emergency alert when needed. Our architecture is composed of three main components: (1) the context aware manager, (2) interaction manager and (3) emergency manager (Fig. 1).

The sensing devices measure information using a skin temperature sensor, a respiration sensor, a geolocation sensor, etc. The sensing devices sense the raw data of the patient and his context and then transfer the raw data to the sensor engine. The sensor engine receives raw data from the sensing devices then matches them to the context ontology.

A patient can interact with the system using different modalities (e.g. speech); these modalities will be captured by the multimodal engine and used in the context ontology.

To explore the potential capabilities of context-awareness, we opt for ontologies. The context ontology models the physical and environmental context of the patient; it classifies entities into lined graph that captures relationships between them. The context ontology is fed by the data provided by the interaction manager component.

The Inference Engine infers the patient context ontology, on the basis of context information collected through the interaction manager, then generates an emergency status if needed.

The last step in our architecture is the emergency notification. When an emergency status is declared as true by the inference engine, the emergency manager will first locate the patient and find the nearest hospital, thus, sends an emergency notification along with the patient's location in order to reach them.

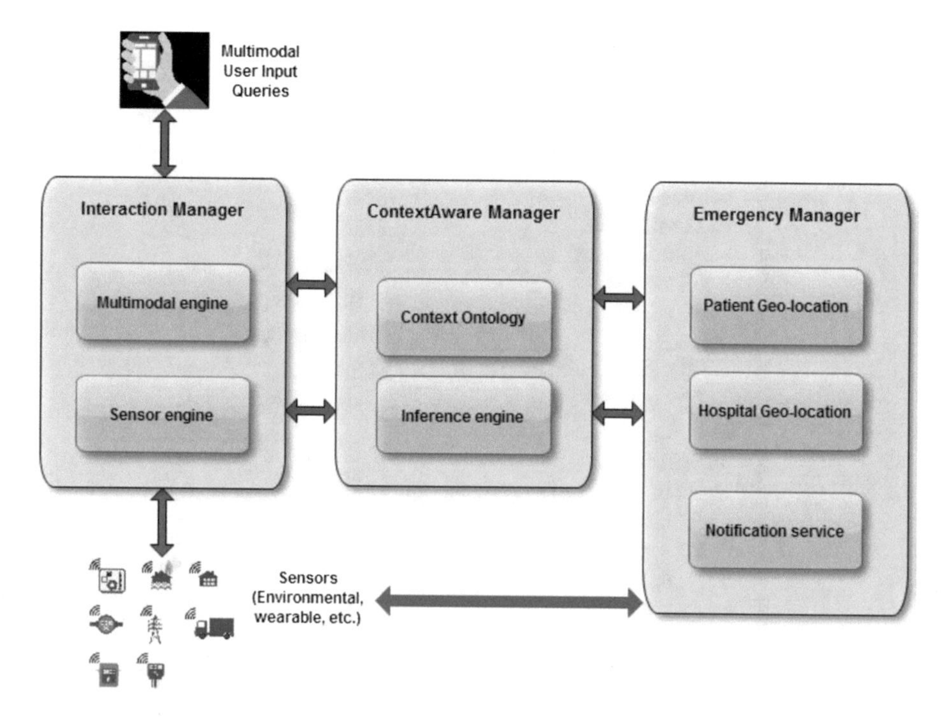

Fig. 1. System architecture

3.1 Context Aware Manager

In order to utilize the information generated from different sources, context information models are needed, and context information models are defined by using the most effective method among the model representation methods. We propose semantic knowledge representation trough ontology. To apply this model to the chronic disease emergency alerting service, inference rules are required to infer designed Ontology.

A. Context Ontology
Many knowledge modeling techniques exist, namely graphical modeling, object-oriented modeling and ontology-based modeling. The ontology-based modeling is very powerful and applicable in the context aware solutions. It has the advantage of sharing knowledge, logic inference and the reuse of knowledge.

The ontology is a specification of a conceptualization that describes the concepts and relationships existing in a domain. The ontology enables applications without the overhead of traditional data integration. Figure 2 illustrates a snapshot of our proposed context ontology for chronic disease patient.

In the Patient context ontology, relevant context items include patient health context (i.e. heart and respiration rate values, etc.), the patient's geolocation and activity, etc. These data can be used by the system to automatically infer the patient critical health status and detect possible emergency alert situations.

The *profile* class describes the personal information of the patient including age, sex, weight and height. The *ChronicDisease* class some of chronic diseases a patient

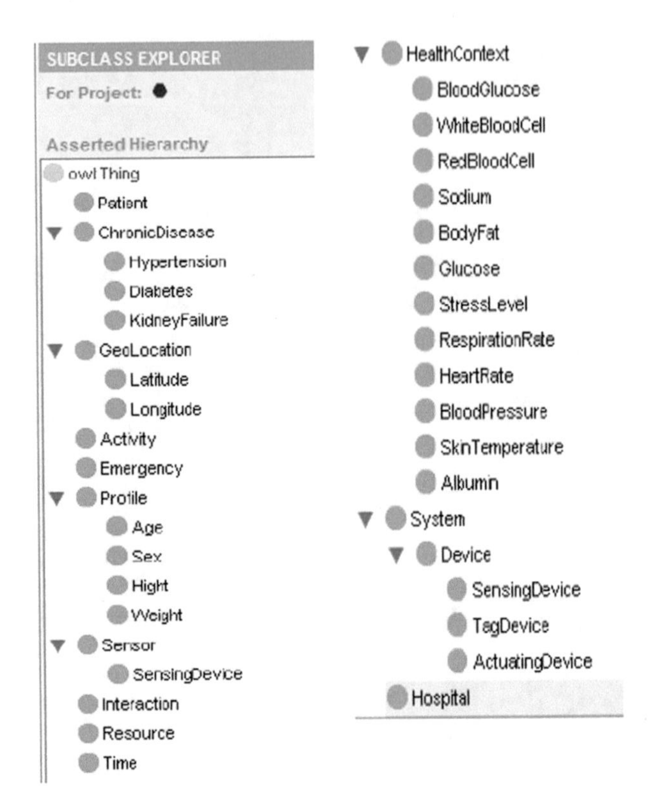

Fig. 2. A snapshot of the proposed context ontology

may face (e.g. hypertension, diabetes, etc.). The *HealthContext* defines the specific details of the health status of the patients. The *GeoLocation* class specifies the geo-location of the patient; it is defined by the latitude and longitude values. The *System* class represents parts of sensing infrastructure. The *Device* class is a subclass of system, it represents three types of devices; *SensingDevice*, *TagDevice* and *ActuatingDevice*.

To retrieve the data stored in an ontology there are several query languages, the most common is called SPARQL [11]. In the following Fig. 3, an example of a SPARQL query asking for the patient's geo-location.

B. Inference Engine

Context information necessary for the emergency service is derived by inferring the context ontology. In order to improve the expressiveness of the proposed ontology and enable the definition of if-then statements; we used the rule based formalism *Semantic Web Rule Language* (SWRL) [12]. Figure 4 shows a rule example used in our system.

This rule indicates if the patient has a heart rate upper to 100, a respiration rate upper to 30 and is age is more than 80 years old, then the emergency status takes the value true.

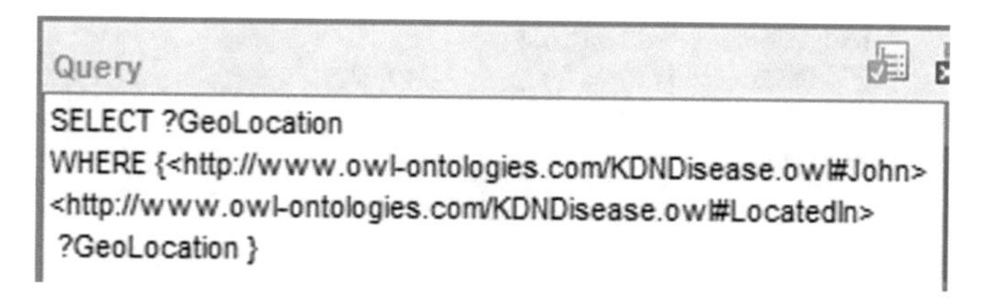

Fig. 3. Geo-location SPARQL query

```
hasValue(?HeartRate>100) ∧ hasValue(?RespirationRate>30)
∧ hasAge(?Age >80)
 → (?Emergency , true)
```

Fig. 4. SWRL rule example

3.2 Interaction Manager

The interaction manager is a main component of our architecture; it enables the collection of raw data from different sources. The interaction manager is composed of two modules; multimodal engine and sensor engine.

A. Multimodal Engine
There are many multimodal services integrated in devices such as; the HandWriting Recognition (HWR), Speech Recognition (SR) and EmotionML for user emotions recognition. The patient input modalities are represented with EMMA language. EMMA is an XML markup language which provides mechanisms for capturing and annotating the various stages of processing of users inputs [13].

The following Fig. 5 shows an EMMA interpretation of a spoken word "help".

In order to integrate data provided by the multimodal engine to our knowledge model, we proposed algorithm (Fig. 6) that aims at mapping the EMMA description which contains the user inputs modalities along with the OWL description which describes the patient context.

The algorithm takes as inputs the EMMA annotation and the OWL description; it gets and compares all nodes from both EMMA and OWL descriptions. When similarities get identified, it takes the data from EMMA nodes and fills it into OWL nodes. Finally, the result is returned in the OWL file.

B. Sensor Engine
The sensor engine is an important component in our architecture; it receives the raw data from sensing devices and transforms them to semantic descriptions.

Sensor data needs to be shared, processed and interpreted. Delivering sensor data as Linked Data enables discovery, access, query and interpretation of it.

The sensed and observed data are encoded through JSON annotation, thus, transformed to semantic descriptions through ThingSpeak[1] platform. The semantic

[1] https://thingspeak.com/.

```
<emma:medium="acoustic"
emma:mode="voice"
emma:function="dialog"
emma:verbal="true"
emma:start="1241035886246"
emma:end="1241035889306"
emma:source="smm:platform=iPhone-2.2.1-5H11"
emma:signal="smm:file=audio-416120.amr"
emma:signal-size="4902"
emma:process="smm:type=asr&version=asr_eng2.4"
emma:media-type="audio/amr; rate=8000"
emma:lang="en-FR"
emma:grammar-ref="gram1"
emma:model-ref="model1">
 <emma:interpretation id="int1"
 emma:confidence="0.75"
 emma:tokens="help">
 <flt><interaction>help</interaction>
 </emma:interpretation> <emma:info>
 <session>E50DAE19-79B5-44BA-892D</session>
 </emma:info>
 <emma:grammar id="gram1" ref="smm:grammar=help"/>
 </emma:emma>
```

Fig. 5. EMMA interpretation example

Algorithm : EmmaToOwlMappingData()	
Inputs	Owl : OWL file Emma : EMMA file
output	Owl file
1.	***Ems***= Emma.getAllElements() ; // get all nodesfromemma file
2.	***owls***= Owl.getAllElements() ; // get all nodesfromOWL file
3.	***if***Ems.containtsLocaltion***then***
4.	loc_1=Ems.getLocation;
5.	***if*** !owls.isLocationDifined***then***
6.	defineLocationClass(Owl)
7.	***end if***
8.	loc_2=owls.getNodeLocation();
9.	loc_2.setLocation(loc_1)
10.	owls.setNodeLocation(loc_2)
11.	***en if***
12.	lng_1=Ems.getLang();
13.	***if*** !owls.isLangDifined***then***
14.	defineLangClass(Owls)
15.	***end if***
16.	lng_2=owls.getNodeLang();
17.	lng_2.setLang(lng_1)
18.	owls.setNodeLang(lng_2)
19.	updateOWL(owls)
20.	return ***owl***

Fig. 6. Multimodal algorithm

annotations become semantic descriptions encoded through the JSON-LD notation. The following example describes a sensor of geo-location (Figs. 7 and 8).

```
{
"@id":"gps_shield",
"@type": "KDNDisease: sensor",
"observes": {
"@id":"geo-location",
"@type":"KDNDisease: geo-location"
        }
}
```

Fig. 7. Geo-location sensor description

```
{
"@id":"geo-location",
"@type": "KDNDisease: geo-location",
"observedData":{
"latitude":{
"@id":" KDNDisease: latitude",
"@type":"xsd: double",
"@value":"33.030908"
       }
"longitude":{
"@id":" KDNDisease: longitude",
"@type":"xsd: double",
"@value":"-7.616505"
       }
                    }
}
```

Fig. 8. Geo-location observation description

In order to collect raw data from sensors, process them and fill them to our proposed ontology, we proposed the following algorithm (Fig. 9).

The algorithm takes as inputs the JSON-LD and the OWL descriptions. It starts by getting data from JSON-LD (e.g. sensor name, longitude and latitude values, etc.). Thus, checks if JSON-LD description contains the required sensed values, if yes, the OWL description will be filled with the collected values.

3.3 Emergency Manager

Once a fall is detected, an alert should be sent to the nearest hospital containing the location of the patient. The emergency manager is composed of three modules: (1) the patient geo-location which specifies the patient real-time location, (2) the hospital geo-location in order to find the nearest hospital to the patient location and (3) the notification service for emergency alert. The following algorithm describes the process of the emergency alert (Fig. 10).

Algorithm JASONLD_to_OWL()	
input	jld: JSON-LD file, owl : owl file
output	owl : final owl file

```
1.   sensor=jld.getSensor();  // get sensed data from JSON-LD
2.   lat=jld.getLatitude();
     long=jld.getLongitude();

     //testing if json-ld contains values (data) collected from sensors
3.   if  lat != "" and long != "" and sensor != "" then
4.       owl.setSensor(sensor); // fill sensed values into Owl
5.       owl.setLatitude(lat);
6.       owl.setLongitude(long);
7.   end if

8.   return owl;
```

Fig. 9. Sensor algorithm

Algorithm : ***EmergencyAlert()***	
inputs	em: emergency manager owl: ontology

```
1.   emergency=false;
2.   geoP=null;
3.   hos=null;

4.   emergency=em.getEmergencyStatus();
     //gets the emergency status from the emergency manager

5.   if emergency=true then
6.   geoP=owl.getPatientGeolocation();
     //gets the geolocation of the patient
7.     if geoP!=null then
8.       hos=owl.getNearbyHospital(geoP);
     //gets the closest hospital to the patient
9.           if hos!=null then
10.          em.sendAlertToHospital(hos,geoP);
     //sends an alert to the closest hospital along with the geolocation
      of the patient
11.          end if
12.     end if
13.  end if
```

Fig. 10. Emergency alert algorithm

The algorithm takes as inputs the emergency manager and the ontology description. It starts by getting the emergency status from the emergency manager. If the returned status is true, it gets the patient geo-location and check the closest hospital to the patient location through *getNearbyHospital()* service. Thus, an emergency alert has to be sent along with the location of the patient in order to reach them.

4 Conclusion

In this paper, we proposed a knowledge representation through an ontology for emergency notification system. Our system allows the prediction of the patient real-time context, analyzing and processing their health conditions to better execute decision notification.

There remains more work to be carried out for covering all the aspects of our proposed approach and for improving our emergency alert system by integrating cloud computing for service continuity. Another work aims to build a context-based agent architecture in which the various components are implemented as autonomous agents to make our proposed framework more generic and distributed.

References

1. Solanas, A., Patsakis, C., Conti, M., Vlachos, I.S., Ramos, V., Falcone, F., Martinez-Balleste, A.: Smart health: a context-aware health paradigm within smart cities. IEEE Commun. Mag. **52**(8), 74–81 (2014)
2. Liu, M., Ma, J., Lin, L., Ge, M., Wang, Q., Liu, C.: Intelligent assembly system for mechanical products and key technology based on internet of things. J. Intell. Manuf. **28**(2), 271–299 (2017)
3. Venkatesh, J., Aksanli, B., Chan, C.S., Akyurek, A.S., Rosing, T.S.: Modular and personalized smart health application design in a smart city environment. IEEE Internet Things J. **5**, 614–623 (2017)
4. Zamanifar, A., Nazemi, E., Vahidi-Asl, M.: DSHMP-IOT: a distributed self healing movement prediction scheme for internet of things applications. Appl. Intell. **46**(3), 569–589 (2017)
5. Venkatraman, S.: User-centric ontology for smart holistic health information systems. Int. J. Ser. Multidiscip. Res. (IJSMR) **3**, 23–37 (2017). (ISSN: 2455-2461)
6. Azimi, I., Rahmani, A.M., Liljeberg, P., Tenhunen, H.: Internet of things for remote elderly monitoring: a study from user-centered perspective. J. Ambient. Intell. Hum. Comput. **8**(2), 273–289 (2017)
7. Muhammad, G., Rahman, S.M.M., Alelaiwi, A., Alamri, A.: Smart health solution integrating IoT and cloud: a case study of voice pathology monitoring. IEEE Commun. Mag. **55**(1), 69–73 (2017)
8. Gruber, T.R.: Toward principles for the design of ontologies used for knowledge sharing? Int. J. Hum Comput Stud. **43**(5), 907–928 (1995)
9. Kim, J., Kim, J., Lee, D., Chung, K.Y.: Ontology driven interactive healthcare with wearable sensors. Multimed. Tools Appl. **71**(2), 827–841 (2014)
10. Ko, E.J., Lee, H.J., Lee, J.W.: Ontology-based context modeling and reasoning for u-healthcare. IEICE Trans. Inf. Syst. **90**(8), 1262–1270 (2007)
11. W3C: SPARQL 1.1 Query Language, W3C (2013). https://www.w3.org/TR/2013/REC-sparql11-query-20130321/. Accessed 19 Oct 2016

12. Horrocks, I., Patel-schneider, P.F., Boley, H., Tabet, S., Grosof, B., Dean, M.: SWRL: a semantic web rule language combining OWL and RuleML. W3C Member Submission, 21 May 2004, pp. 1–20 (2004)
13. Johnston, M.: Building multimodal applications with EMMA. In: Proceedings of the 2009 International Conference on Multimodal Interfaces, pp. 47–54. ACM, November 2009

Personalized Healthcare System Based on Ontologies

Chaymae Benfares[1(✉)], Younès El Bouzekri El Idrissi[1], and Karim Hamid[2]

[1] Department of Systems Engineering Laboratory, ENSA, Ibn Tofail University, Kenitra, Morocco
benfaress.chaimae@gmail.com, y.elbouzekri@gmail.com
[2] Center for Oncology and Hematology, University Hospital Center of Mohammed VI Marrakech, Marrakech, Morocco
hk.psychologue@gmail.com

Abstract. Depression and anxiety disorders are common mental health issues that affect our ability to work and our productivity. In this paper, we propose an architecture of a surveillance system, that provides personalized and intelligent services to medical teams that monitor the psychic state of the patient, in the field of mental health, using knowledge of health services and an interactive context of patients between doctors and mental health professionals, we base on an automatic and homogeneous evaluation of the patient's needs in terms of prevention and detection of depressive tendencies. We use ontologies and recommender systems to provide patients with a climate of well-being and ubiquitous follow-up. Our case study is the prevention and screening of depression and anxiety disorders in cancer patients, the unit of psychology, at the center of ontology and hematology of the University Hospital Center "CHU" of Marrakech.

Keywords: Healthcare · Ontology · Service · Personalization · Depression · Recommender systems

1 Introduction

E-health has become a highly sought-after field in the last few years because of the new information and communication technologies that play a vital role in the health care field for the world's population. Besides, the World Health Organization promotes and supports the development of new smart solutions to address health issues.

On the one hand, and according to WHO's Mental Health Action Plan [1], 2013–2020, mental well-being is an essential component (the WHO definition). Good mental health enables people to self-actualize, to overcome the normal stresses of life, to do productive work and to contribute to the life of their community. This comprehensive plan of action emphasizes the critical role of mental health in achieving the goal of health for all. It is based on a lifelong approach which aims to achieve equity through universal health coverage and stresses the importance of prevention. On the other hand, mental disorders often have an influence on other diseases. For example cancer,

M. Ezziyyani (Ed.): AI2SD 2018, AISC 914, pp. 185–196, 2019.
https://doi.org/10.1007/978-3-030-11884-6_18

cardiovascular diseases. In particular, the situation becomes very alarming in patients with cancer because depressive disorders have been frequently encountered. During routine oncology care, their screening, assessment and treatment are of paramount importance in psychosocial management. Depressive symptoms have a decisive impact on the quality of life for patients, tolerance and their adherence to cancer therapeutics. In addition, morbidity and the possible influence of depression on prognosis represent a huge challenge when it comes to prevention. To overcome barriers and bridge the gap between resources and needs in the treatment of mental disorders, and to reduce the number of years of disability and death associated with these disorders, WHO states the need to set up technologies and information systems in the field of coats disorders. Concerning the objectives of its action plan [1], it stresses four main objectives: to achieve more effective leadership and governance in the field of mental health; provide comprehensive, integrated and responsive mental health services and social protection services in a community setting; implement promotion and prevention strategies; and strengthen information systems, gather more evidence and develop research. Therefore, health care aims to lead the population to valuable assistance in the application of democracy in addition to reducing exclusion and social disparities, and to organize health services around the needs and expectations of the population. (Populations service delivery reforms).

Our approach aims to provide architecture of an intelligent system of adaptive services to the context and needs of patients, based on the hybrid approach of the recommendation system and ontologies. It is also based on an automatic and homogeneous evaluation of the patient's needs in terms of prevention and detection of depression tendencies in order to offer a climate of well-being. In this research, we rely on a diagnostic test, of the Psychological Center of Oncology and Hematology, of the University Hospital Center "CHU" of MOHAMED VI Marrakech. in addition to the Hospital Anxiety and Depression scale "HAD" (to improve the quality of forecasts). The purpose is to have relevant and personalized results for each person.

This document is organized as follows: Sect. 2 describes some related work, Sect. 3 presents Theoretical Framework. As well as Sect. 4, presents mainly the architecture of the personalized health care system that we use in our research. Section 5, details each layer of the system.

2 Related Work

E-health helps to provide answers that will preserve the fundamentals, of the health system while increasing its added value for professionals and patients, through services using new technologies of communication and information, Let's mention the recommendation systems and the semantic web, which open new ways of innovative applications, in the field of health, Faced with the enormous quantity and the heterogeneity of data, in the databases in the field of the health.

In recent years, a lot of research has been done in the field of e-health [2], for example the author proposes [3], an Information Technology (IT) prototype that focuses in accelerating the process for breast cancer detection is proposed. This methodology was used in order to develop the s-Health solution presented [4]. This paper presents the software requirements specification (SRS) of an e-health solution to improve the cardiology healthcare quality and efficiency in Morocco. The authors [5], studies the Big Data e-Health Service to fulfill the Big Data applications in the e-Health service domain. The authors describes [6], The challenges wearable technologies for implementation in healthcare services, and how new developments drive a change in healthcare delivery models and the relationship between patients and healthcare providers. Many research projects had used semantic ontology-based approaches to improve access and integration of information, to overcome the problem of heterogeneity of semantic data of from various sources [7], because ontologies provide formal and structured representations of knowledge, especially in the field of health [8]. This paper [9], propose a solution of personalized recommendation in online health communities with heterogeneous network mining. More, different techniques of the recommendation system have been applied in the field of health. In general, there are three main types of recommender system. The authors [10] propose collaborative filtering method for top-recommendation task by bicustering neighborhood approach, and [11] the authors, present an improved assumption of pairwise preferences, over mixed-type item-sets, by defining the preference on two item sets with different type instead of on a simple item set.

3 The Approach Overview (Healthcare Personalized Services)

In this work, we present a service personalized approach, based on ontologies and intelligent algorithms, we adopted the tools of recommendation systems such as content-based recommendation system and decision support tools “the decision tree”. Domain knowledge representation occurs through ontologies. In this way, the system can provide both services to patients, and at the same time offers decision support to doctors and professionals. In more detail, the proposed approach aims to automate and personalize the selection of relevant services, based on patient profile modeling and the knowledge base, of our health care system (which is represented by ontologies) and extracted with the help of mental health professionals. We used relevant data and tools with the help of experts and clinicians in the field of depression.

As a first step, we formally define the patient’s file that contains:

- Personal data.
- A diagnostic test.
- Self questionnaire: “HAD” scale.

In this approach, professionals have a knowledge base containing all the information on disease symptoms according to patient context. To make decisions about the selection of services, the professionals make inferences, based on the information they have on the entire profile and context of the patient in order to obtain relevant recommendations. We have adopted relevant data and tools to help following depression clinicians:

- The diagnostic test: We used the "CHU" diagnostic test to know the symptoms of each patient.
- "HAD" scale: We used the "HAD" questionnaire associated with the recommendation of good practice for screening of depression and anxiety.

4 Theoretical Framework

4.1 The Semantic Web and Ontology

Ontology is a central concept of the semantic Web. The semantic Web is a set of technologies whose main objective is to make available to the machines the meaning (semantics) of the data present on the Web.

The Semantic Web offers many opportunities, one can cite [12]:

- Optimization of the cooperation between the machines: The use of a common language makes it possible to reinforce the interoperability between the machines.
- Inference reasoning: It is an operation to draw a conclusion from of known data.

An ontology is a specification of a conceptualization Basically, it means that an ontology formally describes concepts and relationships which can exist between them in some community [13]. A concept in an ontology can represent a variety of things. A domain ontology describes the terminology and relationships between the terms of a specific domain. The ontologies can be written in different programming languages [14], to provide a formal description of concepts, terms, or relationships of any domain. These languages are RDFS (Resource Description Framework Schema) and OWL (Web Ontology Language). We have used ontology in your system in order to standardize and define the system domain, in order to ameliorate the personalization of services.

4.2 Recommender System

The development of the web world is becoming an area where the obligation to looking for relevant information is always a challenge [15], however a recommendation system aims to provide a user with relevant resources according to their preferences. The latter sees reduce its search time, but also receive suggestions from the system to which he would not have spontaneously paying attention [16]. The rise of the Web and its popularity has notably contributed to the establishment of such systems as in the field of e-commerce. Recommendation systems can be seen initially as a response to users who have difficulty making a decision in the context of use of an information search system "classic".

Collaborative Filtering

Collaborative filtering models use the collaborative power of the ratings provided by multiple users to make recommendations. The main challenge in designing collaborative filtering methods is that the underlying ratings matrices are sparse.

The basic idea of collaborative filtering methods is that these unspecified ratings can be imputed because the observed ratings are often highly correlated across various users and This similarity can be used to make inferences about incompletely specified values. Most of the models for collaborative filtering focus on leveraging either inter-item correlations or inter-user correlations for the prediction process. Some models use both types of correlations. There are two types of methods that are commonly used in collaborative filtering, which are referred to as memory-based methods and model-based methods:

- Memory-based methods

Memory-based methods are also referred to as neighborhood- based collaborative filtering algorithms, there are two types:

- Collaborative filtering based on the user
- Item-based collaborative filtering.

- Model-based methods

Model-based methods have been incorporated into recommendation systems to address the problems of memory-based methods [17]. To deal with these two problems, the methods model-based techniques use dimensionality reduction techniques or clustering in order to exclude users or non-representative items. Model-based filtering is based on machine learning techniques, such as: clustering, decision trees, bayesian networks, etc.

Content-Based Filtering

Consist of matching a user's preferences with items. CB is based on the content and relevant profiles to generate personalized recommendations, the in order to decide its relevance to the user [18]. In general, content-based recommendation systems depend on three main substances [11].

- User Profile, Item-profile and User utility function: to find the relevance between the user profile and the item profile. If the relevance is high, the item may be recommended to the user.

Hybrid Recommender Systems

This approach addresses the problems of both approaches: collaborative filtering and content-based filtering. Because each of the approaches to the recommendation has advantages and disadvantages. Therefore, the hybrid approach is a solution consists of combining advantages of the two approaches mentioned above.

According to Burke [19] Hybrid recommender systems can be classified as (see Fig. 1).

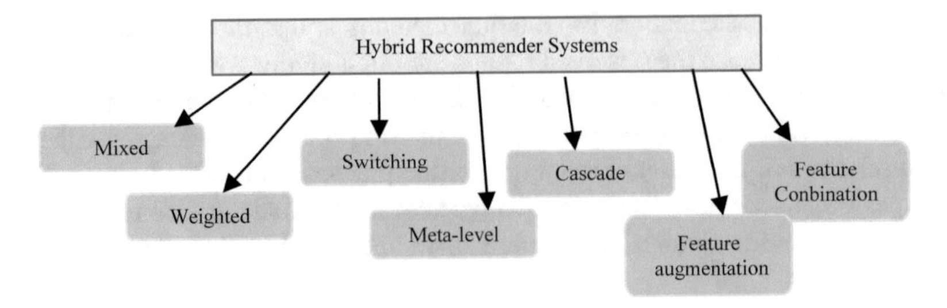

Fig. 1. Hybrid recommender systems

5 System Architecture

In this work, we propose an approach based on the ontology, and the hybrid approach of the recommender system, in order to personalize the services of the mental health, in the matter of screening and the prevention of the tendencies of depression and anxiety in the patients of cancer, at the center of oncology and hematology "CHU" of Marrakech. Personalization is based on the use of ontologies services and profile that records for each person. Our proposal is based on the main architecture that is presented below (see Fig. 2), which is divided into three layers, (we will then explain each layer of the architecture):

- Patient profile layer
- Recommendation layer
- Layer of representation of the system knowledge base.

The first step is the interaction of the patient with the system:

- The patient explicitly filled in his personal data.
- The patient passes a diagnostic test and a self-questionnaire "HAD" Scale,
- The system models the patient profile as a semantic network.
- All the required patient information will be stored in the profile database.

The second phase is to analyze the data from the patient. The recommender system is responsible for calculating the most relevant service recommendations, that best meet the needs of patients (using the patient's profile) by the following steps:

- Calculate similarity between the patient's profile and the knowledge base of the system, based on a content-based recommendation system. Output of this step will be weighting.
- Creation of a self-questionnaire decision tree "HAD" scale, to calculate the second weighting to confirm the diagnosis, based on a model-based recommendation system.
- Finally, the system generates the two weights (we use the hybrid approach of recommendation system.) in order to make the best decision.
- The system recommends to the patient the most relevant services according to his profile.

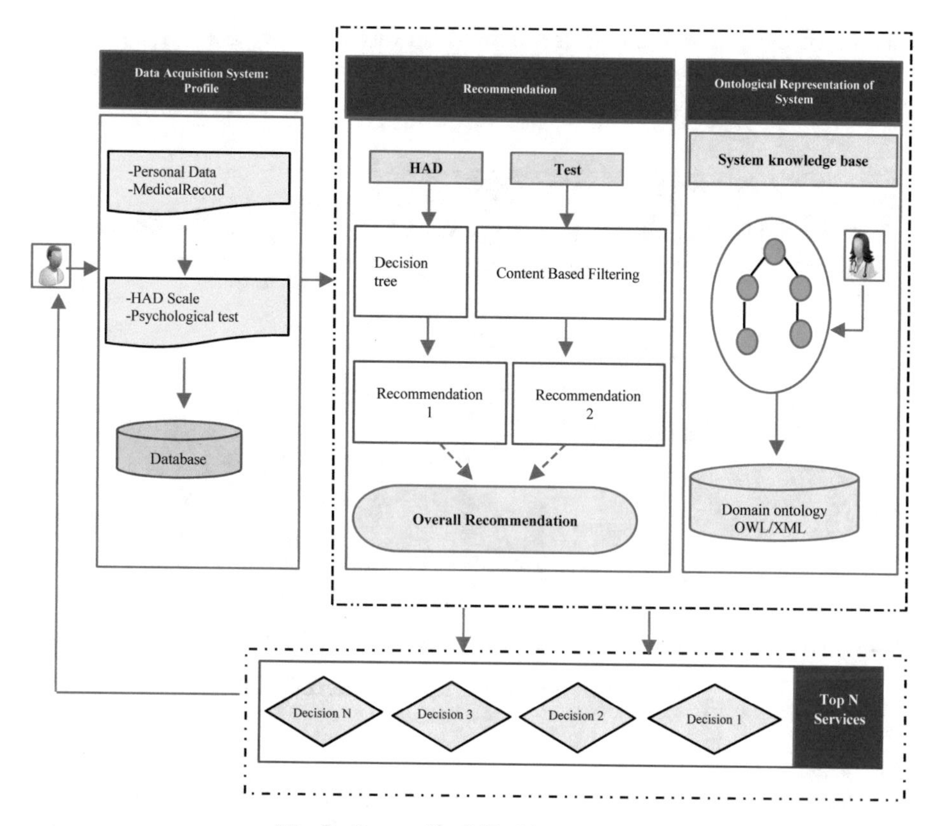

Fig. 2. Personalized Healthcare System

5.1 Profile Layer

Personnel Profile

The patient's profile contains all the information needed to design a relevant diagnosis, in order to personalize their services according to their needs. The patient profile contains:

- Personal data.
- The test.
- Auto questionnaire the "HAD" scale.

In our case, the collection of data is explicit handling, that is to say the patient filled in his personal data, and go through a test in order to extract its symptoms and its general context. In addition the patient completes a self-questionnaire The "HAD" scale, which is an instrument, allows to detect a depressive disorder. So that clinicians and doctors interpret it and conclude its degree of depression. In this work, patient modeling is based on the ontology, OWL, Web Ontology Language (language used to define and instantiate Web Ontologies). To model the profile of the patient we adopted: the semantic network that allows to store the meaning of the words and a more precise learning of the patient's profile (see Fig. 3). In this work, we used Protégé for the modeling of ontologies of the concepts that it is the profile or the base of knowledge, protégé is a free open-source ontology editor and framework [20].

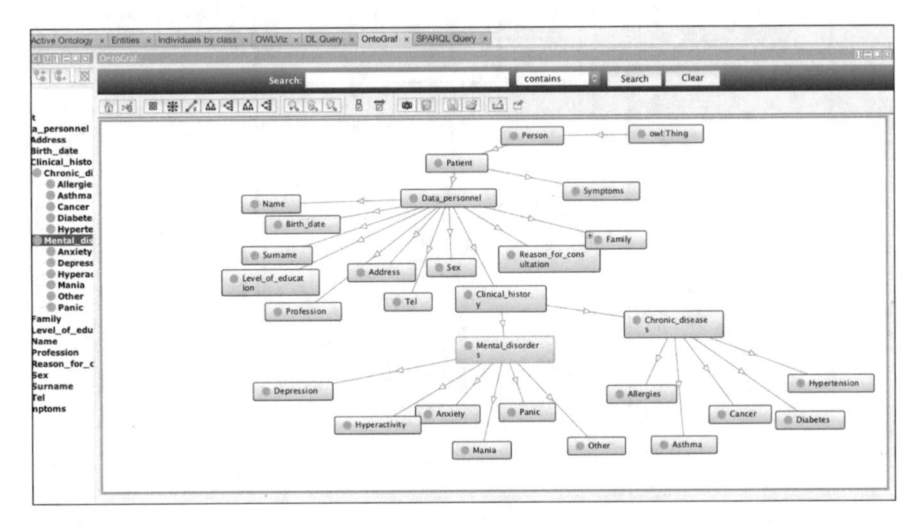

Fig. 3. Protege OntoGraf representation of profile

Diagnostic Test

The following figure (see Fig. 4) shows, example of the symptoms extracted by the diagnosis test of depression and anxiety of "CHU". We modeled the symptoms as a data graph.

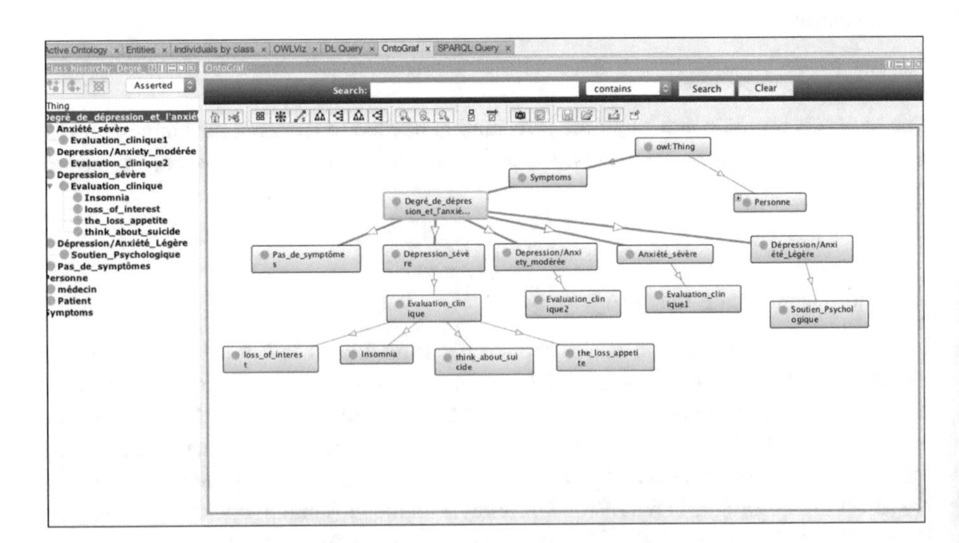

Fig. 4. Ontology model of symptom

Scale HAD

Rating scale of anxiety and depression, is a self-questionnaire completed by the patient. The "HAD" scale is an instrument for detecting anxiety and depressive disorders. It comprises 14 items rated from 0 to 3. Seven questions relate to anxiety (total A) and seven others to the depressive dimension (total D), thus allowing two scores to be obtained (maximum score of each score = 21) [21].

To detect anxious and depressive symptoms, the following interpretation can be proposed for each of the scores (A and D):

- 7 or less: no symptomatology
- 8 to 10: doubtful symptomatology
- 11 and above: certain symptomatology.

5.2 The Knowledge Base Layer

The knowledge base of our system (Personalized Healthcare System) is modeled by the domain ontology of depression and anxiety, using the Protégé tool. It contains all the necessary knowledge:

- The clinical symptoms of the patient.
- Clinical history.
- The health problems of the patient.
- Services and procedures of treatment.

Recommendation Layer

- Phase Similarity Data
  - Similarity content-based filtering

To calculate the similarity between the patient's profile and the knowledge base, we used the content-based recommendation system. The calculation of the similarity between two concepts makes it possible to determine if they are equivalent or independent semantically. we used the following similarity function, in order to calculate a similarity between the patient's symptoms and the knowledge base of the system (the symptoms):

$$GSim(C_i, C_j) = \sum\nolimits_{(K=1,\ldots,Card(A))} \prod\nolimits_{ik} \mathrm{Sim}(Attribut_{ik}, Attributs_{jm}) \tag{1}$$

- Decision Tree

A decision tree describes graphically the decisions to be made, the events that may occur, and the outcomes associated with combinations of decisions and events. Probabilities are assigned to the events, and values are determined for each outcome. A major goal of the analysis is to determine the best decisions, A decision tree describes graphically the decisions to be made, the events that may occur, and the outcomes associated with combinations of decisions and events [22]. A Decision tree models include such concepts as nodes, branches, and attributes.

In this paper, we used the decision tree to generate the weighting across the "HAD" scale, to help clinicians specified of depression and anxiety hang an excellent decision. (see Fig. 5) shows a decision tree that represents the result of the "HAD" scale auto questionnaire. The decision tree has three given services ((green), (yellow), (orange)), on each node a test is performed by a well specified criterion that ultimately reflects a service.

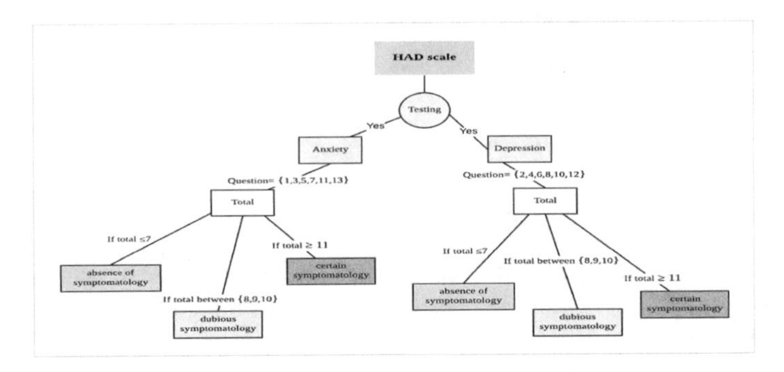

Fig. 5. Decision tree for auto questionnaire "HAD scale"

In the tree, above, the first test is on the test type specification, either "depression" or "anxiety", the second level of the decision tree displays the criteria for each test question, third level is to test and evaluate the service, according to the ranking of, for example:

- If the (total $\leq$ 7) the service is: "absence of symptomatology".
- If total (between {8,9,10}) the service is "dubious symptomatology".
- If (total $\geq$ 11) the service is "certain symptomatology".

– The equation calculates, a value of the probability that a patient belongs to a class of the HAD Scale:

$$Pr(v|u_a, i_k) = \sum_z Pr(v|i_k, z)Pr(z|u_a) \tag{2}$$

– Thus, the prediction is calculated by the following equation:

$$Pred(v|u_a, i_k) = \sum_v \left(v * \sum_z Pr(v|z, i_k)Pr(z, u_a) \right) \tag{3}$$

- Overall Recommendation of Personalized Healthcare

In this paper, we adopted the "Weighted" hybrid approach of recommendation system, by combining two weights obtained, to generate the unified global recommendation, by the formula below, the first prediction is the similarity of content-based filtering to evaluate services according to the symptoms, the second is a test "HAD" filter based on the decision tree of model-based method, in order to obtain a better decision of personalization of health care services, adapted to profile and needs of each patient.

$$hybrid - recom - pred = \beta * pred_{CB} + (1 - \beta) * pred_{CFB} \quad (4)$$

$pred_{CB}$: The weight of content-based filtering algorithm.
$pred_{CFB}$: The weight of collaborative filtering algorithm (Model-based method: decision tree).

6 Conclusion

The personalization of intelligent services has become a fundamental element in the different areas. In this article, we have proposed a hybrid approach to personalize the health care services, in the field of mental health, in the detection of trends of depression and anxiety, at the oncology and hematology center of "CHU" of Marrakech. The future work of this approach is to develop the proposed architecture using a framework implemented in Java language, that will be composed of several intelligent agents that allows to separate each layer of the architecture, also, we will use real data (from CHU databases) in order to simulate our approach and then we will discuss the obtained results.

References

1. OMS: Plan d'action global pour la santé mentale 2013–2020. Organ. Mond. la Santé, 49 (2013)
2. Azimi, I., Anzanpour, A., Rahmani, A.M., Liljeberg, P.: Self-aware early warning score system for IoT-based personalized healthcare. In: eHealth 360°, vol. 181, pp. 49–55 (2017)
3. Avalos, M., Salazar, P., Cities, A.S.: Powered by Leading Edge Cognitive Services Consumed in the Cloud (2016)
4. Ouhbi, S., Idri, A., Hakmi, R., Benjelloun, H., Fernandez-Aleman, J.L., Toval, A.: Requirements specification of an e-health solution to improve cardiovascular healthcare services in Morocco. In: 11th International Conference on Intelligent Systems: Theories and Applications, SITA 2016, pp.16–21 (2016)
5. Liu, W., Park, E.K.: Big data as an e-health service. In: International Conference on Computing, Networking and Communications, ICNC 2014, pp. 982–988 (2014)
6. Lewy, H.: Wearable technologies – future challenges for implementation in healthcare services. Healthc. Technol. Lett. **2**, 2–5 (2015)

7. Kanaan, H., Mahmood, K., Sathyan, V.: An ontological model for privacy in emerging decentralized healthcare systems. In: Proceedings of IEEE 13th International Symposium on Autonomous Decentralized System, ISADS 2017, pp. 107–113 (2017)
8. Cardoso, S., Aimé, X., Felipe, L., Mora, M., Grabli, D., Meininger, V., Charlet, J.: cadre des maladies neurodégénératives. dans le cadre des maladies neurodégénératives, 1 (2016)
9. Jiang, L., Yang, C.C.: Personalized Recommendation in online health communities with heterogeneous network mining. In: IEEE International Conference on Healthcare Informatics, pp. 281–284 (2016)
10. Alqadah, F., Reddy, C.K., Hu, J., Alqadah, H.F.: Biclustering neighborhood-based collaborative filtering method for top-n recommender systems. Knowl. Inf. Syst. **44**, 475–491 (2015)
11. Gao, S., Guo, G., Lin, Y., Zhang, X., Liu, Y., Wang, Z.: Pairwise preference over mixed-type item-sets based bayesian personalized ranking for collaborative filtering. In: IEEE 15th International Conference on Dependable, Autonomic and Secure Computing, 15th International Conference on Pervasive Intelligence and Computing, 3rd International Conference on Big Data Intelligence and Computing and Cyber Science and Technology Congress, pp. 30–37 (2017)
12. Benfares, C., El Bouzekri El Idrissi, Y., Abouabdellah, A.: Recommendation semantic of services in smart city. In: Proceedings of the 2nd International Conference on Big Data, Cloud Application – BDCA 2017, pp. 1–6 (2017)
13. Synak, M., Dabrowski, M., Kruk, S.R.: Semantic web and ontologies. In: Semantic Digital Libraries, pp. 41–54 (2009)
14. Akundi, P.: Reliable semantic systems for decision making: defining a business rules ontology for a survey decision system. In: Semantic Web, pp. 153–172. Springer, Cham (2016)
15. Benfares, C., El Idrissi, Y., Amine, A.: Smart city: recommendation of personalized services in patrimony tourism. In: 4th IEEE International Colloquium on Information Science and Technology (CiSt), 24 October 2016, pp. 835–840. IEEE (2016)
16. Béchet, N.: Etat de l'art sur les Systèmes de Recommandation. Bechet. Users. Greyc. Fr (2012)
17. Pheniics, S.: `se de Doctorat Th e de l' Universit e ´ par e ´ e a pr e l' Universit e Structure des noyaux les plus lords : spectroscopie du noyau 251 Fm (2016)
18. Sulieman, D., Syst, D.S.: Syst`emes de recommandation sociaux et s´emantiques (2014)
19. Mokhtar, B., Mokhtar, A.-B.: Une Technique Hybride pour les Systèmes de Recommandation (2016)
20. protégé. https://protege.stanford.edu/
21. Échelle HAD: Hospital Anxiety and Depression scale, pp. 3–4 (2014)
22. Trees, D.: Introduction to Decision Trees 14. Event (London)

Survey on the Use of Health Information Systems in Morocco: Current Situation, Obstacles and Proposed Solutions

Houssam Benbrahim(✉), Hanaâ Hachimi, and Aouatif Amine

BOSS-Team, GS Laboratory,
National School of Applied Sciences, Ibn Tofail University, Kenitra, Morocco
houssam.benbrahim@uit.ac.ma

Abstract. In order to evaluate the use of Health Information Systems in Morocco, we have contributed an online survey of 199 participants. This survey was based on 27 questions that allow to provide the necessary information about this subject. The results of this study showed that 52.8% of the participants consider that the health services in Morocco are mediocre, 88.4% do not use an Electronic Health Record and 85.9% want to follow their medical situation using Information Systems. Thus, it was found that the majority of the participants think that the Information Systems help to improve the quality of health services, and they have a good knowledge of a new computer technologies like Big Data with a percentage of 61.6%. Also, 83.9% of the contributors are agree with the implementation of a new Health Information System that facilitates the management, control and analysis of health data in Morocco. Concerning the obstacles, we have noticed that the most of participants link the barriers to the lack of the laws and the norms in the first degree, and to the lack of funding in the second degree. We have elaborated this study, first to discover the current situation of the Health Information Systems in Morocco, and to know the different obstacles that are related to this topic. Our second objective is to make available a series of possible solutions to improve the health sector in Morocco.

Keywords: Survey · Health information Systems · Morocco · Electronic health record · Big Data

1 Introduction

Health Information Systems (HIS) mean any system that captures, stores, manages, analyses, controls, secures or transmits health knowledge regarding individuals or the activities of organizations operating within the field of health [1]. The HIS plays an essential role in reducing costs and improve individual and public health outcomes, and research [2]. It aims also to improve the quality of care services, to influence policy and decision-making [3]. Health data are too huge, complex and different in type. It is very difficult to use traditional software to manage, secure and exploit the health data. Actually, the new technology that is taking a big importance by IT experts in all fields and more specifically by the health sector is the Big Data. This technology offer to the health field a positive opportunity, because the tools and the advanced platforms used

M. Ezziyyani (Ed.): AI2SD 2018, AISC 914, pp. 197–204, 2019.
https://doi.org/10.1007/978-3-030-11884-6_19

to ensure multiple and important results as the improvement of the quality of the services of the health, the reduction of the costs, and the predictive analysis. Exploiting health data with big data concept can give to this sector incredible solutions for several problems, including the proposition of new ideas, methods and approaches [4].

The current health situation in Morocco remains marked by a number of problems, particularly in the level of provision of services to individuals, which makes the health system unattractive to the citizen. But this sector has several achievements which show a real willingness to improve the situation [5]. Morocco has launched several projects to strengthen this field, among them we can cite:

- The Sector Strategy “Health” for the period 2012–2016 is a part of the implementation of the Moroccan government’s program. In its development, the Ministry of Health has taken into account the need to consolidate the achievements of previous strategies and to respond to new needs [6].
- The World Health Organization (WHO) strategy of cooperation with Morocco, which represents a medium-term strategic plan for collaboration. For Morocco, this strategy covers the period 2017–2021 and aligns with the sustainable development goals and the strategic directions for health [7].

Our research article is based on an internet survey, its purpose is to evaluate the use of information systems in the health sector in Morocco. Survey research is one of the most important areas of measurement in applied social research. The broad area of survey research encompasses any measurement procedures that involve asking questions of respondents [8].

In this article, we will first present our survey study on internet to gauge the use of health information systems in Morocco. Then we provide and discuss the results collected. Finally, we will propose some solutions to improve the current health situation in Morocco.

2 Materials and Methods

To evaluate the use of information systems in the health sector in Morocco, we released a survey via the internet between December 2017 and April 2018 [9]. As a result, we used 27 items in a survey completed by 199 participants. A survey was created with multiple choices to tick obligatorily to avoid losing data. The survey was developed on google forms, and shared on social networks like Facebook and LinkedIn, as well as we sent the survey by email. The target population is patients as well as healthcare professionals in Morocco such as doctors, nurses, staff of a scientific research laboratory, staff of a pharmaceutical entity, staff of a laboratory medical analyzes, health insurers, and the administrative staff of a health service in Morocco.

The survey allowed us to collect the necessary information about the participants: age, gender, status, as well as the answers to the questions. Most of the questions were formulated using yes/no, in other questions we chose mentions of: excellent, very good, good, average and mediocre. In another, we used mentions: no change, evolving and getting worse. And for one question, the participants were given the choice between: lack of human resources, lack of funding, lack of laws and standards or no idea.

To analyze the results obtained from the survey, we entered into a Microsoft Excel all the data, and we used the Statistical Package for Social Sciences (SPSS) software for Windows version 20.

3 Results and Discussion

During the survey period, we received 199 responses. Our results showed that: 55.1% of participants are women and 44.9% are men, so it can be said that the most of our target population are female. Among the 199 participants, we noticed that the age group that answered a lot on the survey is between 20 and 30 years old with a percentage of 68.9%, after we have 11.2% between 31 and 40 years old, in the third place we have 6.6% between 41 and 50 years old, the fourth is the age group between 51 and 60 years old with 5.6%, the penultimate is the ages that are less than 20 years old with 5.1%, and the last place belongs to the participants who are over 60 years old.

Regarding the status of participants to the survey, we have 11.7% of doctors, 1.5% are nurses, 57.1% of patients, 24.5% are Staff of a scientific research laboratory, 0.5% are Staff of a pharmaceutical entity, 1.5% Staff of a medical analysis laboratory and 3.1% are Administrative staff of a health service. The total absence of health insurers was noted, and no information was received from them. In the survey, 24 questions were completed by health actors. Table 1 groups all the questions proposed.

Table 1. The 24 questions of the survey.

Questions	Signification
Q1	Do you have health insurance?
Q2	Have you ever had a medical consultation?
Q3	Do you have internet access?
Q4	Do you use social networks (like Facebook)?
Q5	Do you know that social networks sell your personal data to multiple companies (like Marketing and Advertising companies)?
Q6	Have you already booked a medical appointment via the internet?
Q7	Have you ever ordered a medical product via the internet?
Q8	How do you see the quality of health services in Morocco?
Q9	Do you have (or do you use) an electronic health record?
Q10	Do you have (or do you use) a health application on your smartphone?
Q11	Do you have (or do you use) a health application on your PC?
Q12	Do you ever have to go back to the doctor to see your medical results?
Q13	Do you like to monitor your health situation using computer applications?
Q14	Do you think that the information systems help improve the quality of health services in Morocco?
Q15	Do you know Big Data?

(continued)

Table 1. (*continued*)

Questions	Signification
Q16	Do you think that health data is not data like any other and must be the subject of special management?
Q17	Are you with a health information system that facilitates the management, control and analysis of data in Morocco?
Q18	Have you ever benefited training on the use of information systems?
Q19	Do you think that the use of information systems in the health sector will change the doctor's decision on healthcare?
Q20	Do you already need (or do you use) health data for a study?
Q21	How do you qualify information technologies in Morocco?
Q22	In your opinion, what are the obstacles for the use of health information systems in Morocco?
Q23	Do you think that Morocco really needs a government law that will determine the use of health data with information systems?
Q24	How do you see the health sector in Morocco in 10 years?

This study shows that 68.3% of participants said Yes for Q1 and 31.7% said No. So, the vast majority have one or more health insurance, which means a generation of important health data. Health insurers store significant information about patients (pharmaceuticals, medical tests, hospitalizations…), these data that can be very useful for some studies and analysis [10]. For the question Q2 we have 93.5% Yes and 6,5% No, this question proves that the number of medical consultations is very high, which translates into a very large production of health data in Morocco. We asked the question Q3 to see if the participants in our survey used the internet or not, and we found that 97,5% said Yes and 2.5% No, we can deduce that there is no problem with the use of the internet. Regarding Q4 we found that 94,5% said Yes and 5,5% said No, the use of social networks shows that our target population is not offline from the evolution of the Web, and that our population have the notion of sharing personal information without any problem, with a significant degree of protection. In fifth question Q5 we have noticed that we have 74,9% Yes and 25,1% No, in our study, we proposed this question to test if that our population has a knowledge about marketing done with the personal data on social networks [11], but most know what's going on, so they have no problem with the reuse of their data for other interests. We have seen that the majority of our population using the internet, so we want to know if that the participants have the notion of booking medical appointments and even the purchase of medical products via the internet. The question Q6 shows that 10,6% said Yes and 89,4% said No, and for the question Q7 we have 13,6% Yes and 86,4% No. We need several efforts to get the target population accustomed to using the internet for medical reasons.

The use of the EHR is so important in the health sector. It allows us to gain a traceability on the medical situation of the patients, to collect information, and to analyze medical data with very advanced tools such as Big Data analytics that will allow us to improve the health care. Participants answered the question Q9 by 11,6%

Yes and 88,4% No, this result shows that Morocco really needs a solid, reliable and efficient EHR. Now we want to test the use of health applications, the target population was answered by 34,2% Yes and 65,8% No on the question Q10, and 11,6% Yes and 88,4% No on the question Q11. So, we can say that the use of health applications is inferior to the medium. For the question Q12 we have 79,9% Yes and 20,1% No, that means the most of the participants are forced to go back to the doctor to see their medical results. For that the question Q13 was asked to see if the participants are motivated to follow their medical situation using computer applications, 85,9% said Yes and 14,1% said No, so the majority of the population are for. The results show that 89,4% said Yes and 10,6% said No for the question Q14, these responses show that the participants have trusted in health information systems. As well as, we have 61,8% of answers Yes and 38,2% No for the question Q15, so our target population follows the evolution of technology such as big data, and show a full awareness of everything that goes on around the world of computing. The special management of health data takes a great interest to the participants, as the results we have 89,9% Yes and 10,1% No for the question Q16.

About the question Q17 we have 83,9% said Yes and 16,1% said No. It can be said that the ease of management, the control and analysis of health data in Morocco that's what prefers our participant. A powerful system able to extract information from health data in order to improve the situation of this sector in Morocco. Concerning the question Q18 we have 52,3% Yes and 47,7% No, we still need the trainings on the use of information systems in Morocco. 73,4% said Yes and 26,6% said No on question Q19, so the majority of the target population said that the new technologies are important tools for improving health care. The question Q23 gives us 87,9% Yes and 12,1% No. So, the presence of a government law that will determine the use of health data with information systems in Morocco is a mandatory request for the participants of our survey. Figure 1 shows the results of the questions asked with Yes or No answers.

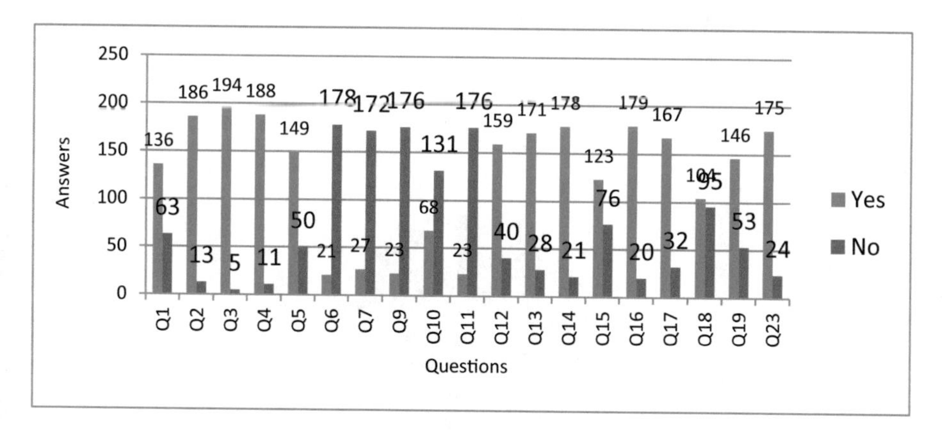

Fig. 1. The survey questions with Yes or No answers.

The answers on the question Q8 show that 52.8% of the target population see that the quality of health services in Morocco is mediocre, 40.7% medium, 6% good, 0.5% very good and 0% excellent. These results can be interpreted that the participants have a very negative view on the health services in Morocco, the thing that requires a direct, strong, and major intervention to change this situation, to improve the quality of services, and that will push this sector to be very enlightened to the near future. The data in the question Q21 show that the target population responded with 1% excellent, 5.5% very good, 40.2% good, 44.7% medium, and 8.5% Mediocre. We can deduce that the participants have a 91.5% confidence in the information technologies in Morocco, the thing that encourages the IT experts and the scientific researchers in Morocco to mount their innovation, their creativity and their support to modify, change and enhance the health situation in Morocco. Figure 2 corresponds to the results of two questions Q8 and Q21.

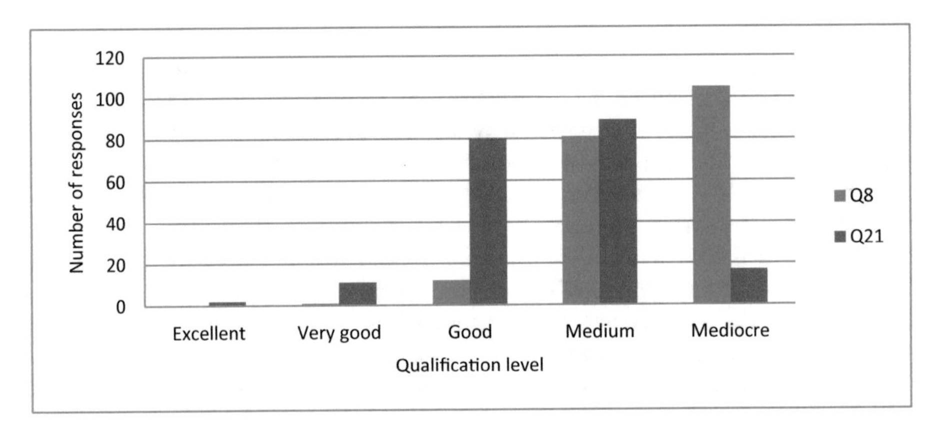

Fig. 2. The answers of the two questions Q8 and Q21.

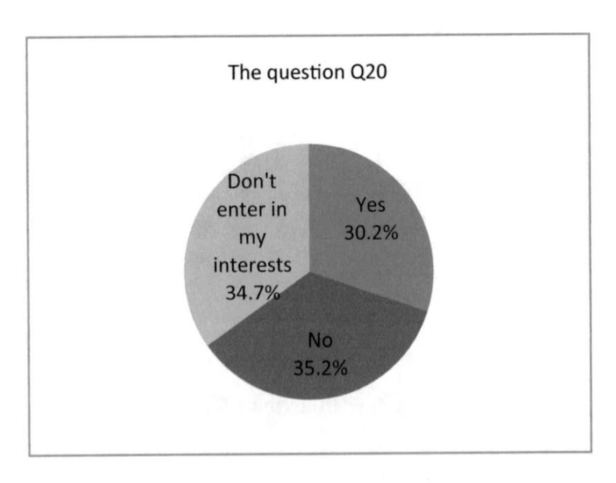

Fig. 3. The answers to the question Q20.

For the question Q20, 30.2% of the participants use health data for studies and research, 35.2% say No, and 34.7% do not enter into their interests. Here we can say that we have a large number of participants who are interested in health data that means they reuse them for studies and research. Important information can be extracted from these data. The results are represented in the Fig. 3.

About the question Q22 we have 36.2% say that the obstacles to the use of the information systems in the health in Morocco are lack of laws and standards, 29.6% lack of financing, 14.1% lack of human resources and 20.1% have no idea. From these results it can be concluded that the majority of stakeholders in the health sector encircle the obstacles to the use of information systems in health in Morocco between: lack of laws and norms and lack of funding. This requires immediate government intervention to create a law that describes how to use health data and to invest significant funding for this sector.

Question Q24 shows that 46.7% of the participants in our survey, see that the health sector in Morocco in change within 10 years, 31.2% say that this sector will stay without any change, and 22.1% say that it will worsen. It is clear that the participants in our survey have a positive vision on the future of the health services' situation in Morocco.

4 Proposed Solutions

We conducted this survey to discover the current situation of health services and more specifically the use of health information systems in Morocco. Moreover, this study is made to detect the main constraints around our subject. In the analytical part of the data collected from the survey, it can be deduced that the health sector in Morocco suffers from several problems. And to overcome its complication we propose multiple solutions to implement in order to improve this sensitive sector in Morocco:

- A powerful, robust and effective EHR will be guaranteed the traceability of the patient's medical situation. The latter must be shared by all the health actors who can attribute to the improvement of the situation of the patients as well as to the evolution of the health sector in Morocco in general.
- The implementation of a health information systems based on techniques, platforms and advanced tools of big data. The latter will ensure the storage, management, control, analysis and security of all information circulating in the health sector in Morocco.
- To overcome the constraints, firstly we must apply a national law that describes the rules, norms, and the way in which the health data must be used, while guaranteeing the anonymity of the personal data. Secondly, to develop the health services, the Moroccan state must provide significant funding, and must seek national and international investors who are interested in this area, and who have a strong will to change the current situation of the health in Morocco. Finally, this sector must be strengthened by experienced, young and active human resources who accept change and the application of new technologies easily. Thus, to make trainings on health information systems for the health professionals.

5 Conclusion

In this study, we analyzed the use of health information systems in Morocco with a survey published on the internet. Our goal is to collect as much information as possible to evaluate the current situation of the health sector, to know the different obstacles and to propose some application and innovative solutions.

During the analysis phase, we noted that the target population has a very negative view of the current state of health services in Morocco. This requires a very advanced intervention to improve and strengthen this area, either by providing the necessary human resources, by significant funding or by the creation of laws and standards. Thus, it was noted that the most of participants haven't used an electronic health record, so, we miss an important source of information because the data collected by the EHR will help us to understand the behavior of the diseases, the state of patients, and the health sector in general. In addition, we can say that the most of the participants in our survey with a health information system that facilitates the management, control and analysis of data in Morocco. This answer gives us a clear idea that the participants have an evolutionary spirit that is why they said that the health sector in Morocco will evaluate in 10 years.

In the last part of this article, we have proposed several solutions to develop the field of health in Morocco, and similarly to guarantee a positive, powerful, and effective change, and moreover we propose to apply the advanced techniques of big data in the health sector in Morocco. The Big Data technology will provide us with an active, solid and evolving environment.

References

1. Health Metrics Network, World Health Organization: Framework and Standards for Country Health Information Systems (2008)
2. Agarwa, R.: The role of information systems in healthcare: current research and road ahead. Inf. Syst. Res. **22**, 419–428 (2011)
3. Koppel, R.: Electronic health records and quality of diabetes care. N. Engl. J. Med. **365**(24), 2338 (2011)
4. Raghupathi, W.: Big data analytics in healthcare: promise and potential. Health Inf. Sci. Syst. **2**(1), 3 (2014)
5. Bouhriz, M.: Big Data Security and Privacy in the Healthcare Recommandations et Proposition de Stratégie dans le Contexte Marocain, Ibn Tofail University, Morocco (2015)
6. Ministry of Health (Morocco), Stratégie Sectorielle de Santé 2012–2016 (2012)
7. Regional Office for the Eastern Mediterranean, WHO-MOROCCO 2017–2021 Cooperation Strategy (2016)
8. opentextbc, Overview of Survey Research. https://opentextbc.ca/researchmethods/chapter/overview-of-survey-research/. Accessed 10 June 2018
9. Google Forms, Etude sur l'utilisation des systèmes informatisés dans le secteur de la santé au Maroc. https://docs.google.com/forms/d/e/1FAIpQLScXLmWXykjhP7subZg67Q-4Jb4vxIdiBu59ECuPszHY6GT_aw/viewform
10. Chen, H.: Business intelligence and analytics: from big data to big impact. MIS Q. **36**, 1165–1188 (2012)
11. Harris, L.: Social networks: the future of marketing for small business. J. Bus. Strategy **30**(5), 24–31 (2009)

Smart System for Monitoring Apnea Episodes in Domestic Environments with Sound Sensor

Javier Rocher[1], Lorena Parra[1], Sandra Sendra[1,2], and Jaime Lloret[1(✉)]

[1] Instituto de Investigación para la Gestión Integrada de zonas Costeras, Universitat Politècnica de València, Valencia, Spain
{jarocmo,loparbo}@doctor.upv.es, ssendra@ugr.es, jlloret@dcom.upv.es

[2] Dep. de teoría de la señal, telemática y comunicaciones, ETS Ingenierías Informática y de Telecomunicación, Universidad de Granada, Granada, Spain

Abstract. The Obstructive Sleep Apnea (OSA) is a disorder that causes frequent pauses in breathing during sleep. This disorder can cause early death, hypertension, etc. Approximately the 4% of the population suffers this disorder. In order to diagnose, it is required a polysomnography (PSG) which s is an expensive test and requires the patient's hospitalization for at least one night This paper presents a system able to detect the OSA during sleep. Our system consists of a sound sensor, a vibrating element and a microcontroller to process the collected data. The sound sensor is placed in the pillow and includes a vibrating element that wakes the user when the OSA event is too long. The sensor and actuator are connected to a microcontroller which includes an IEEE 802.11 interface to be connected to an Access Point (AP). The collected values are processed and sent to a database. The system works analyzing the sound of snoring. Our system can difference 5 different types of snoring: (I) no snoring, (II) movement (III) normal snoring, (IV) snoring before OSA, and (V) OSA. After that, the values of OSA events are checked by the doctor to take, if needed, the appropriate actions. The results show that we can differentiate the different snoring types thanks to the sound level and the distribution curve. Finally, the system has been verified with a patient with OSA diagnosis and our results coincide with the type of diagnosis and type of snoring that the patient received in his medical report.

Keywords: Obstructive Sleep Apnea · Wireless Sensor Network (WSN) · Snore · E-health

1 Introduction

The World Health Organization (WHO) [1] defines Obstructive Sleep Apnea (OSA) as a clinical disorder that consists of frequent pauses in breathing while a person sleeps which is, in most cases, accompanied by loud snoring. This disorder is caused by a repetitive pharyngeal collapse during sleep [2]. OSA is related with hypertension, coronary artery, diabetes mellitus, and with patients under 70 years old [3, 4]. The OSA increases the risk of early death [4]. This disorder affects up to 4% of the population.

M. Ezziyyani (Ed.): AI2SD 2018, AISC 914, pp. 205–215, 2019.
https://doi.org/10.1007/978-3-030-11884-6_20

People with OSA stop breathing repeatedly during the sleep periods with many pauses of 10 s to 30 s along the night [5].

There are some risk factors that increase the possibility of suffering OSA. These are: (I) Increasing age, (II) Male, (III) Obesity, (IV) Alcohol consumption, (V) Menopause, (VI) Craniofacial abnormalities, (VII) Genetics, and (VIII) Nasal obstructions [6]. This disease could be treated with (I) Positive airway pressure and (II) Surgical intervention, although it is possible to enhance the OSA symptoms for cases that are not extremely serious following some recommendations such as (I) sleep posture and sleep hygiene (II) weight loss, (III) not drinking alcohol, or (IV) discouraging the use of sedatives [3, 6], among others. The OSA diagnosis is realized by a polysomnography (PSG). This test consists of simultaneously monitoring different patients' parameters while sleeping. The standard PSG records and evaluates the sleep stages and awakening. Some of the measured parameters are the limb movements, snoring, breathing, oximetry, cardiac rhythm disturbances, etc. [7]. The PSG needs a physician specialist in these disorders and a laboratory or special hospital room to perform it. However, currently, we can find some systems to perform this test at home [7]. This implies a high cost and long waiting lists to perform this kind of medical tests. And sometimes, the patient cannot fall asleep during the test due to the generated stress due to the test itself, the environment, etc.

The strong snoring sound can be used for determining obstruction episodes and predicting the response of surgery in patients [8, 9] demoted that intensity of snoring increase according to the severity of OSA. In [10], authors proposed measuring the snore at home for determining the probability that the person suffers OSA. Although, the use of acoustic analysis of snoring is relatively accurate for determining the OSA, it is not a strong method for diagnosing [11]. Therefore, we can use the snore as a preliminary test for the OSA diagnosis and check its evolution at home. To do it, we can use sensor for continuously monitoring the patient [12]. The wireless sensor network (WSN) in health [13] have been used for monitoring the environment, the patient constants, etc. [14]. For example, Garcia et al. [15] used sensors for monitoring temperature, humidity, luminosity, and noise in domestic environments. These parameters were utilized to monitor the wellness state of people using the Likert's scale. Yan et al. [16] proposed a WSN for constant monitoring, using both fixed and mobile sensors. The system was able to detect two types of situations, the normal situation and the abnormal situation. In an abnormal situation, the system generated an alarm while the normal situations comprised daily tasks as taking medicine, having lunch, turning off the microwave oven etc.

In this paper, we propose a smart system based on an acoustic sensor for detecting the OSA events by monitoring the snore. The system accounts the OSA events during sleep hours and according to the Apnea–Hypopnoea Index (AHI), it establishes the patient severity. Depending on the severity of the OSA, the system is able to takes some decision, i.e., f the system detects an OSA event that takes more than 60 s, the system will activate a vibrating element to wake the patient. The system could be used in two scenarios. On the one hand, due to the low-cost of the system and its simplicity, it could be used for estimating the severity of OSA. A more exhaustive monitoring should be carried out in a hospital. On the other, hand, our proposal could be used for monitoring the evolution of OSA in patients at home, i.e., patients who have been diagnosed and do not have the treatment yet but its evolution should be controlled. In addition, it can be used to determine the improvement after changes in the patients' habits.

The rest of the paper is structured as follows; Sect. 2 presents some related work where similar approaches are presented. Section 3 presents the architecture and algorithm of our system. The results of our system are presented in Sect. 4. Finally, Sect. 5 details the conclusion and future work.

2 Related Work

This section presents different works on sleep monitoring and OSA events detection.

Veiga et al. [17] proposed an Internet of Things (IoT)-based sleep quality-monitoring pillow. The system measured temperature, humidity, luminosity, sound, and vibration. These parameters were used to determine the actions of the Ambient Assisted Living (AAL) [18] for improving the sleeping quality. These actions were focused on adjusting temperature, closing/opening curtains and activating the sound of a fly to generate a movement in the person to try and eliminate the snoring. The system used a sound sensor. However, the authors did not measure the intensity and form of the sound wave to determine the OSA events.

Santos-Silva et al. [19] validated a portable system (Stardust II) based on 4 sensors (airflow, respiratory movements, oxyhemoglobin saturation and heart rate) for diagnosing the OSA. They used 80 patients, 70 with a suspicion of having OSA and 10 subjects without suspicion of OSA. They monitored these patients with the Stardust II and carried out. The results confirmed that the portable system was reliable for OSA evaluation. In addition, the patients did not present problems using the system at home. The system takes into account some more parameters than our system which can difficult the measuring process although it does not include a system for communicating the results to the physician.

Nakano et al. [20] studied the use of a smartphone for measuring the snore and detecting the OSA in a laboratory. They checked a high relation with snore and OSA events. Nevertheless, the results showed this technique cannot be used in type 4 OSA because the reliability of measurements can be affected by environment. Azadeh et al. [21] proposed a system based on sensing the snore and blood's oxygen saturation level (SaO2). Authors classified the noise signal in breath, snore, and noise and analyzed the SaO2 for detecting rises and drops. They combined these two values for determining apnea with and accuracy higher than 91%. These papers presented the way of measuring OSA by the snore monitoring. However, their systems are not able to generate alarms to warn the users and inform the health personnel.

Bsoul et al. [5] Proposed a low cost and real-time sleep apnea monitoring system. This system worked by the measurement of the electrocardiogram (ECG) to take values and classify the OSA by a support vector classifier. This system differs from our system in the use of ECG. Castro et al. [22] presented an evaluation of the use of contactless capacitive-coupled electrocardiography (ccECG) for monitoring the OSA events. Authors compared the ccECG with a reference ECG. The experiments were carried out with 15 patients in a sleep environment in different positions. The results demonstrated that ccECG offers similar results of ECG for detection OSA events. In this case, ECG is in non-contact with the subject. This fact will reduce the sleeping discomfort. However, we think that if the subject suffers nightmares they can alter the results. Finally, these systems do not allow to remotely monitoring the patients.

As we showed in this section, there exist many solutions for monitoring the OSA events. Some works are focused only in the OSA events' monitoring. However, they are not able to remotely monitor the patients and transmit the data to the physicians. In addition, our system can wake the patient in the case of too long OSA event. In this paper, we present a system based on sound sensors which is controlled by an algorithm to count the OSA events and wake the patient, if needed.

3 System Description

This section describes the proposed system, including its architecture and control algorithm.

3.1 Architecture

The proposed system is based on the system described in [17]. In our case, the sound sensor is placed in the pillow in order to gather the sound data from snores. A vibrating element is included in the pillow. This vibrating element will acts as an alarm system to wake the patient if it is need. The sensor and actuator are connected to the node which is wirelessly connected to an access point (AP). The data gathered is locally processed by the node and the results are sent thought the WiFi connection.

The system can be used in two different modes. The first one can be used as a pre-diagnosis test. In this case the system is use during one night. The data is recorded in a SD card and the results of the local analyses are used to activate the alarm. The number of generated alarms is recorded. In this case, the system is not connected to the AP. After the sleep period the pillow is returned to the hospital where the data is downloaded from the node. The second operation mode is used for continuous domestic monitoring. The patient uses the pillow during longer time periods. In this case the node, gathers data during the sleep period, locally analyses the data and activates the vibrating element if it is needed. After the sleep period, the pillow activates the WiFi connection with the AP and sends the results, but not the data. In this way, we can minimize the energy consumed during the data transmission and reduce the bandwidth consumption in the local network. The data gathered, which is saved in the SD, is stored during one week before to be erased. During this period, the medical center can recover the data from the pillow if it is needed for further analyses by artificial intelligence systems of by specialists. The architecture for the second mode can be seen in Fig. 1.

3.2 Control Algorithm

According to preliminary measurements, we are able to detect the differences between regular snores and snores occurred just before an apnea episode. The first difference is

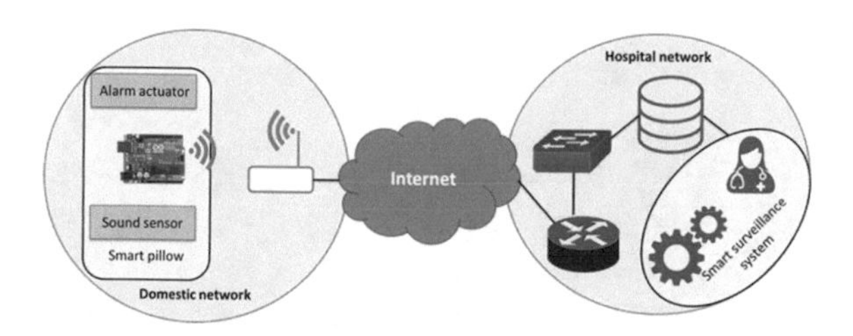

Fig. 1. Proposed architecture

the reached sound pressure level which is higher in the snores occurred before the apnea. However, using the data from the instantaneous sound pressure level is not enough to determine if the person is moving, having regular snores or having snores that are announcing an apnea episode.

So that, we need to analyze the changes in the sound pressure levels with the time. After studying some gathered data, the sound pressure level in dB, during regular snores, follows a normal distribution. They present a first stage when the sound pressure level increases. Then, it reaches its maximum and there is a second period when the sound pressure level decreases. For a snore before the OSA event, the pattern changes. The sound pressure level does not follow a Gaussian distribution, i.e., it presents two maximum peaks. This change in the pattern can be used to differentiate the snoring type. During the night, the person can move and this movement will generate a random pattern of sound, with several peaks and high sound pressure level in few seconds. However, the patient can also be quiet without snoring. Then, the sound pressure level will be low and with a random distribution. Nevertheless this pattern, low sound pressure level and random distributions can indicate a OSA. During the OSA, the patient is not breathing. So no sound is generated. In order to differentiate between both situations, it is need to consider the pattern previous to the silence. If previous to the silence period, the patter indicates a snoring before OSA, it is highly probable that the silence indicates an OSA.

The algorithm to control our proposed system is presented in Fig. 2. First, the system is activated when the person goes to the bed. In this moment, the sensor starts to gather data from sound pressure level and stores it in the flash memory of the node. After 30 s, the microprocessor analyses those 30 s of data and determines if the data corresponds to (I) not snoring, (II) movement, (III) regular snoring, (IV) snoring before OSA or (V) OSA. After analyzing the collected data, the event type determined from the data gathered is stored in the SD card and the data type is stored in flash. If the data type is OSA and the data type of the previous 30 s was OSA the vibrating element is triggered to wake up the patient. For the proposed algorithm, we consider that an OSA of 30 s is not enough to wake up the patient. Nevertheless more than 60 s without breathing can be dangerous for the health and it is need to wake up the person to ensure its breathing. When the person finishes its sleeping period, he/she will press the turn off button. In this moment, the system will send the data types saved in the flash card to the medical centre. Finally, the system will delete the gathered data from the SD card from 7 days ago and will stop the system.

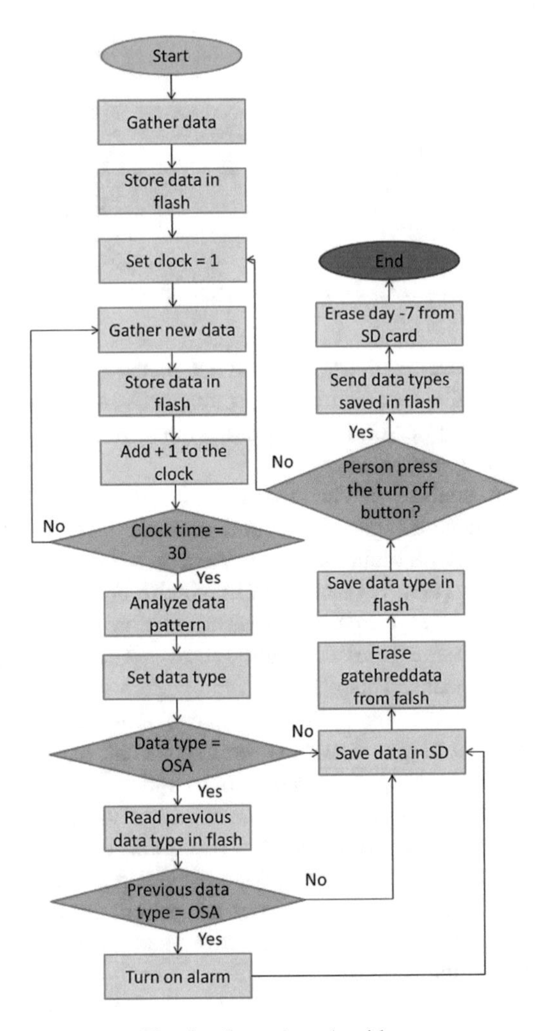

Fig. 2. Operation algorithm.

4 Results

In this section, we present the gathered results and its analyses.

The snores have been measured with a sound sensor Arduino KY-038 and an Arduino Uno module. The sensor was placed at 20 cm from the patient. We differentiated 4 types of sounds: (I) Not snoring, (II) Movement, (III) Normal snoring, (IV) Snoring before OSA and (V) OSA events. Figures 3, 4 and 5, show some of the different sounds related to different snoring types.

In Fig. 3(a) and (b), we can see the sound pressure level reached when the patient is not snoring and it is not moving. In this case, the sound pressure level is low with levels of 35 dB. These levels are background noise and indicate that the patient does not suffer OSA. So, there is no obstruction in the respiratory tract.

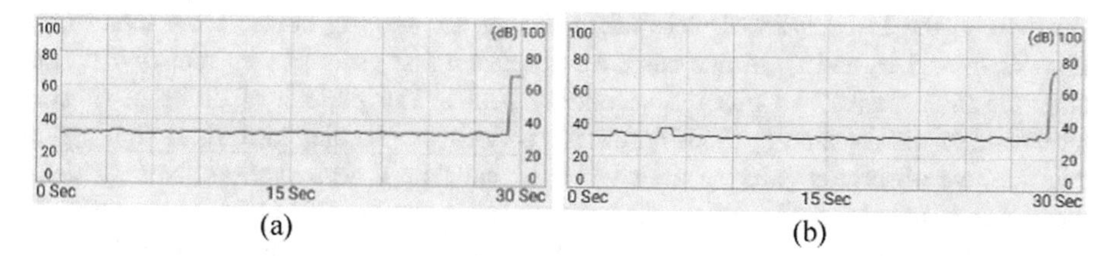

Fig. 3. Not snoring

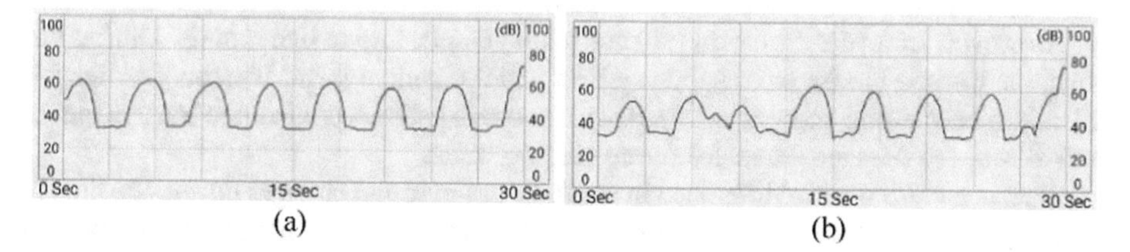

Fig. 4. Normal snoring

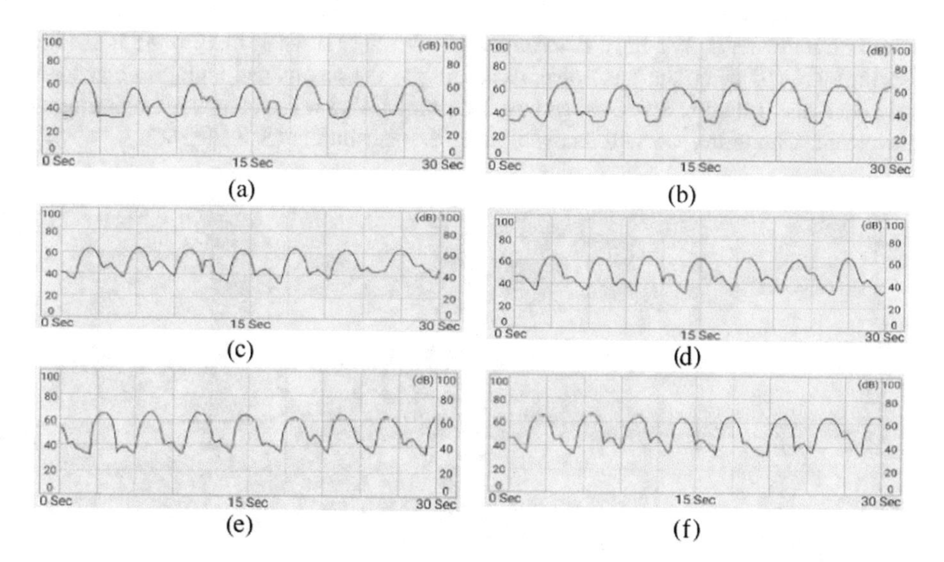

Fig. 5. Snoring before OSA.

Figure 4(a) and (b) represents normal snoring sound levels. In this case, we observe a fast increase and decrease (similar to a Gaussian curve) of dB values. The snoring have approximately the same period between the snore and after the snore and the dB values are the same as background sound The values of dB in the peaks have a value around of 60 dB. In this case, there exists an obstruction in the respiratory tract but the breath is not interrupted.

Finally, the last measures were taken during the snoring before OSA event (See Fig. 5a, b, c, d, e, and f). In this case, we observe a fast grow like normal snoring but after the main peaks, we observe secondary peaks. The periods of different snoring have similar values among them and these periods are similar to normal snoring. In addition, we observe a value of dB slightly higher than a normal snore. Nevertheless, these values are not sufficiently differentiated to determine this phase alone with dB level. In this case, the respiratory tract is partially obstructed but the breath is not interrupted. However, the OSA event is close to happen.

During an OSA event, there is a strong snore followed by a silence period that can last between 10 s and 20 s in a normal case.

However, in severe cases, this silence period can last up to one minute. During this time, the trachea blocks the respiratory tract and the patient is not breathing. After this silence, a new strong snore is detected. This snore is generated when the trachea moves and allows the passage of air for the respiratory tract.

Because there is a big difference in the form of the sound changes during the time in the different type of snoring, the system can be used for determining some the type of snore. In Fig. 6, we can observe the snores during two minutes in the middle of the night. In Fig. 6a, we observe the values of sound detected by the sensor. We have divided this period into 4 parts of 30 s each one. In Fig. 6b, we have analysed the sound pressure level. We have determined two levels; (I) when there is no noise (no snoring) and (II) when there is noise. According to the results and taking into account only the sound pressure level, we cannot determine if that noise comes from snoring or movement. Therefore, we will analyse the noise distribution (See Fig. 6c).

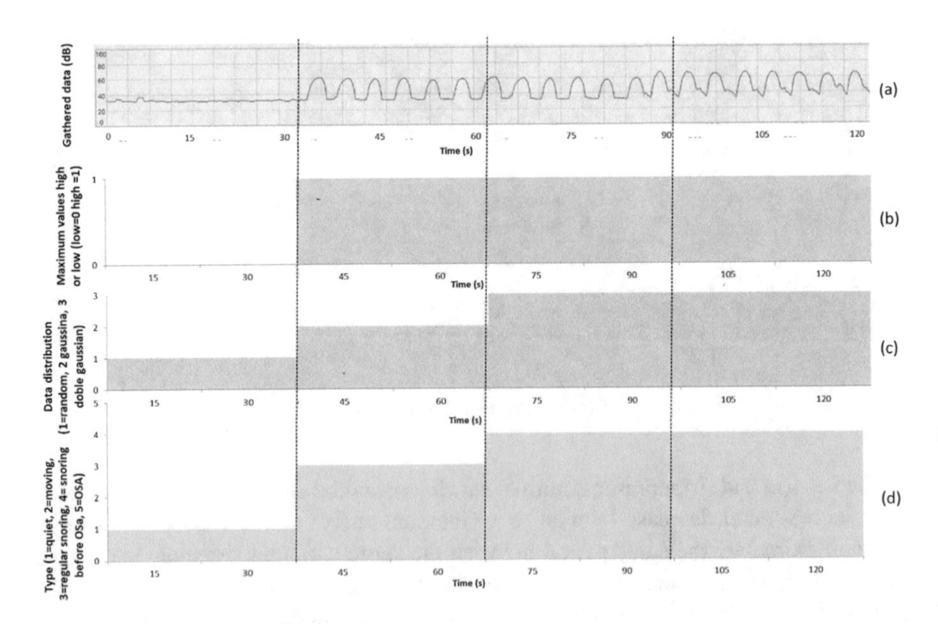

Fig. 6. Simulation of sensor in a night

We tagged the results on three categories:

- Random distribution where the sound does not follow a concrete distribution, as if it is seen in the Fig. 3. In this case the random distribution can be caused by two situations: not snoring or moving.
- Gaussian, the sound follows a distribution similar to Gaussian curve (See Fig. 4). In this case, a regular snoring is being produced.
- Double Gaussian (See Fig. 5). In this case, a snoring occurs and then another smaller. These snores are indicating a forthcoming OSA event. In the third part, 60 to 90 s, the sound is tagged as a double Gaussian distribution because of the last snore is detected with this distribution. Finally, the tag of snoring will occur if there is noise or not and the distribution of noise follow a double Gaussian curve, see Fig. 6d.

As a summary, if we detect a sound, we will analyse it and depending on distribution, we will be able to classify the snoring type.

5 Conclusion and Future Work

The OSA is a disorder that causes stops in the breathing while sleeping. This disorder causes serious health problems such as hypertension, problems in coronary artery or early death, among others. In this paper, we have showed a system for monitoring the OSA events in domestic environments. The system is based on a sound sensor for detecting the sound pressure levels; a vibrating element that acts as an alarm when an OSA event lasts more than 60 s and a microcontroller for registering the values of sound and sending the data to the medical staff. The system firstly analyses the presence of noise. If no noise is detected, it means that the patient is not snoring. In case of detecting noise, the system analyzes the distribution followed by the registered noise. If it does not follow any patron, the noise does not come from the snoring. However, if there is a Gaussian type pattern, it means that there is a normal snore. Finally, if a double Gaussian pattern is detected, the system will determine it is a snoring before OSA events.

As future work, we want to test the sensor in more patients in order to confirm the accuracy of our system to monitor OSA events in domestic environments and evaluating other systems how raspberry pi [23] and add more sensors to monitor sleep quality and quality of life as shown in [24].

Acknowledgment. This work has been partially supported by the "Conselleria d'Educació, Investigació, Cultura i Esport" through the "Subvenciones para la contratación de personal investigator de carácter predoctoral (Convocatoria 2017)" Grant number ACIF/2017/069, by the "Ministerio de Educación, Cultura y Deporte", through the "Ayudas para contratacion predoctoral de Formación del Profesorado Universitario FPU (Convocatoria 2014)". Grant number FPU14/02953.

References

1. World Health Organization: Obstructive sleep apnea syndrome. http://www.who.int/respiratory/other/Obstructive_sleep_apnoea_syndrome/en/. Accessed 20 Apr 2018
2. Malhotra, A., White, D.P.: Obstructive sleep apnea. Lancet **360**(9328), 237–245 (2002)
3. Grunstein, R.R., Hedner, J., Grote, L.: Treatment options for sleep apnea. Drugs **61**(2), 237–251 (2001)
4. Franklin, K.A., Lindberg, E.: Obstructive sleep apnea is a common disorder in the population-a review on the epidemiology of sleep apnea. J. Thorac. Dis. **7**(8), 1311–1322 (2015)
5. Bsoul, M., Minn, H., Tamil, L.: Apnea MedAssist: real-time sleep apnea monitor using single-lead ECG. IEEE Trans. Inf. Technol. Biomed. **15**(3), 416–427 (2011)
6. Gharibeh, T., Mehra, R.: Obstructive sleep apnea syndrome: natural history, diagnosis, and emerging treatment options. Nat. Sci. Sleep **2**, 233–255 (2010)
7. American Association of Sleep Technologists: Technical Guideline - Standard Polysomnography, pp. 1–19, July 2012
8. Lee, L.A., et al.: Snoring sounds predict obstruction sites and surgical response in patients with obstructive sleep apnea hypopnea syndrome. Sci. Rep. **6**, 1–11 (2016)
9. Kim, J.W., Lee, C.H., Rhee, C.S., Mo, J.H.: Relationship between snoring intensity and severity of obstructive sleep apnea. Clin. Exp. Otorhinolaryngol. **8**(4), 376–380 (2015)
10. Alakuijala, A., Salmi, T.: Predicting obstructive sleep apnea with periodic snoring sound recorded at home. J. Clin. Sleep Med. **12**(7), 953–958 (2016)
11. Jin, H., et al.: Acoustic analysis of snoring in the diagnosis of obstructive sleep apnea syndrome: a call for more rigorous studies. J. Clin. Sleep Med. **11**(7), 765–771 (2015)
12. Oller Arcas, T., Lopez Rubio, J., Alcober Segura, J., Tarín, G., Rosas, L., Garcia, J.: Adherence to a treatment of cranial deformities with a sensorised brace device. Netw. Protoc. Algorithms **8**(1), 73–89 (2016)
13. Liu, J., Han, W., Xiao, Y.: Enhancements of temporal accountability in medical sensor networks. Ad Hoc Sens. Wirel. Netw. **37**(1–4), 71–93 (2017)
14. Bri, D., Garcia, M., Lloret, J., Dini, P.: Real deployments of wireless sensor networks. In: 3rd International Conference on Sensor Technologies and Applications, SENSORCOMM 2009, IARA, Athens/Glyfada, Greece, pp. 415–423 (2009)
15. García, L., Parra, L., Romero, O., Lloret, J.: System for monitoring the wellness state of people in domestic environments employing emoticon-based HCI. J. Supercomput., 1–25 (2017)
16. Yan, H., Huo, H., Xu, Y., Gidlund, M.: Wireless sensor network based E-health system: implementation and experimental results. IEEE Trans. Consum. Electron. **56**(4), 2288–2295 (2010)
17. Veiga, A., García, L., Parra, L., Lloret, J., Augele, V.: An IoT-based smart pillow for sleep quality monitoring in AAL environments. In: 3rd IEEE Fog & Mobile Edge Computing (FMEC 2018), Barcelona, Spain (2018)
18. Rghioui, A., Sendra, S., Lloret, J., Oumnad, A.: Internet of Things for measuring human activities in ambient assisted living and e-health. Netw. Protoc. Algorithms **8**(3), 15–28 (2016)
19. Santos-Silva, R., et al.: Validation of a portable monitoring system for the diagnosis of obstructive sleep apnea syndrome. Sleep **32**(5), 629–636 (2009)
20. Nakano, H., et al.: Monitoring sound to quantify snoring and sleep apnea severity using a smartphone: proof of concept. J. Clin. Sleep Med. **10**(1), 73–78 (2014)

21. Yadollahi, A., Giannouli, E., Moussavi, Z.: Sleep apnea monitoring and diagnosis based on pulse oximetery and tracheal sound signals. Med. Biol. Eng. Comput. **48**(11), 1087–1097 (2010)
22. Castro, I.D., Varon, C., Torfs, T., van Huffel, S., Puers, R., van Hoof, C.: Evaluation of a multichannel non-contact ECG system and signal quality algorithms for sleep apnea detection and monitoring. Sensors **18**(2), 1–20 (2018)
23. Vilches, R., Oller, T., Alcober, J.: Pervasive sensors network for wellness based-on Raspberry Pi. Netw. Protoc. Algorithms **6**(3), 1–17 (2014)
24. Ammari, H.M., Gomes, N., Jacques, M., Maxim, B., Yoon, D.: A survey of sensor network applications and architectural components. Adhoc Sens. Wirel. Netw. **25**(1–2), 1–44 (2015)

Adverse Drug Reaction Mentions Extraction from Drug Labels: An Experimental Study

Ed-drissiya El-allaly(✉), Mourad Sarrouti, Noureddine En-Nahnahi, and Said Ouatik El Alaoui

Laboratory of Informatics and Modeling, FSDM, Sidi Mohammed Ben Abdellah University, Fez, Morocco
{eddrissiya.elallaly,mourad.sarrouti,noureddine.en-nahnahi, said.ouatikelalaoui}@usmba.ac.ma

Abstract. Adverse Drug Reactions (ADRs), unintended and sometimes dangerous effects that a drug may have, are a serious health problem and a leading cause of death. Therefore, it is of vital importance to identify ADRs properly and in a timely manner from drug labels. In this paper, we explore both machine learning and deep learning approaches in extracting adverse reaction mentions and modifier terms such as negation, severity, and drug class from drug labels. We investigated Conditional Random Fields (CRF) as a machine learning method, and both Recurrent Neural Network (RNN) and Bidirectional Recurrent Neural Network (Bi-RNN) as deep learning methods. These methods are widely used in biomedical named entity recognition. Experimental evaluations performed on the publicly available datasets SPL-ADR-200db, provided by the TAC 2017 ADRs challenge, show that Bi-RNN achieves good performances compared with RNN and CRF. Bi-RNN outperforms RNN and CRF by an average of 4% and 4.7% in terms of F1-score, respectively.

Keywords: Adverse Drug Reaction · Recurrent Neural Network · Bidirectional Recurrent Neural Network · Conditional Random Fields · Biomedical Named Entity Recognition · Natural Language Processing

1 Introduction

Adverse Drug Reactions (ADRs) represent a serious problem worldwide that refer to drug-associated adverse effects which can complicate a patient's medical condition or contribute to increased morbidity [1]. Therefore, automatic extracting adverse drug reaction is of utmost importance to minimize the potential health risks in a timely manner. The traditional mechanisms for ADRs detection have included clinical trials and spontaneous reporting systems such as Food and Drug Administration (FDA) [2]. However, these methods suffer from important limitations. For instance, clinical trials are not able to detect rare ADRs since they have constraints on scale and time [3]. Spontaneous reporting systems which are

M. Ezziyyani (Ed.): AI2SD 2018, AISC 914, pp. 216–231, 2019.
https://doi.org/10.1007/978-3-030-11884-6_21

composed of suspected ADR reports from patients and healthcare providers suffer from time-consuming to ensure safe use of drugs and receive a low number of reports [4].

Among the source analyzed in ADRs is the content of drug labels in a standard format called Structured Product Label (SPL) [2]. However, the SPL format provides structure only for the sections of the label (e.g., Indications and Usage, Warnings and Precautions, Adverse Reactions) [5]. The content of the individual sections still in an unstructured form (i.e., in natural language), which makes its automated processing increasingly difficult. Thus, an efficient access to ADR related information is challenging. In this context, the Text Analysis Conference (TAC) organized a shared task called "Adverse Drug Reaction Extraction from Drug Labels" [6], which aimed to test various Natural Language Processing (NLP) approaches on extracting ADR information from drug labels. The shared task consists of four sub-tasks which the purpose of the first one is to extract AdverseReactions and related mentions from drug labels.

The task of recognizing ADRs mentions in a textual data is similar to the task of Biomedical Named Entity Recognition (BNER). Due to the importance of the BNER in many biomedical texts mining applications such as biomedical text categorization [7], information retrieval [8], and question answering [9–15], recently, this task has witnessed a growing interest among NLP researchers.

In this work, we focus on the identification of ADR mentions from drug labels. Indeed, recognizing ADR mentions from drug labels remains one of the most important tasks of ADR extraction systems which allows for further extraction of relationships and other information between them by identifying the key mentions of interest. The ADR mentions include [6]:

- AdverseReaction: reported ADRs that can be associated with use of the drug or any of its components. This may include signs and symptoms, worsening medical conditions, etc.
- Severity: measurement of the severity of a specific AdverseReaction. This can be qualitative (e.g., "major") or quantitative (e.g., "grade 1").
- DrugClass: the class of drug that the specific drug for the label belongs to.
- Negation: trigger word for event negation.
- Animal: animal species utilized during drug testing in which an AdverseReaction was observed.
- Factor: any additional aspect of an AdverseReaction that is not covered by one of the other mentions listed above.

For instance, given a sentence "*Adverse reactions were all mild to moderate in severity and were predominantly isolated occurrences (<= 2 patients) of one of the following reactions: dizziness, rash, pruritus, flushing or injection site hemorrhage*", the following mentions can be identified: "*mild*" and "*moderate*" as Severity, "*dizziness*", "*rash*", "*pruritus*", "*flushing*" and "*injection site hemorrhage*" as AdverseReaction.

In this paper, we present an evaluation of a machine learning based method and deep learning-based methods for extracting adverse reaction mentions and modifier terms such as Severity, DrugClass, Negation, Animal and Factor from drug labels. We experimented with Conditional Random Fields (CRF) as a machine learning method, and both Recurrent Neural Network (RNN) and Bidirectional Recurrent Neural Network (Bi-RNN) as deep learning methods. These methods are widely used in biomedical named entity recognition. Experimental evaluations performed on the publicly available datasets SPL-ADR-200db [16], provided by the TAC 2017 ADRs challenge, show that Bi-RNN outperforms RNN and CRF by an average of 4% and 4.7% in terms of F1-score, respectively.

The remainder of this paper is organized as follows. In Sect. 2, we provide an overview of BNER approaches. Section 3 describe the CRF based machine learning method. Section 4 presents RNN based deep learning method. Section 5 reports the experimental results where evaluation metrics, datasets and experimental settings are provided. Finally, Sect. 6 concludes this paper with future work.

2 Related Work

In biomedical domain, named entity recognition has attracted much attention for identification of entities such as genes, proteins and disease. Several text mining methods and tools have been developed to solve the BNER problem which can generally be categorized as dictionary-based, rule-based, machine learning based and deep learning based methods [17].

Dictionary-based method matches the entities with a dictionary that contains all the known entities to detect whether the candidate belongs to a defined mention or not. In other word, if the word or sequence of words from the text matches with the term from the dictionary, it is identified as mention occurrence. Dictionary-based approach is considered as the fundamental approach in BNER systems [18,19]. The major issue with this approach is that it is not possible to have a limited list of entities in dictionaries since new entities are introduced by researchers and scientists around the world making most of them out-of-date and has a poor recall due to spelling mistake, character-level and word-level variations [20].

Rule-based method identifies entities by a group of written orthographic and morphological rules, which are manually done by the domain scientists with linguistic knowledge. Rule-based approaches are said to achieve better performance when compared to dictionary-based approaches for BNER [21,22]. However, it is hard and time-consuming as rules are mainly handcrafted. Moreover, this method cannot identify new named entities since new entity names are frequently coined in the biomedical domain.

Machine learning based method uses a statistical classifier to extract the features (orthographic feature, lexical feature, vowel feature, etc.) that are able to recognize the appropriate mentions. It considers biomedical NER as a sequence labeling problem that find the best mention sequence for a given input sentence. Traditional machine learning approaches include Hidden Markov Models (HMMs) [23,24], Conditional Random Fields (CRFs) [25,26], Support Vector Machine (SVM) [27,28], etc. Settles et al. [25] have used a framework for simultaneously recognizing occurrences of gene and protein mentions in biomedical abstracts by using CRF with a variety of feature sets such as orthographic and semantic features. Zhao et al. [23] have introduced a HMM approach for BNER, with a word similarity-based smoothing to get word formation, prefix, suffix and abbreviation information automatically from biomedical texts. The best results were obtained by systems using CRFs because they are robust for sequence labeling tasks such as BNER [29]. Although the machine learning based approaches have made BNER systems practical by outperforming the rule or dictionary based methods, their performance depends heavily on the quality and quantity of the selected features and the training set which require considerable manual effort and make them much complicated.

Deep learning based method has shown great success for many text mining and NLP tasks to address the aforementioned limitations. Recurrent Neural Network (RNN) [30] has shown promising results in various sequence prediction problems such as general and biomedical domain of NER with little feature engineering [31,32] and relation classification [33,34]. RNN is a class of artificial neural networks which utilizes sequential information and maintains history through its hidden layers. RNNs consider BNER as a sequence labeling problem where the goal is to find the best label sequence (most of the time as BIO (Begin, Inside, Outside) format) for a given input sentence. In such models, words only need to be assigned to low-dimensional dense embedding vectors, and during training the RNN is able to learn improved representations for them. For training, RNN use back-propagation algorithms such as Back-propagation Through Time (BPTT) [35]. Song et al. [36] have proposed a simple and efficient system for genes and proteins recognition based on RNN where complex hand-designed features are replaced with word embeddings. Stanovsky et al. [37] have proposed an ADR recognizing mentions system from social media by using RNN transducer integrated with knowledge graph embeddings of DBpedia, a large-scale cross-domain multilingual knowledge base extracted from Wikipedia. Sahu et al. [38] have proposed various end-to-end RNN models for the tasks of disease name recognition and their classification into four pre-defined categories by using word and character embeddings.

3 Conditional Random Fields

CRF [39] is a probabilistic model to segment and label sequence data which offers several advantages over HMM, a consequence of their conditional nature that results in relaxation of the independence assumptions [39,40]. CRF follow two-stage process for BNER task as shown in Fig. 1: feature engineering and classification. The first stage represents the sentence by numeric vectors using the appropriate feature set while the second classifies each entity into a corresponding mention. The two stages are described sequentially in the following subsections (cf. Sects. 3.1 and 3.2).

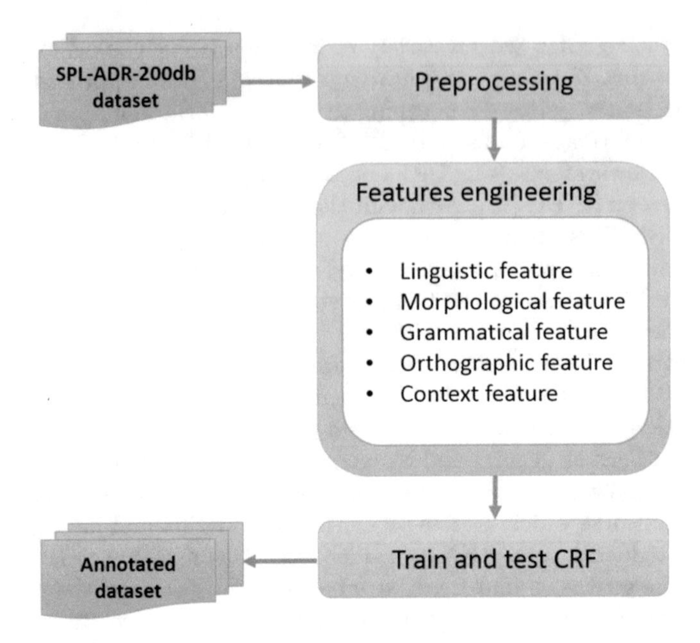

Fig. 1. CRF based machine learning method architecture

3.1 Feature Engineering

Feature engineering is the first stage of machine learning based method, since the predictions will be performed based on the information that they encode. Thus, the definition of a rich and carefully selected set of features is required in order to properly represent the target mentions [40].

- Linguistic features: the most basic internal feature is the word itself.
- Morphological features: reflect common structures of characters among several mention names such as suffixes and prefixes.
- Grammatical features: which associate each word with a particular grammatical category based on its context. The Part-of-Speech (POS) tagging is used for this purpose.
- Orthographic features: capture knowledge about word formation such as whether the word is in uppercase or lowercase or contains digits and special character (e.g. hyphen).
- Context features: consist of adding features of preceding and succeeding tokens as features of each token.

As the input to the CRF model, each feature should assume the value “1” if it is present on the current entity or “0” otherwise.

3.2 Classification

The classification stage of CRF based machine learning method aims to predict the corresponding mention of each entity name. Given a sentence $s = \{w_1, ..., w_n\}$ consisting of n entities. Let $y = \{m_1, ..., m_n\}$ be the sequence of mentions that correspond to the labels assigned to entities in the input sentence s (e.g. AdverseReaction, Severity, etc.). Linear-chain CRFs define the score of a sequence of mentions y given an input sentence s by using Eq. 1:

$$score(y|s) = \sum_{i=1}^{n} \sum_{j=1}^{m} \lambda_j f_j(y_{i-1}, y_i, s, i) \tag{1}$$

where $f_j(y_{i-1}, y_i, s, i)$ is one of the m functions that describes a feature, which takes as input a sentence s, the position i of the entity in the sentence, the mention y_i of the current entity and the mention y_{i-1} of the previous entity. λ_j is a learned weight for each such feature function which should be positive for features that are correlated with the target mention, negative for features that are anti-correlated with the mention, and near zero for relatively uninformative features.

Then, the probability for the sequence y then is defined by a softmax function over all possible mentions by using Eq. 2:

$$P(y|s) = \frac{exp(score(y|s))}{\sum_{\hat{y} \in Y} exp^{score(y|s)}} \tag{2}$$

where Y denotes all the possible mentions. To encourage the model to produce a valid sequence of mentions, the conditional log likelihood of labeled sequences is maximized in training process using Eq. 3.

$$LL = \sum_{i=1}^{n} log\left(P(y_i|s_i)\right) - \sum_{j=1}^{m} \frac{\lambda_j^2}{2\sigma^2} \tag{3}$$

Finally, the mention with highest probability for each entity is calculated by Eq. 4:

$$\hat{y} = argmax(P(y|s)) \tag{4}$$

4 Rccurrent Neural Network

Recurrent neural networks (RNNs) are a powerful model for modeling sequential data which have a recurrent connection and allow a form of memory. This makes them capture information about what has been calculated so far. RNN is considered to be more suitable for NLP tasks as textual data is inherently sequential. In fact, when reading a sentence, the previous words will help to understand the current word. The whole system includes three main layers: the embedding layer as input which to generate representation of each entity in a sentence, recurrent layer which returns another representation sequence that captures the context information of each entity in this sentence, and softmax classifier layer as output to make tagging decisions. The three layers are described sequentially in the following subsections (cf. Sects. 4.1, 4.2 and 4.3).

4.1 Embedding Layer

The embedding layer is the first component of RNN based method. Given a sentence $s = (w_1, ..., w_n)$, the embedding layer produces an embedding vector denoted by $(e_1, ..., e_n)$ for each word by projecting discrete word to low-dimensional dense word vectors. Most of AdverseReaction related mentions are multi-word. In order to represent them, many previous studies have used different segment representations such as BIO (Begin, Inside, Outside). However, the word's position may differ from one entity to another. For instance, a word belonging to the beginning of one entity may appear in the middle of another entity. In this work, we use the following technique: each multi-word entity is converted to one token by adding whitespace punctuation to separate all words in the entity. Then, the resulting token is projected to low dimensional dense vectors as the same as single word entity.

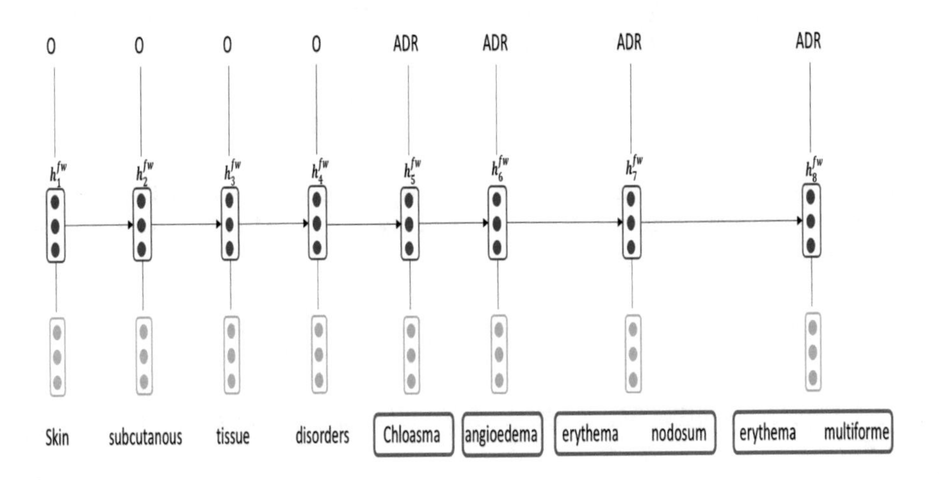

Fig. 2. RNN based deep learning method architecture

4.2 Recurrent Layer

The second component of RNN is the recurrent layer. We start from a simple one-directional forward RNN. The entity vectors $(e_1, ..., e_n)$ are put to the recurrent layer step by step as shown in Fig. 2. For each step t, the network accepts the entity vector e_t and the output at the previous step h_{t-1}^{fw} as the input, and produces the current output h_t^{fw} by a linear transform followed by a non-linear activation function, given by Eq. 5:

$$h_t^{fw} = tanh(W_{fw}e_t + U_{fw}h_{t-1}^{fw} + b_{fw}) \tag{5}$$

$h_t^{fw} \in \mathbb{R}^M$ can be regarded as local segment-level features produced by the entity where M is the dimension of the hidden layer. $W_{fw} \in \mathbb{R}^{M\times D}$, $U_{fw} \in \mathbb{R}^{M\times M}$ and $b_{fw} \in \mathbb{R}^{M\times 1}$ are the model parameters where D is the input vector dimension. The hyperbolic function $tanh(.)$ is used as the non-linear activation function, which can help back-propagate the error more easily due to its symmetry.

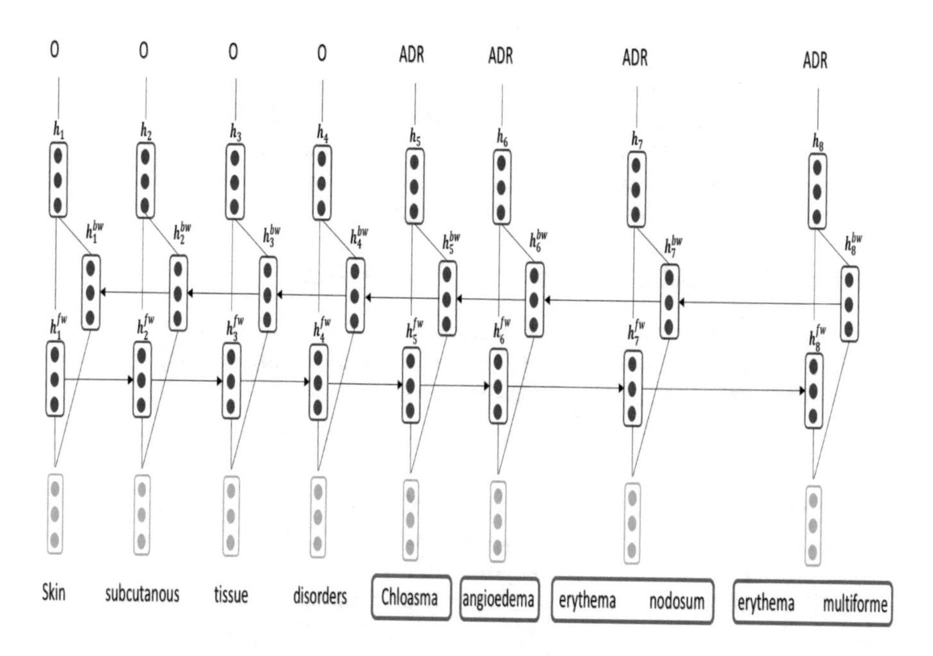

Fig. 3. Bidirectional RNN based deep learning method architecture

One limitation of the one-directional forward RNN is that the information of future entities is not fully utilized when predicting the semantic meaning in the middle of a sentence. In other words, the effective features between adverse reaction mentions might appear in the future entities which can play a part role in the training process. An efficient solution to overcome this problem is to use a bidirectional architecture that makes predictions based on both the past and future words as shown in Fig. 3. With the bidirectional RNN architecture, the prediction at step t is obtained by simply concatenating the output of the forward RNN with the backward RNN, formulated by Eq. 6:

$$h_t = [h_t^{fw}, h_t^{bw}] \tag{6}$$

where $h_t^{bw} \in \mathbb{R}^M$ is the output of the backward RNN by reversing the words in the sentence which possesses the same dimension as defined by:

$$h_t^{bw} = tanh(W_{bw}e_t + U_{bw}h_{t+1}^{bw} + b_{bw}) \tag{7}$$

where $W_{bw} \in \mathbb{R}^{M\times D}$, $U_{bw} \in \mathbb{R}^{M\times M}$ and $b_{bw} \in \mathbb{R}^{M\times 1}$ are the parameters of the backward RNN. At the beginning, h_0^{fw} and h_0^{bw} are initialized randomly.

4.3 Softmax Classfier Layer

The softmax classifier layer calculates the probability distribution over all mentions given by Eq. 8 and chooses the mention with highest probability for each entity.

$$\hat{y} = softmax(W_o h_t + b_o) \tag{8}$$

where W_o and b_o are the RNN output parameters. RNN uses cross-entropy cost function as the training objective function. The RMSprop (Resilient Mean Square Propagation) [41] is used to optimize the parameters of RNN model with respect of the objective function since it is empirically an appropriate optimization algorithm for learning the RNN based model.

5 Experimental Results and Discussion

In this section, we present the performance of adverse drug reaction mention recognition task by evaluating the CRF based machine learning and RNN based deep learning methods on SPL-ADR-200db datasets.

5.1 Datasets

We evaluated the performance of the studied methods on SPLADR-200db datasets [16]. SPL-ADR-200db was generated from TAC 2017 ADRs challenge into two formats: the Brat format and CSV format. Although both forms of SPL-ADR-200db have the same coding information, the first format is intended for the development of NLP applications such as BNER, while the second is intended for building datasets similar in the future.

The SPL-ADR-200db Brat annotation format consists of 101 labels for training set and 99 labels for test set. Each set consists of two types of files: text files which have the following name: "DRUGNAME_SectionName.txt" and the Brat files have the following name: "DRUGNAME_SectionName.ann" where section name can be Boxed Warning, Warnings AND Precaution or Adverse Reactions. For ADR mentions recognition, the Brat files define six predefined mentions: AdverseReaction, Severity, DrugClass, Negation, Animal and Factor. In our experimental study, the mention "O" is also added which means "Outside" to represent normal word. The statistics of the predefined ADR mentions are shown in Table I.

5.2 Evaluation Metrics

The evaluation was performed in terms of the precision (P), recall (R) and their harmonic mean, the F1-score (F1). They are based on the number of true positives (TP), false positives (FP) and false negative (FN) as shown in Eq. 9.

$$P = \frac{TP}{TP + FP}, R = \frac{TP}{TP + FN}, F1 = \frac{2 \times P \times R}{P + R} \tag{9}$$

where TP is the number of correct entity mentions that the system returns, FP is the number of incorrect entity mentions that the system returns, and FN is the number of missing entity mentions.

Table 1. Statistics of the ADR mentions

Mention	Training	Test	Total
AdverseReaction	13,795	12,693	26,488
Animal	44	86	130
DrugClass	249	164	413
Factor	602	562	1,164
Negation	98	173	271
Severity	934	947	1,881

5.3 Text Preprocessing

The text files of the SPL-ADR-200db datasets were segmented into sentences using the Genia Sentence Splitter,[1] and tokenized using NLTK toolkit[2] and some heuristic rules to handle the complicated entities. The stop words were removed in the sentences because of the stop words weak discriminative ability in the system performance. The numbers occur frequently in the SPL-ADR-200db datasets. For instance, in the sentence "*The safety of ACTEMRA-IV was studied in 188 pediatric patients 2 to 17 years of age with PJIA who had an inadequate clinical response or were intolerant to methotrexate.*", there are three numbers ("*188*", "*2*" and "*17*"). Replacing these numbers to zeroes won't change the sentence semantic. Therefore, it will reduce the size of the vocabulary and make the embedding more compact.

5.4 Hyper-parameter

The CRF model was implemented using CRFsuite provided by Okazaki [42] since it is fast and provides a simple interface for training and tagging the input features. The RNN model was implemented using Keras library.[3] As there is no separate development or validation set available, the original training dataset was divided into two parts, 90% as training and rest 10% as validation set. Hyper-parameters are tuned using this validation set.

The embedding layer dimension could affect system performance as shown in Fig. 4. The small entity vectors dimension does not contain enough semantics information. Furthermore, these vectors bring much more noise despite their richer semantics with the increase of the dimension. Therefore, we set the embedding layer dimension as 200 in both Bi-RNN and RNN. The number of hidden node of RNN was set as the same size of the input dimension of the RNN layer to simplify our study. For RMSprop optimization, we set the learning rate $lr = 0.005$. To alleviate the over-fitting problem, dropout [43] was set as 0.5 and applied to the RNN and softmax layers.

[1] https://github.com/ninjin/geniass.
[2] http://www.nltk.org/.
[3] https://keras.io/.

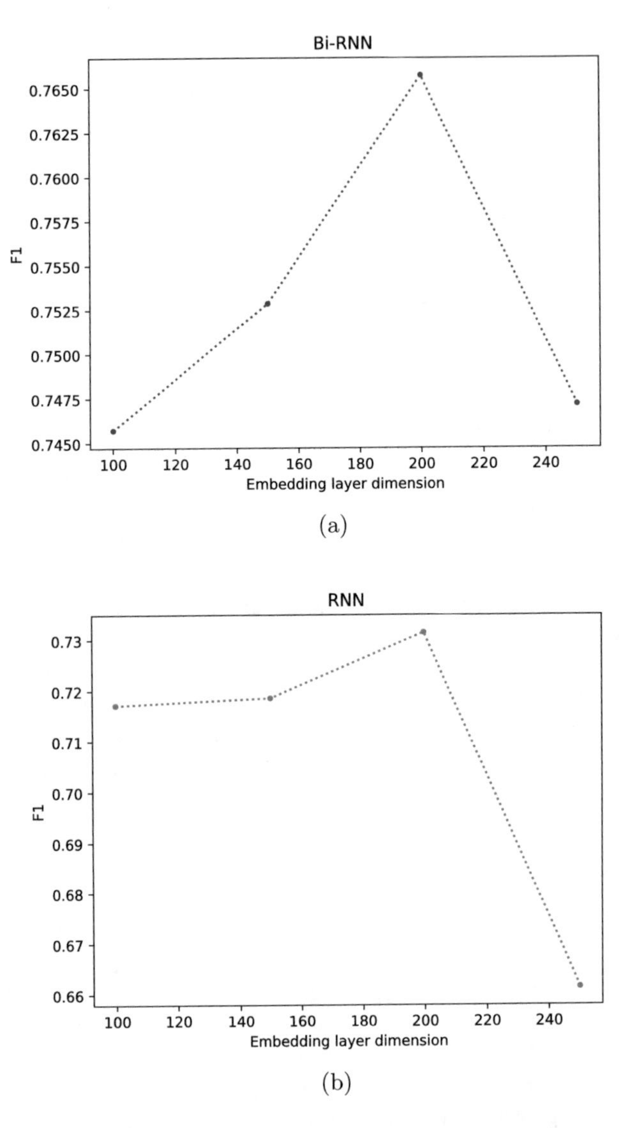

Fig. 4. The effect of embedding layer dimension of Bi-RNN (a) and RNN (b)

5.5 Results and Discussion

We conducted several experiments to evaluate the effectiveness of the studied methods on ADR mentions recognition. For deep learning models, we first evaluated using one-directional forward RNN which is used as the baseline. Then, we added backward RNN to represent bidirectional RNN. Table 2 shows the mention-level evaluation of the studied methods on the test set. The AdverseReaction mention outperforms its related mentions in both CRF based machine learning and RNN based deep learning methods. This may be rational due to

Table 2. Mention-level evaluation of CRF, RNN and Bi-RNN on the test set

Method	Mention	P(%)	R(%)	F1(%)
CRF	AdverseReaction	92	85	88
	Animal	100	16	28
	DrugClass	76	12	21
	Factor	73	60	66
	Negation	82	31	45
	Severity	92	58	71
RNN	AdverseReaction	83	87	85
	Animal	87	63	73
	DrugClass	61	41	49
	Factor	50	44	47
	Negation	35	7	12
	Severity	57	57	57
Bi-RNN	AdverseReaction	83	91	87
	Animal	86	59	70
	DrugClass	32	43	37
	Factor	53	62	57
	Negation	60	27	37
	Severity	65	60	62

the following reasons: (1) there exists the imbalance distribution of each mentions in the datasets as shown in Table 2 where the AdverseReaction is the dominant mention compared to others; (2) The ratio between AdverseReaction related mentions and normal words are really huge which proved a decrease of precision, rappel and F1-score for the rare mentions, such negation; (3) Inconsistency in category assignment may be responsible for the relation between the training size and the category classification performance. We can see from Tables 1 and 2 that the best performing mention, AdverseReaction, has the largest number of mentions instances (13,795). Moreover, RNN based method can identify the greatest number of mentions compared with CRF based method which fails to recognize effectively Animal, DrugClass and Negation mentions (F1-score ranges between 21% and 45%). Compared with RNN, the bidirectional variant achieve the best performance for all mentions which approved the effectiveness of adding the backward direction to represent the future information for predicting the semantic meaning in adverse drug reaction mentions recognition.

Table 3 shows a comparison in terms of precision, recall and F1-score between CRF, RNN and bidirectional RNN. Bi-RNN outperforms all the other methods, achieving an F1-score of 64.1%. It presents a significant improvement of 4% over one-directional forward RNN. Therefore, the bidirectional variant of RNN indeed leads to quality improvements for ADR mention extraction from drug

Table 3. Comparison in terms of precision, recall and F1-score of CRF, RNN and bi-RNN

Method	P(%)	R(%)	F1(%)
CRF	87.2	51.4	59.4
RNN	67.4	56.7	60.1
Bi-RNN	68.3	62.9	64.1

label, for instance, given the sentence "*progressive multifocal leukoencephalopathy [see warnings and precautions (5.9)]*", the Bi-RNN succeed to tag the entity "*progressive multifocal leukoencephalopathy*" as AdverseReaction if it knows the following words are warnings and precautions from the backward direction of the sentence compared with one-directional forward RNN. Moreover, Bi-RNN and RNN present an improvement of 4.7% and 0.7% respectively compared with CRF. Indeed, CRF-based methods rely on hand-crafted features and require a domain-specific knowledge to obtain better performance while RNN-based methods can fully utilize word embedding as input to capture syntactic and semantic information between mentions and extract high-level features for adverse drug reaction mentions recognition task. Moreover, the RNN models can capture variable range dependencies among entity mentions compared with CRF due to the recurrent property that make them to capture long span historical information about what have been calculated so far.

6 Conclusion and Future Work

In this paper, we have presented a comparative study between Conditional Random Fields (CRF) as a machine learning method, and both Recurrent Neural Network (RNN) and Bidirectional Recurrent Neural Network (Bi-RNN) as deep learning methods for adverse drug reaction mentions recognition task. Experimental evaluations performed on SPL-ADR-200db show that Bi-RNN outperforms RNN and CRF by an average of 4% and 4.7% in terms of F1-score, respectively through using little feature engineering.

Although RNNs can achieve good performance and model long-range dependencies, training them is difficult, likely due to the vanishing and exploding gradient problem. In future work, we intend to improve the overall performance of adverse drug reaction mentions recognition by applying the variants of RNN and integrating additional semantic and morphological features of entities as input in deep learning models.

Acknowledgment. The authors would like to thank the TAC 2017 ADRs challenge [6] organizers who provided the datasets used in this study for evaluating ADR mentions extraction methods.

References

1. Ji, Y., Ying, H., Dews, P., Mansour, A., Tran, J., Miller, R.E., Massanari, R.M.: A potential causal association mining algorithm for screening adverse drug reactions in postmarketing surveillance. IEEE Trans. Inf. Technol. Biomed. **15**(3), 428–437 (2011). https://doi.org/10.1109/titb.2011.2131669
2. Segura-Bedmar, I., Martínez, P.: Pharmacovigilance through the development of text mining and natural language processing techniques. J. Biomed. Inform. **58**, 288–291 (2015). https://doi.org/10.1016/j.jbi.2015.11.001
3. Harpaz, R., Callahan, A., Tamang, S., Low, Y., Odgers, D., Finlayson, S., Jung, K., LePendu, P., Shah, N.H.: Text mining for adverse drug events: the promise, challenges, and state of the art. Drug Saf. **37**(10), 777–790 (2014). https://doi.org/10.1007/s40264-014-0218-z
4. Russo, E., Palleria, C., Leporini, C., Chimirri, S., Marrazzo, G., Sacchetta, S., Bruno, L., Lista, R., Staltari, O., Scuteri, A., Scicchitano, F.: Limitations and obstacles of the spontaneous adverse drugs reactions reporting: two "challenging" case reports. J. Pharmacol. Pharmacother. **4**(5), 66 (2013). https://doi.org/10.4103/0976-500x.120955
5. Fung, K.W., Jao, C.S., Demner-Fushman, D.: Extracting drug indication information from structured product labels using natural language processing. J. Am. Med. Inform. Assoc. **20**(3), 482–488 (2013). https://doi.org/10.1136/amiajnl-2012-001291
6. Roberts K., Demner-Fushman D., Tonning J.M.: Overview of the TAC 2017 Adverse Reaction Extraction from Drug Labels Track Background: Adverse Drug Reactions (2017). https://bionlp.nlm.nih.gov/tac2017adversereactions/
7. Rios A., Kavuluru R.: Convolutional neural networks for biomedical text classification. In: Proceedings of the 6th ACM Conference on Bioinformatics, Computational Biology and Health Informatics - BCB 2015. ACM Press (2015). https://doi.org/10.1145/2808719.2808746
8. Wang, Y., Wu, S., Li, D., Mehrabi, S., Liu, H.: A part-of-speech term weighting scheme for biomedical information retrieval. J. Biomed. Inform. **63**, 379–389 (2016). https://doi.org/10.1016/j.jbi.2016.08.026
9. Hu, Z., Zhang, Z., Yang, H., Chen, Q., Zuo, D.: A deep learning approach for predicting the quality of online health expert question-answering services. J. Biomed Inform. **71**, 241–253 (2017). https://doi.org/10.1016/j.jbi.2017.06.012
10. Sarrouti, M., Alaoui, S.O.E.: A passage retrieval method based on probabilistic information retrieval model and UMLS concepts in biomedical question answering. J. Biomed. Inform. **68**, 96–103 (2017). https://doi.org/10.1016/j.jbi.2017.03.001
11. Sarrouti, M., Alaoui, S.O.E.: A machine learning-based method for question type classification in biomedical question answering. Methods Inf. Med. **56**(03), 209–216 (2017). https://doi.org/10.3414/me16-01-0116
12. Sarrouti, M., Lachkar, A.: A new and efficient method based on syntactic dependency relations features for ad hoc clinical question classification. Int. J. Bioinform. Res. Appl. **13**(2), 161 (2017). https://doi.org/10.1504/ijbra.2017.083150
13. Sarrouti, M., Alaoui, S.O.E.: A yes/no answer generator based on sentiment-word scores in biomedical question answering. Int. J. Healthc. Inf. Syst. Inform. **12**(3), 62–74 (2017). https://doi.org/10.4018/ijhisi.2017070104
14. Sarrouti M., El Alaoui S.O.: A biomedical question answering system in BioASQ 2017. In: BioNLP 2017, Association for Computational Linguistics (2017). https://doi.org/10.18653/v1/w17-2337

15. Sarrouti M., El Alaoui S.O.: A generic document retrieval framework based on UMLS similarity for biomedical question answering system. In: Intelligent Decision Technologies 2016, pp. 207–216. Springer, Cham (2016). https://doi.org/10.1007/978-3-319-39627-9_18
16. Demner-Fushman, D., Shooshan, S.E., Rodriguez, L., Aronson, A.R., Lang, F., Rogers, W., Roberts, K., Tonning, J.: A dataset of 200 structured product labels annotated for adverse drug reactions. Sci. Data **5**, 180001 (2018). https://doi.org/10.1038/sdata.2018.1
17. Almas, T., Archana, B.: A survey on biomedical named entity extraction. Asian J. Eng. Technol. Innov. **4**, 25–28 (2016)
18. Rindflesch T.C., Tanabe L., Weinstein J.N., Hunter L.: EDGAR: extraction of drugs, genes and relations from the biomedical literature. In: Biocomputing 2000, World scientific (1999). https://doi.org/10.1142/9789814447331_0049
19. Song, M., Yu, H., Han, W.-S.: Developing a hybrid dictionary-based bio-entity recognition technique. BMC Med. Inform. Decis. Mak. **15**(S1) (2015). https://doi.org/10.1186/1472-6947-15-s1-s9
20. Tuason O., Chen, L., Liu, H., Blake, J., Friedman, C.: Biological nomenclatures: a source of lexical knowledge and ambiguity. In: Biocomputing 2004, World scientific (2003). https://doi.org/10.1142/9789812704856_0023
21. Zeng, Q.T., Goryachev, S., Weiss, S., Sordo, M., Murphy, S.N., Lazarus, R.: Extracting principal diagnosis, co-morbidity and smoking status for asthma research: evaluation of a natural language processing system. BMC Med. Inform. Decis. Mak. **6**(1) (2006). https://doi.org/10.1186/1472-6947-6-30
22. Hanisch, D., Fundel, K., Mevissen, H.T., Zimmer, R., Fluck, J.: ProMiner: rule-based protein and gene entity recognition. BMC Bioinform. **6**(Suppl 1), S14 (2005)
23. Zhao, S.: Named entity recognition in biomedical texts using an HMM model. In: Proceedings of the International Joint Workshop on Natural Language Processing in Biomedicine and its Applications - JNLPBA 2004. Association for Computational Linguistics (2004). https://doi.org/10.3115/1567594.1567613
24. Zhang, J., Shen, D., Zhou, G., Su, J., Tan, C.-L.: Enhancing HMM-based biomedical named entity recognition by studying special phenomena. J. Biomed. Inform. **37**(6), 411–422 (2004). https://doi.org/10.1016/j.jbi.2004.08.005
25. Settles, B.: Biomedical named entity recognition using conditional random fields and rich feature sets. In: Proceedings of the International Joint Workshop on Natural Language Processing in Biomedicine and its Applications - JNLPBA 2004. Association for Computational Linguistics (2004). https://doi.org/10.3115/1567594.1567618
26. Wang, H., Zhao, T., Li, S., Yu, H.: A conditional random fields approach to biomedical named entity recognition. J. Electron. (China) **24**(6), 838–844 (2007). https://doi.org/10.1007/s11767-006-0255-6
27. Takeuchi, K., Collier, N.: Bio-medical entity extraction using support vector machines. In: Proceedings of the ACL 2003 workshop on Natural language processing in biomedicine. Association for Computational Linguistics (2003). https://doi.org/10.3115/1118958.1118966
28. Kazama, J., Makino, T., Ohta, Y., Tsujii, J.: Tuning support vector machines for biomedical named entity recognition. In: Proceedings of the ACL 2002 workshop on Natural language processing in the biomedical domain. Association for Computational Linguistics (2002). https://doi.org/10.3115/1118149.1118150

29. Li, D., Kipper-Schuler, K., Savova, G.: Conditional random fields and support vector machines for disorder named entity recognition in clinical texts. In: Proceedings of the Workshop on Current Trends in Biomedical Natural Language Processing - BioNLP 2008. Association for Computational Linguistics (2008). https://doi.org/10.3115/1572306.1572326
30. Elman, J.L.: Finding structure in time. Cogn. Sci. **14**(2), 179–211 (1990). https://doi.org/10.1207/s15516709cog1402_1
31. Yao, L., Liu, H., Liu, Y., Li, X., Anwar, M.W.: Biomedical named entity recognition based on deep neutral network. Int. J. Hybrid Inf. Technol. **8**(8), 279–288 (2015). https://doi.org/10.14257/ijhit.2015.8.8.29
32. Unanue, I.J., Borzeshi, E.Z., Piccardi, M.: Recurrent neural networks with specialized word embeddings for health-domain named-entity recognition. J. Biomed. Inform. **76**, 102–109 (2017). https://doi.org/10.1016/j.jbi.2017.11.007
33. Zhang, D., Tan, X.: Relation Classification via Recurrent Neural Network (2015). CoRR abs/1508.01006
34. Luo, Y.: Recurrent neural networks for classifying relations in clinical notes. J. Biomed. Inform. **72**, 85–95 (2017). https://doi.org/10.1016/j.jbi.2017.07.006
35. Werbos, P.: Backpropagation through time: what it does and how to do it. Proc. IEEE **78**(10), 1550–1560 (1990). https://doi.org/10.1109/5.58337
36. Song, D., Shuang, L., Jin, L., Huang, D.: Biomedical named entity recognition based on recurrent neural networks with different extended methods. Int. J. Data Min. Bioinform. **16**(1), 17 (2016). https://doi.org/10.1504/ijdmb.2016.079799
37. Stanovsky, G., Gruhl, D., Mendes, P.: Recognizing mentions of adverse drug reaction in social media using knowledge-infused recurrent models. In: Proceedings of the 15th Conference of the European Chapter of the Association for Computational Linguistics (vol. 1, Long Papers). Association for Computational Linguistics (2017). https://doi.org/10.18653/v1/e17-1014
38. Sahu, S., Anand, A.: Recurrent neural network models for disease name recognition using domain invariant features. In: Proceedings of the 54th Annual Meeting of the Association for Computational Linguistics (vol. 1, Long Papers). Association for Computational Linguistics (2016). https://doi.org/10.18653/v1/p16-1209
39. Lafferty, J.D., McCallum, A., Pereira, F.: Conditional random fields: probabilistic models for segmenting and labeling sequence data. In: International Conference on Machine Learning (ICML) (2001)
40. Campos, D., Matos, S., Luis, J.: Biomedical named entity recognition: a survey of machine-learning tools. In: Theory and Applications for Advanced Text Mining, InTech (2012). https://doi.org/10.5772/51066
41. Tieleman, T., Hinton, G.: Lecture 6.5—RmsProp: Divide the gradient by a running average of its recent magnitude. COURSERA: Neural Netw. Mach. Learn. (2012)
42. Okazaki, N.: Crfsuite: a fast implementation of conditional random fields (crfs) (2007). http://www.chokkan.org/software/crfsuite/
43. Hinton, G.E., Srivastava, N., Krizhevsky, A., Sutskever, I., Salakhutdinov, R.: Improving neural networks by preventing co-adaptation of feature detectors (2012). CoRR abs/1207.0580

Early Childhood Education: How Play Can Be Used to Meet Children's Individual Needs

Rachid Lamrani(✉), El Hassan Abdelwahed, Souad Chraibi, Sara Qassimi, and Meriem Hafidi

Computer Systems Engineering Laboratory,
Faculty of Sciences Semlalia Marrakech FSSM,
University of Cadi Ayyad, Marrakesh, Morocco
{rachid.lamrani,meriem.hafidi}@ced.uca.ac.ma,
{abdelwahed,chraibi}@uca.ac.ma,
sara.qassimi@ced.uca.ma

Abstract. Education provides useful social life skills in order to prepare future proficient leaders. In this regard, a pedagogical scenario is needed to maximize children's learning in terms of apprehending the knowledge, improving their attitudes, etc. Wherefore, why we don't benefit from the natural way of learning? Playing, represent a natural and privileged mode for children expression. It is an integral part of their daily lives, which allows them to experiment and acquire new social, cognitive, and emotional skills. Accordingly, several research, analysis, and reflections have been conducted to provide a play-based learning mode, such as Montessori pedagogical method. Correspondingly, our study propose some finality games (serious games) in order to enhance and promote a playfully and creative learning. Therefore, we carried out a qualitative systematic analysis and synthesis of the existing literature concerning learning through playing. This paper underlines the contribution of serious games as a learning tool. Based on the Pedagogical Method, set of conceptual designs have been proposed to represent the serious games ideas and their functioning. We have implemented some serious games scenarios to evaluate our proposal. Future works will focus on testing the developed pedagogical applications aiming for better results and feedbacks.

Keywords: Early years education · Preschool skills activities · Serious games · Montessori · Benefits of play

1 Introduction

Education is crucial to give people capabilities such as literacy, confidence, and attitudes [3]. Beyond, it is considered fundamental for the economic, social and cultural development of all societies [1, 2].

However, it remains a challenge in some parts of the world, particularly in developing countries. A majority of children are deprived of their rights due to several causes, such as poverty, tuition fees, or associated costs (uniforms, supplies) as well the lack of security. All those causes might create barriers, pushing some parents to keep their children away from school.

M. Ezziyyani (Ed.): AI2SD 2018, AISC 914, pp. 232–245, 2019.
https://doi.org/10.1007/978-3-030-11884-6_22

Everyone should take full responsibility by gathering all the concentrated efforts for obtaining adequate solutions, to ensure an accessible education allowing a gapless learning.

Morocco sets up several reforms to improve educational access [4]. As an example, this period was marked by the discussion about a strategic vision implementation on 2015–2030 [5, 6]. Conjointly, in response to the learning quality crisis, it's necessary to redefine the objective of the educational system. The valuable pillars of teaching and learning (i.e., the acquired skills, knowledge and attitudes) must reflect and take into account the individuals needs and expectations.

Learning starts in infancy (at the birth), and the first six years are for discovery and exploration. Thus, the parents are the first and the most important child's teachers, because not only it is their primary role, but the education responsibility falls to them [7]. For the upbringing of their children, the parents have to set up intellectual and emotional life bases, to pass suitable and valuable attitudes in order to ensure an active participation for a good pre-school departure [8, 9].

Besides, preschool is regarded as an essential and important step or even compulsory. It ensures the continuity between the family and school. Moreover, the role of the preschool institution does not take the family's place but rather it remedies, compensates and enriches the family's upbringing deficiencies. Thusly, Children who enter kindergarten without foundational early literacy skills remain a risk to reading difficulties throughout their schooling [10].

Furthermore, four factors play a crucial role in increasing learners' intrinsic motivation: challenge, curiosity, control, and fantasy. Thereupon, if we provide an adapted solution to the children's experience, and offer the possibility of reaching a goal so that the child increases his confidence and his skills, but also if we give him the opportunity to define new challenges, his intrinsic motivation will be maintained.

Allowing our children to choose their activities and to establish their own ways of doing things, will give them the feeling of controlling their learning. Therefore, what is the most efficient approach to perform this goal?

Since the beginning of the human history, Play was and still present in all cultures. It is an innate human behavior, which accompanies the human rise. It is has a vital role in the healthy development of the child enabling an open and ludic way of his development, learning, and socializing [11–13]. In fact, whether it is a toddler, teenager, or even a retired person, play is a fantastic tool for learning and development [14].

Additionally, the rapid widespread of technology has reached and involved children in their daily lives. Its influence has changed teaching methods. Information and communications technologies (ICTs) have already expanded access to high-quality educational content, such as textbooks, videos, and distance education with a lower price. ICTs have paved the way for personalized learning, adapted to the pace of each, and have allowed parents and teachers with limited resources to provide learners with better learning opportunities. Thereby, why we do not benefit from these advantages, on aim to create a link between technology, game, and children to improve the educational gap.

This paper presents a methodological approach underlines serious games and the cognitive of playing based on new technologies, in order to offer a research-based solution that makes playtime more stimulating and educational for children.

2 Pillars of Learning: Cognitive Science Point of View

Cognitive science has identified at least four key factors, described as "pillars of learning" [15]. Those pillars might assign a positive role in the speed and ease of all learning types.

Indeed, mobilizing children's attention is a priority goal. The teacher must create attractive materials that do not distract the child from his primary task. Therefore, given the sensitivity of their brain to social cues, the educational counseling attitude is essential: he must focus the child's attention through visual and verbal contact.

Moreover, the active engagement role underscores how important it is for the child to be maximally attentive, and predictive. Accordingly, a care must be taken in order to introduce learning situations that are neither easy nor difficult for the child, adequating to his context. As a matter of fact, teachers and parents must avoid giving a long lecture to preserve child's involvement and engagement. For that matter, they must hold on children's by frequently guiding, and allowing them discovering some aspects by themselves. Consequently, they evolve theirs curiosity rather than discourage it.

Withal, the feedback importance underlines the educational status of the error. The educational accompanist should realize that from the point of view of cognitive neuroscience, far from being a fault or a weakness, the error is normal, inevitable even, and in any case indispensable for learning. Better an active child who is wrong and learns from his mistakes, that a passive child.

Further, the consolidation considered as the knowledge automation. Automation is the act of passing from conscious treatment with an effort, to an automated unconscious treatment.

Correspondingly, the child learns by its emotional intelligence [16, 17] as early as 2 years, he likes the colors, shapes, textures, the sonorities… Then, the link that it develops in the kindergarten with her mistress, make him learn more words and operations. As soon as it grew, he should be initiated at the intelligence logic, which must be implemented by single organizations and visual methods.

In this last epoch, and thanks to the new technology increases, our children have the skill to manipulate brilliantly different objects, such a computer, console games… and those plays normally a formative role in children's development [18]. Intimately, in the rural environment (which we're interested in our study), children's cannot afford to buy textbooks and supplies, wherefore the technological media can be very beneficent if we can provide it.

Beyond, knowledge does not only exist by the paper but also by the image, and one session dedicated to the educational screening of a film could be a big step and a more interesting thing for the learners, especially child's.

On that account, why not exploit children's habit and easiness to the games, based on a pedagogical method and the new technologies as well, to present a ludic, fun, beneficent area basing on the learning pillars, on aims to put the child at the center of the Educational Act.

3 Learning Through Play

3.1 Importance of Games for Child Development

Outdoor Games and Playing are very important for every child's, considered as a legitimate right of the childhood, it represents a crucial aspect of the physical, intellectual and social child development. It's fundamental to their well-being.

When child's play, they develop their skills on several plans: reflection, problems solve, expression, move, cooperation, and a font call to their impressions, as well the exercise of moral conscience [19, 20, 24], but also their development unconsciously increase [21].

Moreover, all play kinds and games can be specified by means of different components. The first component is the *rule* or *gameplay*, which creates the pattern defined through the game rules that connects the player and the game. The second is the *challenge*, which determines the bonuses to reward the good actions or the obstruction and barriers that avoid the player reaching the game goal easily. Challenges are used to create the different difficulty levels of the game in order to encourage enjoyment and motivate the player to spend more time with the game. The third component is the *interaction* which represents the way the player communicates with the game. Interaction refers to any action that is done by to start some activity, it can be visual, listening, physical (typing, mouse, touchpad, button pressing), dialogue exchange, etc. And the last component is the *objective* which is defined as something that one's efforts or actions are intended to attain or accomplish.

3.2 Play, How It Impacts Brain Development

A pioneering researcher and educator Marion Diamond and her colleagues published a paper about brain growth in rats. The neuroscientists had conducted a landmark experiment, raising some rats in boring, solitary confinement and others in exciting, toy-filled colonies.

When researchers examined the rats' brains, they discovered that the "enriched" rats had thicker cerebral cortices than did the "impoverished" rats [22, 23]. Subsequent research confirmed the results—rats raised stimulating environments had bigger brains.

Do these benefits of play extend to humans?

Research shows us that many of the fundamental tasks that children must achieve, such as, exploring, risk-taking, fine and gross motor development, and the absorption of vast amounts of basic knowledge, can be most effectively learned through play. Or rather and for example, when children move over, under, beside and near objects, the child better grasps the meaning of these prepositions and geometry concepts. When children are given the opportunity to physically demonstrate action words as stomp, pounce, stalk or slither, or descriptive words such as smooth, strong, or enormous, word comprehension are immediate and long-lasting. The words are used and learned in context, as opposed to being a mere collection of letters. This is what promotes emergent literacy and a love of language. Similarly, if children take on high, low, wide, and narrow body shapes, they'll have a much greater understanding of these quantitative concepts, than children who are just presented with the words and definitions.

Learning by doing and through play, creates more neural networks in the brain and throughout the body, making the entire body a tool for learning.

Neural pathways are the connections that allow information to travel through the brain – the more pathways, the larger the brain. A newborn enters this world with their brain only 25% formed and 90% of human brain development occurs in the first five years of life.

The way a child's neural pathways form is determined by the type of human contact and interactions they have in their early years. The neural pathways that are developed in a child's first three years act like roadmaps to later learning.

So, play impacts the brain by causing the prefrontal cortex to become bigger and faster. "The experience of play changes the connections of the neurons at the front end of your brain," says Sergio Pellis, a researcher at the University of Lethbridge in Alberta, Canada. "And without play experience, those neurons aren't changed," he says. This is important because the prefrontal cortex is the brain's executive control center. That's where the brain regulates emotions, makes plans, and solve problems.

So, scientists confirm that play is essential to healthy and even exceptional to the brain development.

4 Game with Serious Purposes (SGs)

What does a serious game mean? It's a computer application that combines a serious pedagogical, informative, communicational intent, with playful which it springs from the video game (collaboration, competition, strategy …) [25, 26].

Therefore, it departs from the simple entertainment, proceeding a productive character, thus, its design and use are intended to operate among players a transformation, such as a phenomenon or a mechanism understanding, the apprehension of a concept but also, skills improvement [27].

Relevant serious games applications, have recently been developed in different domains, including training, well-being, advertisement, cultural heritage, interpersonal communication, and healthcare [28].

Likewise, serious games are now part of the educational domain range (domain of concern). Furthermore, the addictive gameplay nature and obsession of the players with digital games, is attempted to be used to facilitate the learning process [29]. Thus, many contributions are directed towards, and we mention for instance this work [30].

Additionally, benefits of serious games usage in preschool (our interest), are too numerous, yet, the studies and works that target them on preschool context still not sufficient enough.

A study that investigates whether preschoolers respond to the mathematical notion of most probable in a probabilistic game designed on the computer. This random-game, named "Shoes and Squares", allowed children to get actively involved and infer the most probable outcome among different conditions with structural changes in the composition of the sample space [31]. Another work presents an effect study. It was conducted in order to evaluate the learning effects of the serious game Mijn naam is Haas (My name is Haas) upon vocabulary growth in children in grade 1 and grade 2 (age 4–7) [32].

On another side, we have already shown SGs interest through: An introduction and a survey, which we had discuss gamificaction, game based learning and the serious games, (applications …), as well, we had unveiled our approach for an educational pervasive adaptive serious game EPASG [33].

In the same way, and in order that Morocco can have an extra entrepreneurial potential, we must help and encourage young people to discover their creative talent to develop their innovative spirit and inspire them to undertake their own business. Another work was presented as a chapter, which aim, to achieve a collaborative platform to promote entrepreneurial thoughts among young people, which we highlight the serious games use [34].

5 Early Childhood Education Importance

The preschool represents for young children an instructive period in the formation of concepts and the constant ideas [35]. It prepares them for the elementary education.

Besides, a child is not a vase that needs to be filled in, but a source that we leave unleashing. Farther, if we will charge to our children a learning system that does not consider the natural levers of their spirit, we put them in ordeal situations. And if we look at how most preschool systems work, we see that the demands we make on children are mostly unsuitable for their way of functioning, and although wired to learn effortlessly, thus, they struggle in class and lose confidence in themselves.

The preschool must be a linguistic gateway allowing the children to develop their mother tongue strengthening their emotional and social development, promoting the early acquisition of behaviors and attitudes.

Also, it must allowing children's to live in the community preparing for the social relationships which make them aware that there are rules to respect and constraints to accept.

6 Pedagogical Approach

Dr. Maria Montessori thought that no human being could be educated by another person. The individual must act himself or he will never make it. She adds that a really educated individual, continues to learn long after hours and the years he spent, because it is motivated by a natural curiosity and love of knowledge.

Maria Montessori was an Italian physician, educator, and innovator. She started her first classroom "Casa dei Bambini" or Children's House in 1907. Through her efforts and the work of her followers, his pedagogical approach "Montessori" was adopted worldwide.

Thence, the purpose of the Montessori approach is: firstly, leaving each child experiment the enthusiasm to learn according to its own choice rather than obligation, and secondly, helping child to refine their natural learning tools.

Dr. Maria has always stressed that the hand was the main teacher of the child. The best way for a child to concentrate and to fix its attention on a task is to accomplish it with his hands (See Fig. 1).

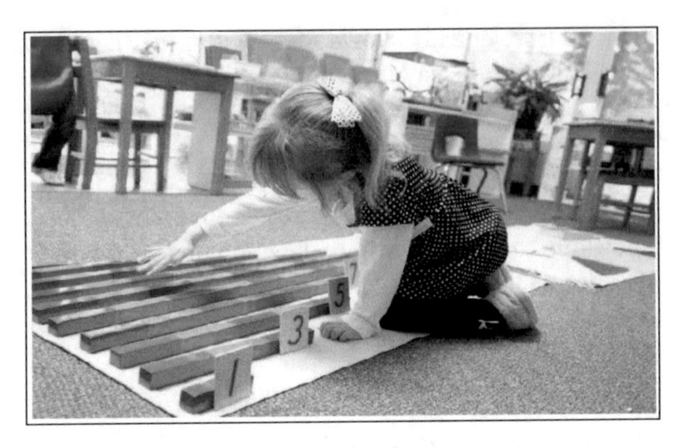

Fig. 1. Illustration of the learning by doing principle [36]

Thus, Montessori has a great introduction to the practical life activities with activities for each of the main areas (see Fig. 2).

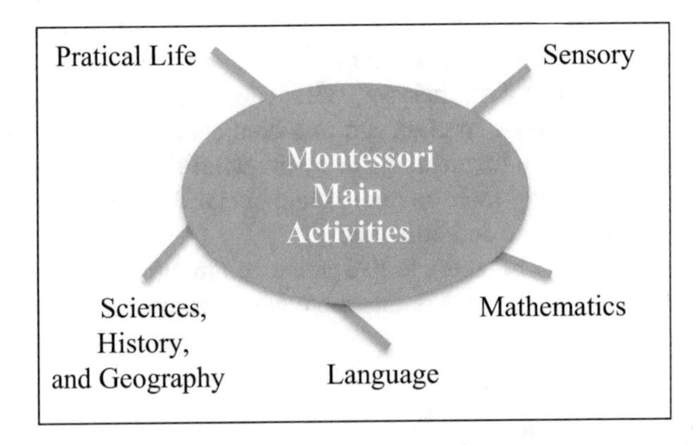

Fig. 2. The Montessori approach main activities

7 Design Methodology and Results

The different objects of the Montessori approach contribute to the child sensory organs development. They furnish and enrich the universe which surrounds it on looking, affecting, listening, smelling and tasting. Therefore, this Approach insists on the choosing environment and the accompaniment persons.

In fact, as an actor of its own development plan, the child is in need of a preparing environment adapted to its demands. This environment must be "wrapped" by a responsible person companionship (the educator). We shouldn't believe that we could let everything to the child, but he always needs the accompaniment, reminding him with benevolence the dangers, prohibitions, respect … and establishing an assistant without too intervene or lead.

In this respect, we underline that we draw inspiration from this method (Montessori) as well we based on a thorough theory (with respect to the pillars of learning reflecting the educational cognitive science point of view), to offer and introduce some games and apps with purpose (serious games), allowing a gamification integration, to manage behaviors or learning, such, mathematics improving and science skills, languages progression … (see Tables).

Thus, our main goal is to propose some finality games (serious games) in order to enhance and promote a playfully and creative learning.

All the serious games we have developed could be used within group of children in the context of an online learning or a blended learning that combines them with traditional classroom methods.

In this regard, we carried out meetings where we have defined each time our needs, we have listed the basic axes depending on our theoretical research (see the comparative table), then we have started the development by always maintaining the Agile Method.

We project to deploy, as quickly as possible, and conduct tests of our approach in a real context in rural preschools near Marrakech. Our aim is to get feedback as earlier as possible relative to user experience and assess the children's acceptance and usefulness of our system. We should mention that in this article, we are presenting just some of developed games, however, we still developing and improving others.

And below some Serious Games and applications that we have already developed (Tables 1, 2, 3, 4, 5 and 6).

Table 1. Preparing children's to understand and to respect the environment

Game Name	Flower
	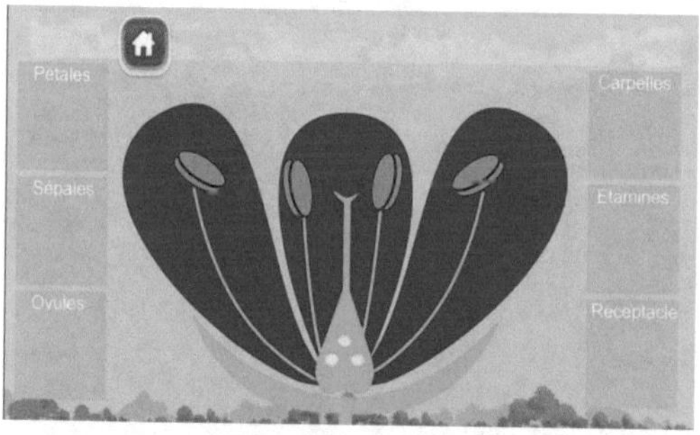
Game Goal	This serious game serves as a double purpose: while the child is making and constructing a puzzle of a flower, he is learning about the parts of a flower such as (the parts names…), thus, we prepare them to respect the environment.

Table 2. Let's learn the language, initialization to the language development

Game Name	Let's learn the language
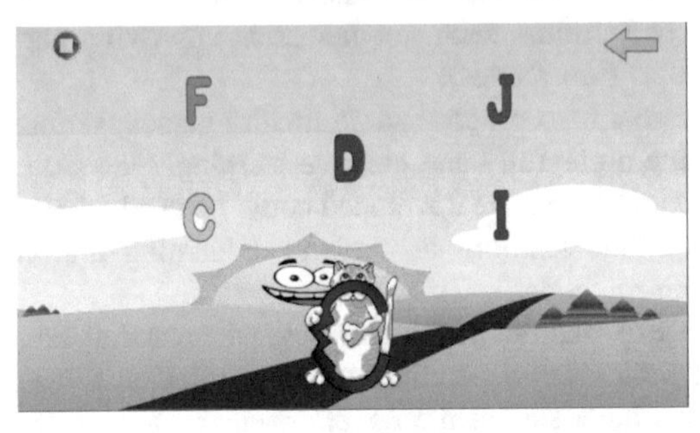	
Game Goal	This serious game serves to learn languages basics (we have started with the French language and we will add other's later). Children listen to an animated character to say the letter and then click on the corresponding it. Other levels are developed, such as word building, etc.

Table 3. MSID 2.0, serious game for some basic mathematical operations with a ludic and fun learning

Game Name	MSID 2.0
Game Goal	Is about numbers and how to use them and apply some basic mathematical operations, such as addition etc... The numbers are represented with fruits in order to add some entertainment, and the levels are represented with a plant that grows after making progress in the game.

Table 4. Let's do it, for tracing alphabets and numbers

Game Name	Let's do it
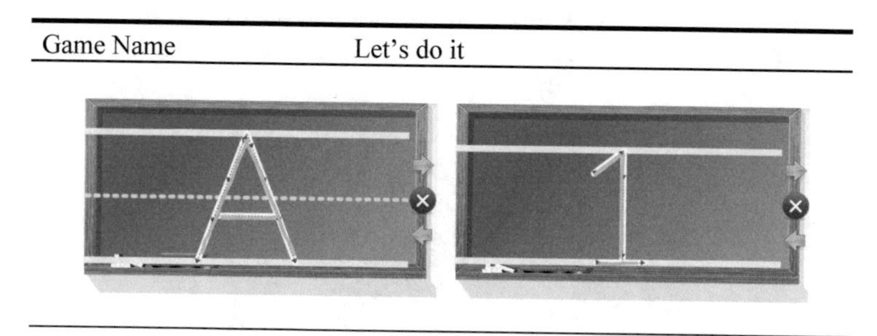	
Game Goal	Let's do it aims to help kids recognizing letter, numbers shapes, associate them with phonic sounds, and put their alphabet knowledge to use in fun exercises.

Table 5. Colors, a ludic child's color's learning

Game Name	Colors
Game Goal	It aims to teach child's colors with their names and pronunciation's.

Table 6. Let's clean, help children develop their memories and to have a sense of responsibility

Game Name	Let's Clean
Game Goal	Called let's clean, with aims, helping child's, to practice their memory, as well the sense of responsibility
Guidelines	A room image is displayed where everything is put right where it has to be. The image is displayed to the child until he feels able to put every single item right at his place once the room is disordered.

We summarize, Abilities wishing developed for children's (Table 7):

P1: Children's arithmetic development
P2: Memorization with understanding development
P3: Recognizing Child Development
P4: Sight child development
P5: The Responsibility Sense
P6: Child's speech and language development.

Table 7. Comparative table of the axes developed by our games/Applications

Games/Apps	P1	P2	P3	P4	P5	P6
Let's do it		✓	✓			
MSID 2.0	✓	✓	✓			
Colors			✓	✓		
Let's clean		✓	✓		✓	
Flowers		✓	✓			
Let's learn the language		✓	✓			✓

8 Conclusion and Perspectives

Play is the main children's source whether on its emotional, social, physical, language or cognitive development. It allows being independent while acquiring manual and communication skills, as well alternatively, the imagination takes a strong stimulation.

Through play, the child discovers the world around him, adopts a positive attitude towards action and increases his skills.

Undoubtedly, Play is not the only human activity that gives pleasure, but it is the only activity where we find pleasure as a central engine.

But apart the pleasure, the goal is to combine the serious aspects such as teaching, learning, communication, with playful springs.

Crucially, our desire is to improve the accessibility and quality of education, especially for the rural environment, since the schooling of rural world children's (especially girls) remains very insufficient.

By this article, we propose an integration of serious games as a facilitating way of learning.

Each of those applications and serious games developed, will help to process the information and implement visual skills through fun exercises, accompanied by ludic and funny designs.

We work out to deploy, as quickly as possible, and conduct tests of our approach in a real context in rural preschools near Marrakech aiming for better results and feedbacks.

Acknowledgment. The authors would like to kindly thank the students Outhmane Lagnaoui and Ilyass Moummad (Bachelor's degree in Computer Science at Cadi Ayyad University) for their insightful contributions for the project completion.

References

1. Every child has the right to an education. https://www.unicef.org/crc/index_73893.html. Accessed 5 Aug 2018
2. Monteiro, A.: The right of the child to education: what right to what education? Procedia Soc. Behav. Sci. **9**, 1988–1992 (2010)
3. Sen, A.: Development as Freedom. Anchor Books, New York (2013)
4. Djeflat, A.: Les efforts du Maroc dans l'économie fondée sur la connaissance. Report (2012)
5. Amel, N., Bakkali, I.: L'usage des TIC à l'école marocaine: état des lieux et perspectives. Hermès La Rev. **78**(2), 55–61 (2017)
6. Csefrs.ma. http://www.csefrs.ma/wp-content/uploads/2017/09/Vision_VF_Fr.pdf. Accessed 5 Aug 2018
7. Landry, S.H.: The role of parents in early childhood learning. In: Tremblay, R.E. (ed.) Encyclopedia on Early Childhood Development (2014)
8. Erola, J., Jalonen, S., Lehti, H.: Parental education, class and income over early life course and children's achievement. Res. Soc. Stratif. Mobil. **44**, 33–43 (2016)
9. Grindal, T., Bowne, J., Yoshikawa, H., Schindler, H., Duncan, G., Magnuson, K., Shonkoff, J.: The added impact of parenting education in early childhood education programs: a meta-analysis. Child Youth Serv. Rev. **70**, 238–249 (2016)

10. Alexander, K., Entwisle, D., Olson, L.: Lasting consequences of the summer learning gap. Am. Soc. Rev. **72**, 167–180 (2007)
11. Yilmaz, R.: Educational magic toys developed with augmented reality technology for early childhood education. Comput. Hum. Behav. **54**, 240–248 (2016)
12. Moreno, M.: Supporting child play. JAMA Pediatr. **170**, 184 (2016)
13. Milteer, R., Ginsburg, K., Mulligan, D.: The importance of play in promoting healthy child development and maintaining strong parent-child bond: focus on children in poverty. Pediatrics **129**, e204–e213 (2011)
14. Miller, J., Kocurek, C.: Principles for educational game development for young children. J. Child. Media **11**, 314–329 (2017)
15. Dehaene, S.: Cognitive foundations of learning in school-aged children. Collège de France. https://www.college-de-france.fr/site/en-stanislas-dehaene/course-2014-2015.htm. Accessed 5 Aug 2018
16. Raver, C., Garner, P., Smith, D.: The roles of emotion regulation and emotion knowledge for children's academic readiness: are the links causal? In: Planta, B., Snow, K., Cox, M. (eds.) School Readiness and the Transition to Kindergarten in the Era of Accountability, pp. 121–147. Paul H Brookes Publishing, Baltimore (2007)
17. Eggum, N., Eisenberg, N., Kao, K., Spinrad, T., Bolnick, R., Hofer, C., Kupfer, A., Fabricius, W.: Emotion understanding, theory of mind, and prosocial orientation: relations over time in early childhood. J. Posit. Psychol. **6**, 4–16 (2011)
18. Plowman, L.: Researching young children's everyday uses of technology in the family home. Interact. Comput. **27**, 36–46 (2014)
19. Hughes, F.: Children, Play, and Development. Sage Publications, Los Angeles (2010)
20. Berk, L.: Child Development. Pearson, Boston (2013)
21. Catron, C.: Early Childhood Curriculum: A Creative Play Model. Pearson, Boston (2008)
22. Diamond, M.: Response of the brain to enrichment. An. Acad. Bras. Ciênc. **73**, 211–220 (2001)
23. Diamond, M., Krech, D., Rosenzweig, M.: The effects of an enriched environment on the histology of the rat cerebral cortex. J. Comp. Neurol. **123**, 111–119 (1964)
24. Vaughan, C., Brown, S.: Play. Avery, New York (2014)
25. Djaouti, D.: Serious games pour l'éducation: utiliser, créer, faire créer? Tréma **44**, 51–64 (2016)
26. Wattanasoontorn, V., Boada, I., García, R., Sbert, M.: Serious games for health. Entertain. Comput. **4**, 231–247 (2013)
27. Giessen, H.: Serious games effects: an overview. Procedia Soc. Behav. Sci. **174**, 2240–2244 (2015)
28. Laamarti, F., Eid, M., El Saddik, A.: An overview of serious games. Int. J. Comput. Games Technol. **2014** (2014). Article ID 358152, 15 pages
29. Romero, M., Usart, M., Ott, M.: Can serious games contribute to developing and sustaining 21st century skills? Games Cult. **10**, 148–177 (2014)
30. Muratet, M., Torguet, P., Jessel, J., Viallet, F.: Towards a serious game to help students learn computer programming. Int. J. Comput. Games Technol. **2009**, 1–12 (2009)
31. Nikiforidou, Z., Pange, J.: Shoes and squares: a computer-based probabilistic game for preschoolers. Procedia Soc. Behav. Sci. **2**, 3150–3154 (2010)
32. Schuurs, U.: Serious gaming and vocabulary growth. In: De Wannemacker, S., Vandercruysse, S., Clarebout, G. (eds.) Serious Games: The Challenge. ITEC/CIP/T 2011. Communications in Computer and Information Science, vol. 280. Springer, Heidelberg (2012)

33. Lamrani, R., Abdelwahed, E.H.: Learning through play in pervasive context: a survey. In: IEEE/ACS 12th International Conference of Computer Systems and Applications (AICCSA), Marrakech, pp. 1–8 (2015)
34. Lamrani, R., Abdelwahed, E.H., Chraibi, S., Qassimi, S., Hafidi, M., El Amrani, A.: Serious game to enhance and promote youth entrepreneurship. In: Rocha, Á., Serrhini, M., Felgueiras, C. (eds.) Europe and MENA Cooperation Advances in Information and Communication Technologies. Advances in Intelligent Systems and Computing, vol. 520. Springer, Cham (2017)
35. Arbianingsih, Rustina, Y., Krianto, T., Ayubi, D.: Developing a health education game for preschoolers: what should we consider? Enferm. Clínica **28**, 1–4 (2018)
36. Alvarez, C.: Les lois naturelles de l'enfant. Les Arènes (2016)

The Right Pricing Between the Econometric Model "Generalized Linear Model" and the Era of Data Science Application on the Basic Health Insurance in Morocco

Karima Lamsaddak[1(✉)] and Driss Mentagui[2]

[1] Department of Applied Mathematics, Operational Research and Statistics Faculty of Sciences, Ibn Tofail University, Kénitra, Morocco
lamsaddak.karima6@gmail.com
[2] Faculty of Sciences, Ibn Tofail University, Kénitra, Morocco

Abstract. The digital revolution, the availability and the immediacy of information are the key factors that define today's consumer. A demanding consumer who can easily judge value for money. As a result, the insurer is obliged to offer the correct rate for these insurance products. For this reason, the aim of this article is to give a basic pricing for the cover of the "disease" risk by the application of the generalized linear model and the proposal of an alternative pricing based on the Data Science.

Keywords: Health insurance · Pricing · Generalized linear models · Data Science · Big Data

1 Introduction

Social security is one of the major challenges that nations are seeking to raise. The concern for equity and solidarity in the access to medical care is a major factor in social cohesion. It is in this sense that Morocco advocates a particular interest in this issue, through the implementation of compulsory health insurance "AMO' in 2005 and RAMED insurance for the poor population in 2011. However, public or private bodies which, at that date, provide their employees with optional medical cover with insurance companies, mutual insurance companies or internal funds, may continue to provide this cover on the condition of bringing the proof to the social security bodies. To model the basic insurance product in Morocco we have selected the medical consumption portfolio in 2013 of the insured population by insurance companies.

Thus, the insurance product is a flagship product of other insurance products. To this end, retaining and attracting potential customers for this product means retaining its portfolio of other insurance products (automobile, fire, etc.). As a result, the actuary is faced with the double constraint of properly valuing his risk through the fair rate and respecting the overall portfolio constraint.

The aim of this article is therefore, to define an approach allowing to build pricing bases for group basic health contracts and to propose a fast and satisfactory pricing alternative for today's customer.

M. Ezziyyani (Ed.): AI2SD 2018, AISC 914, pp. 246–260, 2019.
https://doi.org/10.1007/978-3-030-11884-6_23

The modelled variable is a company's annual medical care consumption. The collective rate is sought for an individual contribution of the insured persons of the company.

Generalized linear models represent a tool well suited to this type of study. For several years now, they have been established in the pricing of non-life insurance contracts as a good alternative to the deterministic methods traditionally used. otherwise, these methods, costly in terms of time, can be judged out of phase with the digital era marked by instantaneity. Therefore, we will propose a pricing alternative based on the Data Science concept.

The work is presented through four parts, the first one presents the generalized linear model (GLM), the second part illustrates our database and work methodology, the third presents the results of GLM and the last part proposes an alternative modeling by Data Science.

2 Theorical Overview GLM

2.1 Presentation of the Model

2.1.1 Definition

Generalized linear models are a generalization of the Gaussian linear model, obtained by allowing other (conditional) laws than the Gaussian law. The possible laws must belong to the exponential family whose density is written in the form (Eq. (1)) [1]:

$$f\ (y/\theta, \varphi) = \exp\left\{\frac{y\theta - b\ (\theta)}{a(\varphi)} + c(y, \varphi)\right\} \tag{1}$$

Where θ, φ are the settings and a, b, c functions.

This family of laws (called exponential) proves to be particularly useful for constructing econometric models much more general than the usual Gaussian model. A sample (Yi, Xi) is assumed, where the variables Xi are exogenous information about the insured or the insured property, and where Yi is the variable of interest.

It is assumed that, conditionally to the explanatory variables X_i, the variables Y_i are independent and identically distributed.

It is also assumed that $g\ (\mu_i) = \eta_i = X_i\beta$ i = 1,…,n for a given g(-) link function and where $\mu_i = E\ (Y_i|X_i)$. The link function is the function that links the linear preacher η_i to the mean μ_i.

Thus, a generalized linear model is composed of three elements, namely:

- Variables to explain Y_i, i = 1, …, n; whose densities are in the form of a density belonging to the exponential family.
- A set of parameters $\beta = (\beta_0, \ldots, \beta_p)^t$ belonging to a non-empty open of $\mathbb{R}^{p+1}$.
- Explanatory variables $X_i = (X_1, \ldots, X_p)$.
- A link function g(.) which is specific for each of the probability laws of the linear exponential family.

2.1.2 Examples of Legislation

The Log-Normal Law:

A variable is called Log-Normal if its logarithm follows a Normal distribution. It has the advantage of being positive, therefore suitable for cost modeling, and allows asymmetric phenomena to be adjusted.

The density of the Log-Normal law takes the following form (Eq. (2)) [1]:

$$f\left(x,\mu,\sigma^2\right) = \frac{1}{x\sqrt{2\pi\sigma^2}}\exp\left(-\frac{(\log(x)-\mu)^2}{2\sigma^2}\right) \tag{2}$$

Applying the maximum likelihood estimation method, we obtain the estimators of the following parameters [3]:

$$\hat{\mu} = \frac{1}{n}\sum_{i=1}^{n}\log(x_i)$$

$$\hat{\sigma}^2 = \frac{1}{n}\sum_{i=1}^{n}(\log(x_i)-\hat{\mu})^2$$

Gamma and exponential law:

The maximum likelihood estimate is less trivial for the Gamma law parameters than for the Log-Normal law.

The density of Gamma law takes the form in Eq. (3):

$$f(x,k,\theta) = x^{k-1}\frac{e^{-x/\theta}}{\theta^k\Gamma(k)} \text{ pour } x,k,\theta > 0 \tag{3}$$

With: If k is a positive integer

$$\Gamma(k) = \int_0^{+\infty} x^{k-1}e^{-x}dx \text{ et } \Gamma(k) = (k-1)!$$

The maximum likelihood estimators are therefore:

$$\hat{\theta} = \frac{1}{k^*n}\sum_{i=1}^{n}x_i$$

$$k \approx \frac{1}{2}\frac{1}{\ln\left(\frac{1}{n}\sum_{i=1}^{n}x_i\right)-\frac{1}{n}\sum_{i=1}^{n}\ln(x_i)}$$

2.2 Model Validation

2.2.1 The Total Deviance

Deviancy is often used to measure the fit quality of a GLM model. Deviancy is calculated by formula in Eq. (4):

$$D = 2 * (\ln \mathrm{L}(\mathrm{Y}|\mathrm{Y}) - \ln \mathrm{L}(\hat{\mu}|\mathrm{Y})) \tag{4}$$

A model is well fitted if it has a minimal deviation.

With $\ln \mathrm{L}(\mathrm{Y}|\mathrm{Y})$ log likelihood.

2.2.2 Akaike Information Criteria: AIC

AIC is one of the most widely used criteria when validating a GLM model. A model is considered efficient if it corresponds to the lowest AIC. The AIC is calculated according to the formula in Eq. (5) [2]:

$$AIC = -2 * \ln \mathrm{L}(\mathrm{Y}|\mathrm{Y}) + (2\mathrm{k} + 1) \tag{5}$$

2.2.3 Residue Analysis

In the conventional linear model, validation is done by checking these assumptions, including the normality of the residuals. However, in the generalized linear model, the notion of residual, as it is conceived in the classical model no longer exists: the explained variable is no longer decomposed into an "explanatory" part and a "residual" part supposed to verify probabilistic properties. On the other hand, we can examine different types of residues that make it possible to measure, for each observation, the error made by the model in estimating the explained variable, that is, the difference between the values observed and the values estimated by the model.

These residues make it possible to highlight outliers and to assess, to a certain extent, the validity of a model.

We propose to present two types of residues [2]:

- Pearson residue (formula (6)):

$$\mathrm{r}_i^p = \frac{y_i - \mu_i}{\sqrt{v(\widehat{\mu_1})}} \tag{6}$$

- Deviance residues (formula (7)):

$$\mathrm{r}_i^d = \mathrm{signe}(y_i - \widehat{\mu_1})\sqrt{d_i} \tag{7}$$

d_i is the component of deviance induced by the ième observation, with $D = \sum_{i=1}^{n} d_i$ model deviation.

Pearson and deviance residues have approximately 0 mean and ϕ variance. These residues should generally not exhibit any trend in mean or variance when plotted against the fitted values μ_i.

In practice, the distribution of Pearson residues is fairly asymmetric around 0, so deviance residues are preferable.

3 Database and Methodology

This work is done based on the data of the health portfolio collected in 2013.

3.1 Variable to Explain Y

The variable to be modelled is the annual consumption by type of beneficiary (Table 1).

Table 1. Medical consumption of beneficiaries in currency units.

Type of beneficiary	Medical consumption average
Insured Man	27
Insured Woman	32
Spouse	27
Child	14

Consumption varies according to the type of beneficiary, insured women consume more than insured men, therefore, a modeling by type of beneficiary will be the subject of the following.

3.2 Variable Explicative X

The variables that can explain medical consumption are: age, sex, limits, reimbursement rate, company size, company activity, annual salary of the insured, profession and region of the insured.

4 GLM Modeling Results

The modelling is done by type of beneficiary, the choice of explanatory variables is made after a correlation and dependence analysis between the variables. Thus, a segmentation was made to create homogeneous segments by explanatory variables.

4.1 Choice of Distribution Law

One of the essential steps in a model, called GLM, is the choice of data distribution. The Q-Q plot, quantile-quantile plot, is a graphical technique that compares the fit of an observed distribution to a theoretical model. Figures (1 and 2) present medical consumption data with the candidate laws of the exponential family.

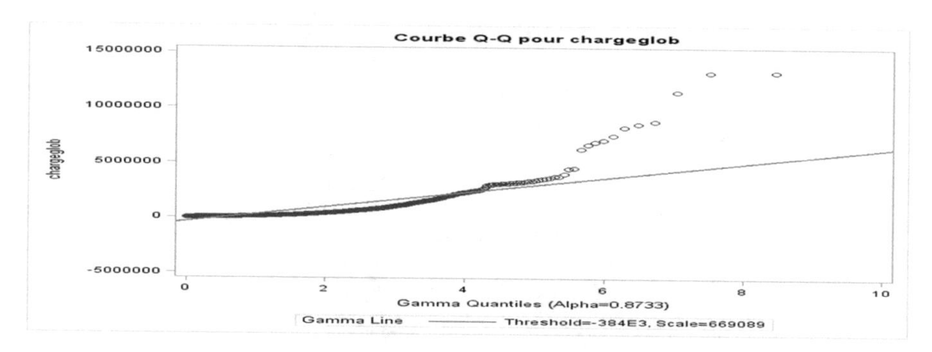

Fig. 1. Q-Q Plot GAMMA Model

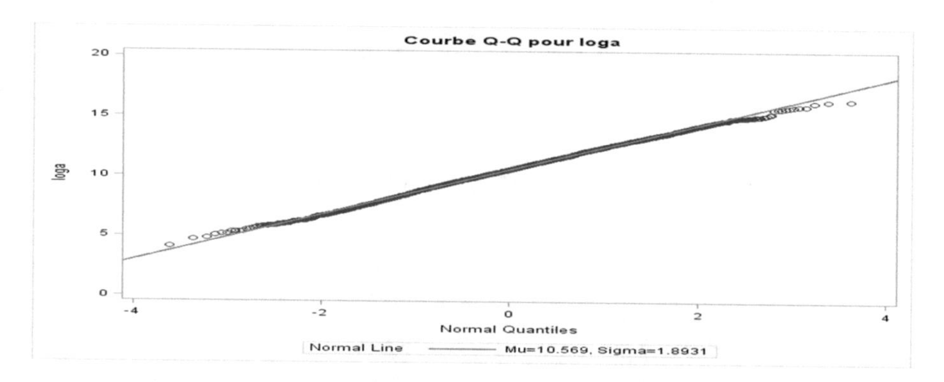

Fig. 2. Q-Q Plot LOGNORMAL Model

From the Figs. (1 and 2), we can see that the log-normal law fits better than the gamma law. On the other hand, modelling will be carried out by the two laws to ensure that the model is chosen.

4.2 Criteria for Assessing Model Is Chosen

We modeled our data on SAS software by the two distribution laws. The criteria for assessing the adequacy of each model are presented in Tables 2 and 3.

Table 2. GAMMA Model deviation creteria.

Critères d'évaluation de l'adéquation			
Critère	DDL	Valeur	Valeur/DDL
Deviance	4221	5692.6064	1.3486
Scaled Deviance	4221	4971.5095	1.1778
Pearson Chi-Square	4221	7968.3267	1.8878
Scaled Pearson X2	4221	6958.9585	1.6487
Log Likelihood		-51826.3581	
Full Log Likelihood		-51826.3581	
AIC (smaller is better)		103684.7161	
AICC (smaller is better)		103684.8450	
BIC (smaller is better)		103786.3381	

Table 3. LOGNORMAL Model deviation creteria.

Critères d'évaluation de l'adéquation			
Critère	DDL	Valeur	Valeur/DDL
Deviance	4221	6494.1737	1.5385
Scaled Deviance	4221	4236.0000	1.0036
Pearson Chi-Square	4221	6494.1737	1.5385
Scaled Pearson X2	4221	4236.0000	1.0036
Log Likelihood		-6915.6154	
Full Log Likelihood		-6915.6154	
AIC (smaller is better)		13863.2307	
AICC (smaller is better)		13863.3596	
BIC (smaller is better)		13964.8527	

Based on all of the criteria presented in Tables 2 and 3, the Lognormal model has better criteria, minimal deviance, AICC, AICC and BIC than the Gamma model. As a result, the Lognormal model was used.

4.3 Deviance Residue Analysis

The deviance residue graphs of the two models, presented in Fig. 3 and 4, show that the appearance of the Lognormal model residues is better, since it shows no particular trend.

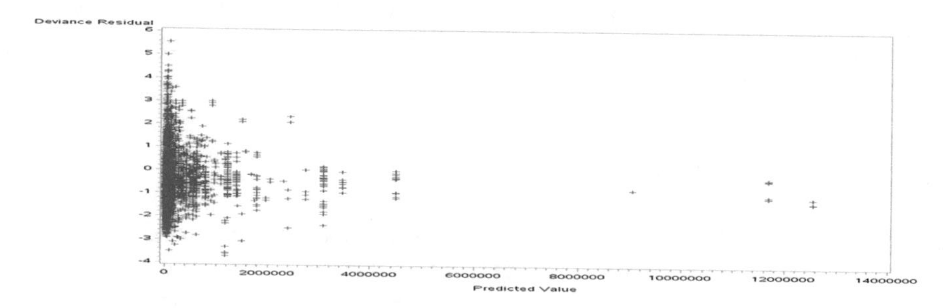

Fig. 3. GAMMA Model deviation residue

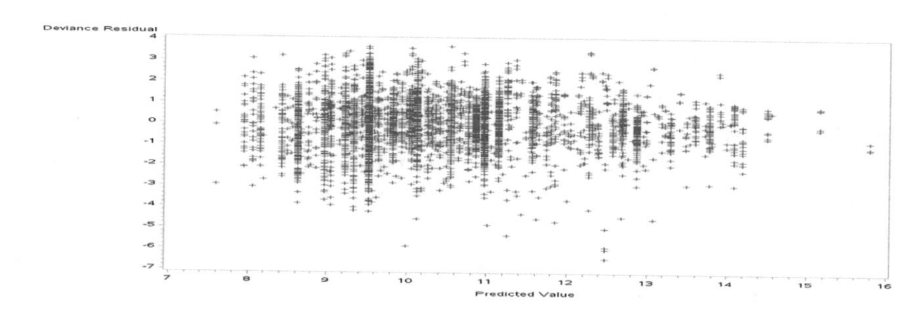

Fig. 4. LOGNORMAL Model deviation residue

Application Example

To properly illustrate the mechanism of operation of our model, we take the following example:

The characteristics of the new company

A new pricing request by a company with the following features:

- Characteristics of the insured population:
  - Employees: 100 insured (50 men and 50 women) with 50 spouses and 80 dependent children;
  - Average age: 40 years for insured men, 35 years for women, 30 years for spouses and 10 years for children;
- Characteristics of the company:
  - Region/City: Casablanca;
  - The activity sector: industry;

- Selected services:
  - Reimbursement rate: 80%;
  - Ceilings: General 100000 DHS, Dental 2000 DHS, Optical 1000 DHS and 3000DHS Maternity Package;

The pure premium obtained by our model is 257.000DH. If we assume that the company will apply the premium in an equitable way between its main insureds, the premium to be paid by its insureds is 2570DH. Management fees must be added to this sum in order to obtain the commercial rate.

5 Alternative Pricing by Data Science

Today, the power of computers and the availability of data (either internal or external) push the actuary to move towards pricing based on the use of available data in order to save time and energy wasted in choosing and adapting an econometric model and capture more factors that can influence claims experience [4].

This section proposes a pricing alternative based on a fair rate simulation algorithm that reflects the available portfolio.

5.1 Modeling Framework

5.1.1 Data Science

"Data Science is a disciplinary mix between data inference, algorithm development and technology, whose objective is the solution of complex analytical problems. At the heart of this great mix are the data, the massive quantities of raw information stored in the companies' data warehouses. In concrete terms, data science allows data to be used creatively to generate value for businesses" [6].

5.1.2 Pricing Tool

In order to exploit the information available in databases, insurers use the purchase of powerful software in data processing. An example is the SAS software (our work tool). However, if the company does not have powerful enough software, the actuary can work with open source software, for example the R language which makes it possible to process databases of more than 2 billion lines.

As a result, the actuary has two types of information:

- The information stored internally through the company's claims history;
- External information: available on open source databases.

5.2 Modeling Approach

It should be noted that the proposed pricing alternative is based on the internal database of insurance companies. Therefore, the proposed model is limited to the variables available in our database.

5.2.1 Rate Variables

Since our approach is based on the use of all the information available on our database. We have retained the majority of available variables (Xi). Its variables are grouped into 3 categories:

Variables relating to the benefits chosen by the company: These are the reimbursement rate, general ceiling, dental ceiling, optical ceiling and maternity package;

Variables relating to the company: Size of the company (man, woman, spouse and child insured employees), sector of activity, region and turnover;

Variables related to the insured population: age, sex, marital status, salary, etc.

Thus, the Fig. 5 presents the tariff variables (Xi) by the type of information offered:

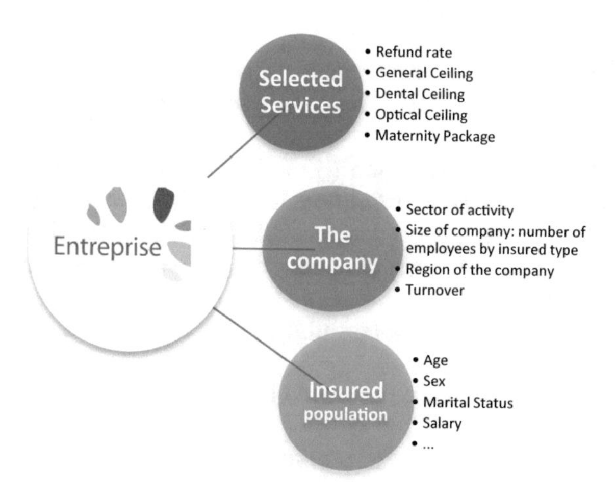

Fig. 5. Rate variables of a company

Our target variable (to be modelled) is the annual consumption of the company Yi.

In order to broaden the field of data exploitation we have created a new actual consumption variable (Y'i):

Y'i = Yi/reimbursement rate: this variable presents the actual consumption of the company's insured and beneficiaries.

5.2.2 Segmentation of Tariff Variables

Before starting modelling, it is first necessary to perform a classification of quantitative explanatory variables to make them qualitative and qualitative variables having a very large number of modality (region variable).

Based on SAS ENTERPRISE MINER software 13.1. We obtained the classes to retain for the quantitative variables in the modeling of the male insured (Table 4):

Table 4. Number of classes by explanatory variable.

Variable	Number of classes
Average Age	3
Number of insured	4
Region	3
Dental Ceiling	4
Optical Ceiling	3
General Ceiling	3
Turnover	3

5.2.3 Pricing Process

The objective of our process is to determine the annual consumption of a new business based on its characteristics, the benefits selected and the demographic characteristics of these employees.

Each line shows the consumption (j) of the insured person (i) employed in the company (k) on date t and the information relating to the insured person (i), i.e. date of birth, region of residence, salary, marital status, etc. Also, the lines contain all the information relating to the act consumed, the ceiling which corresponds to it, the rate of reimbursement…etc.

When the database does not contain all the information deemed useful in pricing, a joint between tables is necessary.

By type of insured, we have a set of consumption lines for the different medical procedures for a given year.

Company k's consumption is the sum of the consumption of all its policyholders and beneficiaries:

$$Z_k = \sum_{i=1}^{n1} Y_i + \sum_{i=1}^{n2} Z_i + \sum_{i=1}^{n3} C_i + \sum_{i=1}^{n4} E_i \tag{8}$$

With:

n1 the number of male insured persons, n2 the number of female insured persons, n3 the number of spouses and n4 the number of children.

(8) presents the company's consumption (k) by summing:

- Annual consumption of all male insured $\sum_{i=1}^{n1} Y_i$;
- Annual consumption of all women insured $\sum_{i=1}^{n2} Z_i$;
- Annual consumption of all spouses $\sum_{i=1}^{n3} C_i$;
- Annual consumption of all children $\sum_{i=1}^{n4} E_i$.

Thus, the consumption of each insured and beneficiary is the sum of the different acts consumed during the year. For example, the insured's consumption (i) is the sum of his consumption during the year (Eq. 9):

$$Y_i = \sum_{j=1}^{n} Y_{i,j} \tag{9}$$

With: n number of medical use in the year.

Pricing Process

The proposed process runs through the following steps (illustrated in the graphic in Fig. 6):

Step 1: Enter the characteristics of the new company;
Step 2: Filtration of four databases (male, female, spouse and child insured) with the characteristics of the new company;
Step 3: Validation of the size of the pricing segment:

1. If the base of each sufficient type the algorithm goes to the next step;
2. Otherwise, step 2 is repeated with fewer selection criteria and the base size is validated until it is big enough;

Note that, when the database is not validated (insufficient size), the reduction of the selection criteria is done in order of important tariff variables.

Step 4: Sum of the consumption lines within the limits of the ceilings chosen by the new insured;
Step 5: Calculation of the average of the actual annual pure consumption;
Step 6: Calculation of the commercial tariff by increase or discount of the pure tariff according to the company's performance indicator, the insured portfolio and the company's environment.

With:

NAH: Number of insured men
NAF: Number of women insured
NC: Number of spouses
NE: Number of children
CM_AH: Average consumption of male insured persons
CM_AF: Average consumption of insured women
CM_C: Average consumption of spouses
CM_E: Average consumption of children

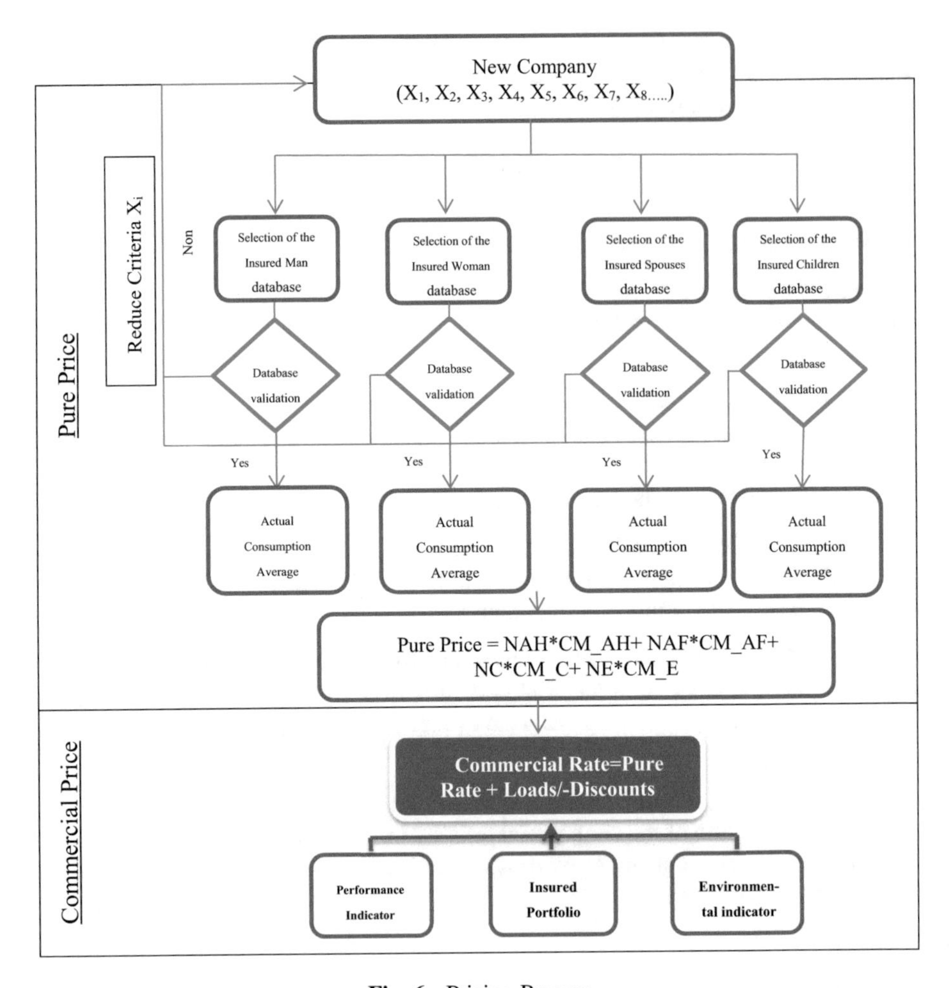

Fig. 6. Pricing Process

Application Example

To properly illustrate the mechanism of operation of our process we take the following example:

Step 1: Enter the characteristics of the new company

A new pricing request by a company with the same example of the GLM part.

Step 2: Filtering four databases

Since our data source is a historical claims database, we assume that the four types of beneficiaries (male insured, female insured, spouse and child) exist in our database.

Step 3: Validation of the size of the pricing segment

In this example it is assumed that the size is validated when: the size of the base is greater than 20 beneficiaries.

Step 4: Summation of the consumption lines within the limits of the chosen ceilings by the new insured person
It is assumed that, in a single year, each beneficiary has 10 records (medical consumption), thus the database contains 200 records. The actual consumption must be summed within the limits of the chosen ceilings by the company (100 000 DHS).
Step 5: Calculation of the average of the actual annual pure consumption
The average annual actual consumption of each beneficiary is calculated. As a result, the pure0020rate is:
Pure Tariff = 50*CM_AH + 50*CM_AF + 30*CM_C + 67*CM_E
The pure Tariff obtained for this company is 271.000Dh. That is 2710 Dhs per insured.
Step 6: Calculation of the commercial tariff
We assume that our company has a large portfolio (possibility of concluding other contracts), good performance indicators and the environment gives good prospects. In this case, the pure rate can be retained, or even discounts can be made to encourage the company to take out the contract.

The pure tariff obtained by the second method is higher than the first tariff. The sources of difference may be due to the treatment of anomalies (and aberrations) made in the first method. The second method calculates an average rate without any processing or deletion of existing data.

6 Conclusion

The use of generalized linear models (GLM) has made it possible to identify, among the available data, those that have the greatest influence on an insured’s medical care consumption, and to quantify this influence. The chosen model is based on the characteristics of the claims history of the used portfolio. This loss experience changes over time according to several factors: the insured population, the way of life, the social climate, the quality of the services offered, the change in drug prices, etc. As a result, the model needs to be updated and adapted over time (and even between years).

On the other hand, the second method, based on the total exploitation of the available information in the databases (internal or external), allows on the one hand an automatic calculation of the tariff and on the other hand the improvement of the algorithm with the integration of new criteria if available.

Thus, it is important to remember that in the second method our algorithm is applied on the database available internally. However, the outlined process presents the major steps for an application in Big Data. Therefore, this work can be complemented by extending the algorithm to other factors that may explain the medical care consumption also on other types of data such as Big Data.

References

1. Wajnberg, E.: Introduction au Modèle Linéaire Généralisé. UE7-Université de Nice Sophia Antipolis, October 2011
2. Monbet, V.: Modèles linéaires généralisés, IRMAR, Université de Rennes 1, December 2016
3. Denuit, M., Charpentier, A.: Mathématiques de l'assurance non vie, Tome II: tarification et provisionnement, Economica (2005)
4. Françoys Labonté Technologie, method et application du Big Data, 20 May 2015
5. Froidefond, E., Chappelleir, S.: BIG DATA et données externs dans les modèles de tarification (2014)
6. https://lebigdata.fr

Deep Learning Algorithm for Suicide Sentiment Prediction

Samir Boukil[1(✉)], Fatiha El Adnani[1], Loubna Cherrat[1], Abd Elmajid El Moutaouakkil[1], and Mostafa Ezziyyani[2]

[1] Laboratory (LAROSERI), Department of Computer, Faculty of Sciences, Chouaib Doukkali University, El Jadida, Morocco
boukilsamir@yahoo.fr, ftheladnani@gmail.com, cherratloub-na2@gmail.com, elmsn@hotmail.com
[2] Faculty of Sciences and Technologies, Abdelmalek Essaadi University, Tangier, Morocco
ezziyyani@gmail.com

Abstract. The increasing use of social media provides unprecedented access to the behaviors, thoughts, feelings and intentions of individuals. We are interested, in this paper, in the detection of notes that express bad feelings that might lead to committing suicide. Our goal is to present an automated detection and prediction system capable of recognizing severe depression through analyzing sentiments and feelings expressed on social networks, blogs, emails and even textual notes. In this work, we have set up a chain of treatments to extract characteristics from notes reflecting the emotional state. We can summarize these treatments in two phases: a pretreatment phase based on the Arabic stemming algorithms, and a phase of construction of feature vectors specific to each word of the corpus based on Term Frequency-Inverse Document Frequency method. Then, we applied a model based on Convolutional Neural Networks to predict the nature of feelings behind the note. The Convolutional Neural Network algorithm is one of many famous algorithms of deep learning field. It is originally created for image processing applications. But recently, it is more and more used in text mining and sentiment analysis field. The originality of the approach is, in one hand, to consider both the nature of the words that individuals used to express themselves. And in the other hand, to use the advantages of the Convolutional Neural Network to automatically extract the most significant and reliable features. A preliminary experiment allowed us to evaluate our approach on real cases of online suicidal notes.

Keywords: Suicide · Depression · Classification · Sentiment analysis · Deep learning · Convolutional Neural Networks · Term Frequency-Inverse Document Frequency

1 Introduction

In the last decade, the online social networks have emerged and increased connectivity between people, its goal was and still is to build and activate living communities in the world, as people share their thoughts, interests and activities through posts, tweets,

M. Ezziyyani (Ed.): AI2SD 2018, AISC 914, pp. 261–272, 2019.
https://doi.org/10.1007/978-3-030-11884-6_24

notes, images, videos and many other forms of expression. Those information and ideas can be spread to a immense number of users in a matter of a blink of eye. Social networks has its advantages and has afforded many benefits to individuals and to society too, it connects the world to each other, it establishes new relationships and consolidate past relationships, it introduces people to each other and remind people of events that friends have, it brings together views and opinions, and it represents a means of exchanging ideas, information and knowledge, developing skills and creative ideas, as well as learning about the culture of other peoples, leading to the development of societies. However, if it was used in a bad and wrong way, this will be reflected on the user life, it might preoccupy the person from his real life, and it may lead to the isolation of people, mental illness and even suicidal tendencies [1]. Suicide behavior is an ancient problem dating back to the dawn of human life and its existence on earth. The World Health Organization (WHO) reported, in 31 January 2018, that every year close to 800 000 people take their own life, which presents approximately 2192 suicides per day, and it mentioned also that suicide represents the second cause of death amidst 15–29-year-olds, after accidents. It is a series of actions by which some individual tries to destroy his own life. It is therefore difficult to establish specific causes of suicide. Many studies [2–4] combined the social, psychological and medical factors among them for the suicide act. As this phenomenon is impossible to control and extract from human behavior. Despite the fact that the rates of diagnosing mental and psychological health have enhanced in the course of recent decades, several cases continue to be undetected. Indications and symptoms related with psychological illness and even suicide are recognizable on social networks, blogs and even emails [5, 6], which leads researchers to increase their works in the analysis of feelings expressed on these social networks to come up with the best automated systems for discovering and predicting severe depression and suicidal thoughts [7], this field of research is presented in the literature as sentiment analysis [8]. Therefore, and for this particular purpose, many researches have been done in order to detect possible online victims to increase the prevention of suicide using social media [6]. However, to date there is limited studies that are especially focused on suicidal ideation based on Arabic suicidal notes [5]. Thus, our work presents a contribution to the literature of predicting suicidal ideations based on Arabic-language notes by (i) creating a new Arabic dataset, containing suicidal and non-suicidal notes, to identify and extract special features which are specific to suicidal intentions, (ii) developing and creating a classifier model capable of recognizing disturbing and suspicious notes and predicting self-harmful ideations of the individual.

The remainder of the paper is organized as follows. Section 2 describes the related work on sentiment analysis topic and especially on suicidal ideations detection. Section 3 describes methodology. Experimental results and discussion are presented in Sect. 4. And finally, Sect. 5 draws conclusions and identify possible perspectives for future work.

2 Related Work

Many studies have focused on the notes left by individuals before committing a suicide. The analysis of these notes led to the development of supervised and unsupervised classifiers in order to identify the topics discussed as well as the emotions and sentiments expressed [9].

More recently, several studies have worked on the evaluation of suicidal risk factors in social media to better understand or prevent suicide by detecting suicidal ideation early. For example, Birjali [5] builds a corpus related to suicide from Twitter using the Twitter4J API. After that, it computes the semantic similarity, based on WordNet, of new tweets and tweets of corpus. Schoene [10] focused on the linguistic features in discourse that are representative of a suicidal state of mind and automatically identifies them based on supervised classification. It used three different datasets: Genuine Suicide Notes (GSN), Love/happiness (LH) and Depression/loneliness (DL). For each dataset, it extracted two types of features: sentiment features and linguistic features. And it executed several experiments on those two types of features using several classification algorithms. The results showed that using a combination of sentiment analysis and linguistic features with the logistic tree regressor algorithm gave the greatest accuracy (86.61%). Singh [11] mixed both morphological evaluation and negative sentiment prediction of Punjabi language text. The pre-processing stage of this work included morphological evaluation and normalization of Punjabi words to their respective canonical forms. The following stage carried out training and testing of deep neural network model on refined Punjabi tokens obtained from the previous stage. The proposed model classified Punjabi tokens into four negative classes based on farmer suicide cases with an average accuracy of 90.29%. Alam [12] tried to classify sentiments from Bangla text corpus. The work consisted of two steps: preprocessor step and model generator step. The preprocessor step cleaned the data, mapped words to numbers and produced input matrices for the CNN model built in the model generator step. The used dataset contains 850 comments, 58.82% were positives comments and 41.18% were negatives. To evaluate the system, a comparison with SVM classifier have been done and the results proved that the CNN model had the best performance with an accuracy of 99.87%. Billot [13] presented a comprehensive process of data mining on a sample of suicidal patients from two European hospitals. The first goal of this work was to identify groups of similar patients and the second goal was to identify risk factors associated with the number of attempts. Unsupervised methods (Multiple Correspondence Analysis: MCA, and Hierarchical Classification on Main Components: HCMC) and supervised methods (classification and regression tree: CART) are applied. The authors reclaimed that the obtained results would make it possible for each patient to obtain a precise level of risk on which the hospital decision would be based. The Durkheim 5 project [14] studies the activities of US veterans on Twitter, Facebook and LinkedIn. The aim of this project is to identify risk behavior signs. It developed prediction models using the notes texts. The results show that suicidal people often express fear and agitation before taking action. The prediction models proposed showed accuracy rates close to 65%. Gunn [15] analyzed the Twitter messages of a girl who had just committed suicide, published the twenty-four hours before her death.

They found an increase in positive emotions and a shift from self-focusing to others when the moment of death approached. The authors also studied a wider range of tweets. For this, they used the Linguistic Inquiry and Word Count (LIWC) software to identify emotionally charged words and cognitive processes in speech. Sueki [16] used an online panel of 250 twenties, regularly using Twitter, to examine the association between suicide tweets and taking action. The authors studied the linguistic characteristics of suicidal thoughts and ideation. For example, sentences such as "I want to commit suicide" are highly associated with suicide attempts, while sentences suggesting suicidal intent such as "I want to die" are less associated. Unlike popular learning techniques, Karmen [17] combined several automatic language processing methods to filter forum users and identify symptoms of depression. These authors matched traditional depression screening questionnaires with a set of symptom-related terms. Then, they detect these terms in the texts and deduce a score at the message level.

Current literature suffers from an immense lacks models for predicting suicide attempts based on Arabic notes. Currently, very few approaches focused on severe depression and suicidal intention of individuals expressing themselves on Arabic language.

3 Methodology of Suicidal Sentiment Analysis

The methodology followed in this work can be resumed in three parts: the first part is the collection of the dataset; the dataset is collected manually from different resources (Twitter, Facebook, Forums, Blogs and Magazines). The second part is the construction of the feature matrix associated to each note. This feature matrix is the vertical concatenation of the feature vectors of all the words in the note. Those feature vectors are obtained with the help of the Term Frequency-Inverse Document Frequency (TF-IDF) method. The third part is about building a Convolutional Neural Network (CNN) model capable of distinguishing the correct suicidal notes from other notes based on the extracted feature matrix. Figure 1, illustrates the architecture of our work.

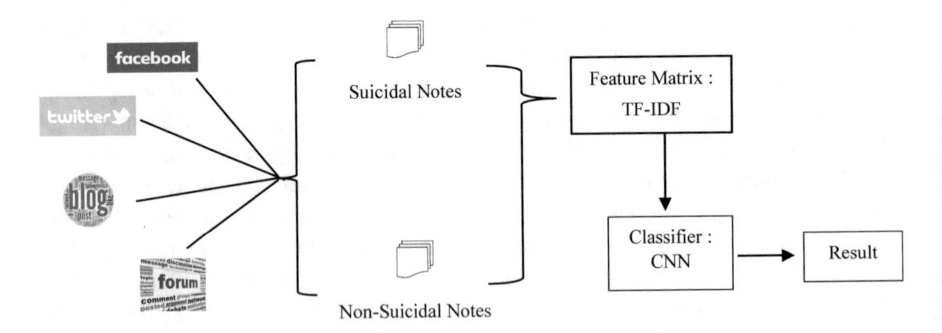

Fig. 1. Architecture of our suicide detection system

3.1 Data Collection

Due to the absence of any online suicidal or depression corpus in Arabic or any other language, and for the purpose of analyzing Arabic suicidal notes, we initially collected notes from several Websites (Facebook, Twitter, Blogs and Forums) written in Arabic. This brought approximately 300 anonymized posts with different length from a couple of words to many sentences. We have some difficulties in collecting these 300 notes, and the reason of that is because the suicide act is considered as a taboo in Arab culture, so we rarely talk about it. and the notes left by the suicidal are, in most cases, hidden and even destroyed, and rarely communicated and posted to the public. All collected notes were annotated manually and categorized into two classes: suicidal and non-suicidal notes. After collecting the corpus, we applied a preprocessing step on the corpora: elimination of punctuations, special characters and stop words [18]. And next, a light-stemming algorithm [19] was applied to remove all extensions from every word.

3.2 Feature Matrix

The classifier cannot deal with the notes directly, so we must represent the notes in a way that the classifier can deal with. That representation is called the Feature Matrix. Each word from each note is represented with a feature vector based on the application of TF-IDF method, and the concatenation of those vectors is the Feature Matrix specific to the note in question.

Basically, TF-IDF calculates the relative frequency of a word in a document compared to the inverse ratio of that word over the whole corpus. Naturally, the TF-IDF proves how important a given word is for a particular document. So, common words in the entire corpus have lower TF-IDF scores, while words that are found in a single or some documents have higher TF-IDF scores. Given a group of documents E, a word w, and an individual document $d \in E$, we calculate $w_{w,d}$ the weight of the word w by applying (1) and (2).

$$w_{w,d} = TF \times IDF \tag{1}$$

$$W_{w,d} = h_{w,d} \times \log(|E| / h_{w,E}) \tag{2}$$

where $h_{w,d}$ is the number of times the word w appears in the document d, $|E|$ is the size of the corpus, and $h_{w,E}$ is the number of documents in which w is found [20].

Let's say that $|E| \sim h_{w,E}$, i.e. the word w appears in all the documents of the corpus E. If (3) is true for some very small constant cte, at that point $w_{w,d}$ will be smaller than $h_{w,d}$ yet still positive.

$$1 < \log(|E| / f_{w,E}) < cte \tag{3}$$

This suggests that the word w is approximately present in all the documents of the corpus E, and yet at the same time presents some significance throughout E. For instance, this could be the situation for extremely basic words such as articles, pronouns, and prepositions.

Finally, imagine that $h_{w,d}$ is large and $h_{w,E}$ is small. At that point, $log(|E|/h_{w,E})$ will be quite large, and so $w_{w,d}$ will obviously be large. We are more interested in this situation, since the words with high $w_{w,d}$ suggest that they are significant in the document d but not common in the corpus E.

Thus, a list of the most descriptive words expressing severe depression and suicide intention is provided with their weight (TF-IDF) and arranged by those values.

3.3 Classification Step: Convolutional Neural Networks

In this section, we reformulate the problem and present our model so that it can be used to monitor suicidal thoughts. Our model is based on the Convolutional Neural Networks (CNN). Moreover, it can be easily generalized regardless of the number of emotional states.

Most of classification algorithms require the construction of a multidimensional feature vector used as input to the algorithm. Therefore, experts become indispensable to define the feature vectors of the desired operation. A different and innovative approach lies in not using an expert to build the feature vector, by automatically extracting it using a learning algorithm. Deep learning algorithms are algorithms that have the ability to automatically learn deep and useful features for the classification task. CNN are variants of those deep learning algorithms. In fact, they are very similar to ordinary Neural Networks, they are made up of neurons that have learnable weights and biases. Each neuron receives some inputs, executes a dot product and it may follow it with a nonlinear function. The entire system still expresses a single differentiable score function: from the inputs to the classes in the outputs. And they still have a loss function on the last layer. CNNs are typically a sequence of successive layers, in which the outputs of every layer are the inputs of the next layer. Those layers are: convolutional layers, pooling layers and fully connected layers [21, 22].

In our proposed CNN model, the typical convolutional layer, pooling layer and fully-connected layer are illustrated in Fig. 2.

Input Matrix. We fixed the input in 80 words, and that's because the larger note in our corpus, after the preprocessing step, has 80 words. The dimension of the word vectors is 300, and that is the total number of documents in the whole corpus. We let s mean the number of words and dw mean the dimension of the word vector, therefrom we now have an input matrix of the shape s $\times$ dw or 80 $\times$ 300.

Filters. One of the advantages of CNN is that it preserves orientation, that's good for us because texts have a one-dimensional structure where the sequence of words in a given text has its importance. Moreover, all words in the corpus are each replaced by a 300-dimensional word vector. Therefrom, one dimension of the filter was fixed for all the filters to match the word vectors, and the region size h was varied from one filter to another. Region size represents the number of rows of the input matrix, which mean the number of words the filter can handle at once. In the Fig. 2, filters represent exactly the filters with their different region sizes, it does not represent the results of filtering operation of the input matrix. We picked here to utilize 3 region sizes, each region recovers respectively 2, 3 and 4 words at once. Furthermore, 2 filters for each region was chosen. Generally speaking, there is 6 filters.

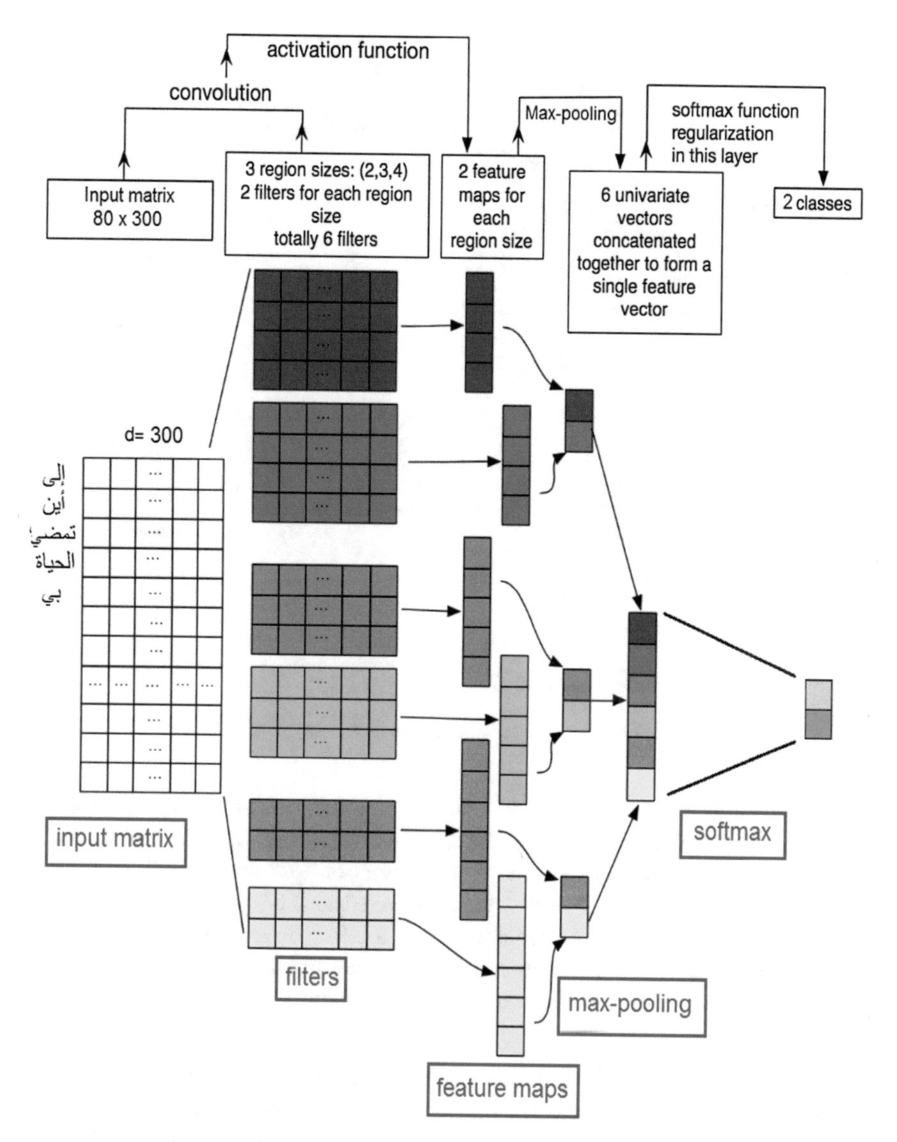

Fig. 2. Illustration of our (CNN) model architecture for depression notes expressed in Arabic language

Feature Maps. In this section, we explain how convolutions/filtering are performed by the CNN. We have filled the input matrix with some results, and the filter matrix also is filtered with some numbers for clarity the explanation. This example is illustrated in Fig. 3.

In the beginning, the two-word filter, represented by the (2×300) yellow matrix w, get over the word vectors of "إلى" and "أين". After that, it calculates an element-wise product for all its (2×300) elements, and then it calculates the sum of these products

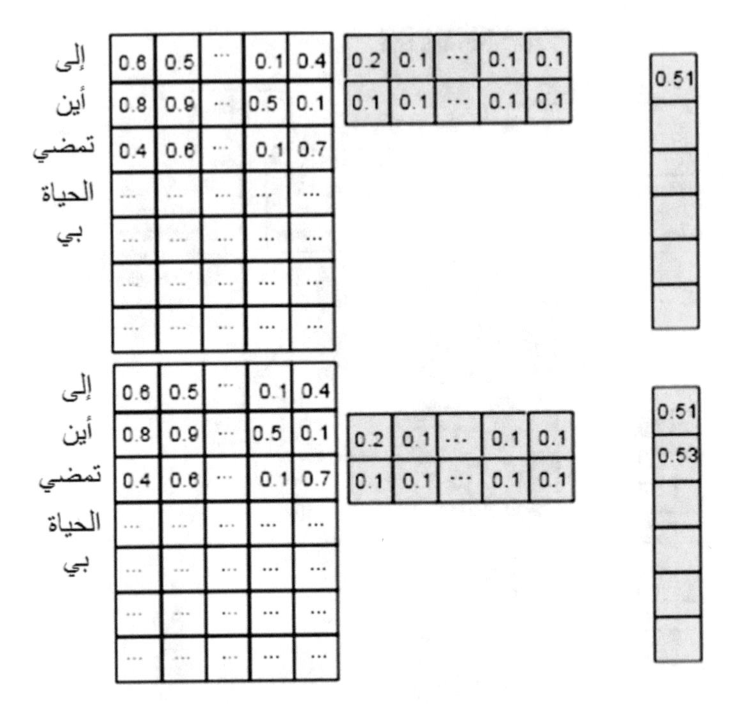

Fig. 3. How convolutions (filtering) work

and get one number ($0.6 \times 0.2 + 0.5 \times 0.1 + \ldots + 0.4 \times 0.1 = 0.51$). 0.51 represents the first element of the output sequence, o, for this filter. At that point, the filter descends by 1 word and get over the word vectors of “أين” and “تمضي” and the same operation is remade to get 0.53. Thus, the new dimensions of o will be ($s - h + 1 \times 1$), in this case (79×1). To get the feature map, c, a bias term is added, and an activation function is applied. The activation function that we chose to apply is the Rectified Linear Unit function (ReLU). The resulting feature map c has the same dimensions as o (79×1).

Max-pooling. The dimensionality of c is reliant both s and h, which mean, it will change through filters of various region sizes. To handle this issue, we used the max-pooling function and pull out just the biggest number from each c vector and drops the rest. This function assumes that the highest number is more significant and has more information than the rest of the vector.

Softmax. After the max-pooling step, the resulting vector has a fixed-length of 6 elements (number of filters). This resulting vector can then be fed into a fully-connected (softmax) layer to achieve the classification task.

4 Experimental Results and Discussion

The work has been done on a MacBook Pro i7 6th Generation (206 GHz), RAM 16 Go, Hard disk: SSD 512 Go, touring on MacOs High Sierra.

4.1 Datasets

The dataset is a collection of Arabic notes written in classical and modern Arabic language. The text contains alphabetic, numeric and symbolic words. The dataset consists of 300 notes and 5550 words structured and categorized into two text files (see Table 1). This dataset was divided into two sections: training dataset and testing dataset. The training dataset represents 70% of each class and it allows us to build the model, while the testing dataset represents the remaining 30% and it helps us to verify the accuracy of our model. Records in the dataset were stored as matrices, where every word is presented as a vector.

Table 1. Number of words and notes in the dataSet

Classes	Notes	Words
Suicide	120	2000
Nonsuicide	180	3550

4.2 CNNs Experiments Setup

The choice of hyper-parameters of CNNs model may influence the performance of the classification. In our experiments we employ stochastic gradient descent (SGD) to train the network and use backpropagation algorithm to calculate the gradients. We initialize the learning rate at 0.001. Likewise, we utilize Dropout [23] to enable the model to better converge (dropout ratio as 0.5).

4.3 Baseline Methods

We use the Weka machine learning libraries [24] to conduct some baselines experiments. We choose two of the most used algorithms in the classification task: Naive Bayes classifier (NB) and K-Nearest Neighbor classifier (KNN). Our choice of the Weka tool is based on its popularity in the machine learning community. It is well adjusted to the field of machine learning algorithms as well as for data mining algorithms. Moreover, it is simple to use, and it supports several types of data formats.

4.4 Results and Discussions

The classification was done multiple of times and the experimental evaluation metrics are the averages of precision, of recall and of F1-Score which were calculated after each classification step.

In Table 2 and Fig. 4, we present the results, in precision, recall and the F1- score, of suicidal and non-suicidal notes prediction performance of baseline and our CNN model. We can notice from those results that our CNNs model has the best performances. Our model presents the highest precision of 82.14%, and in the second place we find the k-nearest neighbor with a precision of 77.04% and in the third place the precision of Naive Bayes with 74.23%. We find the same order in Recall and F1-Score both where our CNN model has always the best results. Those results are quit satisfying despite the fact that they are under the 90%. The reason for that is the relatively small size of the corpus used to build our model (300 notes, 5550 words).

Table 2. Evaluations of NB, K-NN and our CNN model on suspected suicidal notes.

	Precision	Recall	F1-Score
NB	74.23	68.14	71.05
K-NN	77.04	70.77	73.77
CNNs	82.14	75.27	79.07

Compared with the Bag of Words model (BoW) used in the baseline methods, the TF-IDF method gives the best results as a way of reformulating and presenting textual data, which increases the performances of the classification task.

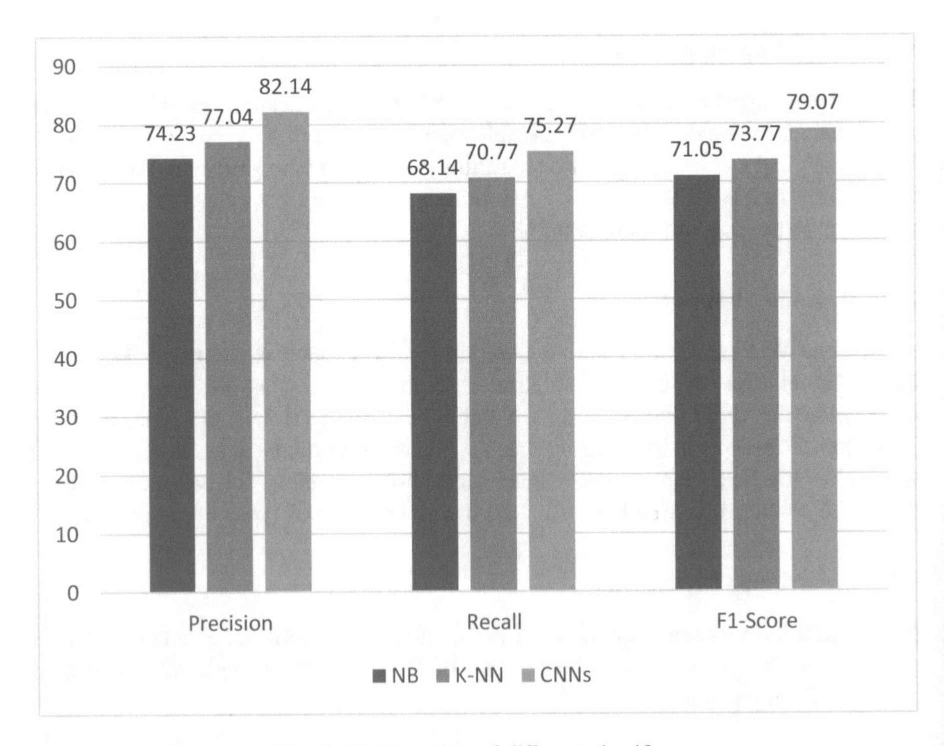

Fig. 4. Performance of different classifiers

The experiment results clearly illustrate that our model obtained the best performance on the suicidal note classification. This indicates that a part of our model is specialized in unsupervised feature extraction, so the noise is extracted from data and the most significant features are chosen. With clean and relevant data, the chances of getting the most accurate results are greater.

5 Conclusion

In this paper we propose an automatic system to extract and predict the suicidal intention of an individual based on textual messages and notes. To build our system, we collected a corpus formed with actual suicidal notes and non-suicidal notes. Those notes are writing in Arabic language, so we use the TF-IDF method to reformulate those notes into a presentation that our system can recognize and understand. And finally, we build up a model based on CNN algorithms to recognize and classify notes that present potential suicidal intention and those that are not.

References

1. Burnap, P., Colombo, G., Amery, R., Hodorog, A., Scourfield, J.: Multi-class machine classification of suicide-related communication on Twitter. Online Soc. Netw. Media J. **2**, 32–44 (2017). https://doi.org/10.1016/j.osnem.2017.08.001
2. Simons, R.L., Murphy, P.I.: Sex differences in the causes of adolescent suicide ideation. J. Youth Adolesc. **14**(5) (1985). https://doi.org/10.1007/BF02138837
3. Cha, C.B., et al.: Examining potential iatrogenic effects of viewing suicide and self-injury stimuli. Psychol. Assess. J. **28**(11), 1510–1515 (2016). https://doi.org/10.1037/pas0000280
4. Chatard, A., Selimbegović, L.: When self-destructive thoughts flash through the mind: failure to meet standards affects the accessibility of suicide-related thoughts. J. Personal. Soc. Psychol. **100**(4), 587–605 (2011). https://doi.org/10.1037/a0022461
5. Birjali, M., Beni-Hssane, A., Erritali, M.: A method proposed for estimating depressed feeling tendencies of social media users utilizing their data. In: Abraham, A., Haqiq, A., Alimi, A.M., Mezzour, G., Rokbani, N., Muda, A.K. (eds.) Proceedings of the 16th International Conference on Hybrid Intelligent Systems (HIS 2016), Marrakech, Morocco. Advances in Intelligent Systems and Computing, vol. 552, pp. 413–420. Springer, Cham (2016). https://doi.org/10.1007/978-3-319-52941-7_41
6. Kasturi, D.V., Nurhafizah, T.: Suicide detection system based on twitter. In: Science and Information Conference, London, UK, pp. 785–788. IEEE (2014). https://doi.org/10.1109/sai.2014.6918275
7. Gualtiero, B., Colombo, P., Burnapa, A., Hodorog, J.S.: Analysing the connectivity and communication of suicidal users on twitter. Comput. Commun. **73**, 291–300 (2016). https://doi.org/10.1016/j.comcom.2015.07.018
8. Gonzalez-Marron, D., Mejia-Guzman, D., Enciso-Gonzalez, A.: Exploiting data of the Twitter social network using sentiment analysis. In: Sucar, E., Mayora, O., Munoz de Cote, E. (eds.) Applications for Future Internet. Lecture Notes of the Institute for Computer Sciences, Social Informatics and Telecommunications Engineering, vol. 179. Springer, Cham (2017). https://doi.org/10.1007/978-3-319-49622-1_5

9. Spasic, I., Burnap, P., Greenwood, M., Arribas, M.A.: A Naïve Bayes approach to classifying topics in suicide notes. Biomed. Inform. Insights **5**(1), 87–97 (2012). https://doi.org/10.4137/bii.s8945
10. Schoene, A.M., Dethlefs, N.: Automatic identification of suicide notes from linguistic and sentiment features. In: Proceedings of the 10th SIGHUM Workshop on Language Technology for Cultural Heritage, Social Sciences, and Humanities, Berlin, Germany, pp. 128–133. Association for Computational Linguistics (2016). https://doi.org/10.18653/v1/w16-2116
11. Singh, J., Singh, G., Singh, R., Singh, P.: Morphological evaluation and sentiment analysis of Punjabi text using deep learning classification. J. King Saud Univ. Comput. Inf. Sci. (2018). https://doi.org/10.1016/j.jksuci.2018.04.003
12. Alam, M.H., Rahoman, M.-M., Azad, M.A.K.: Sentiment analysis for Bangla sentences using convolutional neural network. In: The 20th International Conference of Computer and Information Technology (ICCIT), Dhaka, Bangladesh, pp. 1–6. IEEE (2017).https://doi.org/10.1109/iccitechn.2017.8281840
13. Billot, R., Berrouiguet, S., Larsen, M., Walter, M., Castroman, J.L., García, E.B., Courtet, P., Lenca, P.: Providing data mining for suicidal risk prevention. Apport de la fouille de données pour la prévention du risque suicidaire. In: Proceedings of International Conference on Extraction and Knowledge Management, vol. RNTI-E-34, Magazine of New Information Technologies, Paris, France, pp. 143–154 (2018)
14. Poulin, C., et al.: Predicting the risk of suicide by analyzing the text of clinical notes. PLoS ONE **9**(1) (2014). https://doi.org/10.1371/journal.pone.0085733
15. Gunn, J.F., Lester, D.: Twitter postings and suicide: an analysis of the postings of a fatal suicide in the 24 h prior to death. Suicidologi **17**(3), 28–30 (2012)
16. Sueki, H.: The association of suicide-related twitter use with suicidal behavior: a cross sectional study of young internet users in japan. J. Affect. Disord. **170**(1), 155–160 (2015). https://doi.org/10.1016/j.jad.2014.08.047
17. Karmen, C., Hsiung, R.C., Wetter, T.: Screening internet forum participants for depression symptoms by assembling and enhancing multiple NLP methods. Comput. Methods Programs Biomed. J. **120**(1), 27–36 (2015). https://doi.org/10.1016/j.cmpb.2015.03.008
18. Bahassine, S., Kissi, M., Madani, A.: Arabic text classification using new stemmer for feature selection and decision trees. J. Eng. Sci. Technol. **12**(6), 1475–1487 (2017)
19. Larkey, L.S., Ballesteros, L., Connell, M.: Improving stemming for Arabic information retrieval: light stemming and cooccurrence analysis. In: The 25th Annual International Conference on Research and Development in Information Retrieval (SIGIR 2002), Tampere, Finland, pp. 275–282 (2002)
20. Salton, G., Buckley, C.: Term-weighing approach in automatic text retrieval. Inf. Process. Manag. **24**(5), 513–523 (1988). https://doi.org/10.1016/0306-4573(88)90021-0
21. Krizhevsky, A., Sutskever, I., Hinton, G.E.: ImageNet classification with deep convolutional neural networks. In: Proceedings of the 25th International Conference on Neural Information Processing Systems, NIPS 2012, Lake Tahoe, Nevada, vol. 1, pp. 1097–1105. IEEE (2012). https://doi.org/10.1145/3065386
22. Lecun, Y., Bottou, L., Bengio, Y., Haffner, P.: Gradient-based learning applied to document recognition. Proc. IEEE **86**(11), 2278–2324 (1998). https://doi.org/10.1109/5.726791
23. Al-Zaghoul, F., Al-Dhaheri, S.: Arabic text classification based on features reduction using artificial neural networks. In: The 15th International Conference on Computer Modelling and Simulation (UKSim), Cambridge University, United Kingdom, pp. 485–490. IEEE (2013). https://doi.org/10.1109/uksim.2013.135
24. WEKA: A machine learning tool set. http://www.cs.waikato.ac.nz/ml/weka/index_downloading.html. Accessed 9 Aug 2018

The Role of Recommender System of Tags in Clinical Decision Support

Sara Qassimi(✉), El Hassan Abdelwahed, Meriem Hafidi, and Rachid Lamrani

Laboratory ISI, Cadi Ayyad University, Marrakesh, Morocco
{sara.qassimi,meriem.hafidi,rachid.lamrani}@ced.uca.ma,
abdelwahed@uca.ac.ma

Abstract. The widespread use of the Electronic Health Records EHRs has increasingly emerged in the healthcare industry. The structured and unstructured forms of EHRs are implemented in a Clinical Decision Support System CDSS. The CDSS is an health information technology system designed to provide healthcare professionals with clinical decision support. In this article, we aim to enhance the computer-aided diagnosis in medical imaging by recommending diseases for each patient's medical image. We propose a recommender system of tags based on the tags co-occurrence, the graph of tags and the graph of the community of patients. The proposed approach is called MedicalRecomTags. The tags are the commonly used diseases or pathologies terms. The graphs, namely, the graph of tags and the graph of the community of patients, are derived by analyzing the annotated medical images. The experimental results show the effectiveness of the tag recommendation approach. In future works, the suggested tags will be evaluated by healthcare providers to affirm their relevancy. The intended online evaluation will enrich and enhance the recommender system of tags.

Keywords: Recommender system of tags · Graph-based tag recommendation · Electronic health record · Clinical images · Clinical decision support

1 Introduction

The implementation of the Electronic Health Record EHR has surged in the recent years. An electronic health record contains basic information of a patient including his medical history and detailed clinical data [1]. The healthcare providers use software to store, maintain and share their patients' EHR in structured and unstructured form. This software, called Clinical Decision Support System CDSS, is designed to aid healthcare providers in making clinical decision support including organizations guidelines like patients follow up, reminders, warning systems, and diagnostic suggestions [2]. The CDSS provides effective supports when it has a full access to the EHRs data carrying clinical information, like laboratory results and clinical observation diagnosis notes.

M. Ezziyyani (Ed.): AI2SD 2018, AISC 914, pp. 273–285, 2019.
https://doi.org/10.1007/978-3-030-11884-6_25

Most efforts had been devoted to the structured part of patients' EHRs by improving the process of linking, reusing and accelerating data analysis [3]. Nonetheless, most of the clinicians lean towards textual notes to communicate important information about their patients [4]. In primary care electronic patient records, the free text medical notes have a rich source of information that could be of great use for the CDSS. The clinical text notes incorporate details about symptoms and diseases which enrich and complement structured information [5]. In some cases, the textual notes are the only available health information that activates and triggers the CDSS. For example, the medical history, physical examination, and radiography diagnosis are reported in free-text form [6].

However, the act of typing detailed free-text electronic notes is time-consuming and not easily accessible and readable [7]. Moreover, physicians spend two hours documenting a patient's EHR for one hour of medical consulting [8]. The clinical text notes are characterized by breve and succinct expressions of medical terms. The medical jargon might contain spelling mistakes, abbreviations and ungrammatical constructions which harden the employing of Natural Language Processing (NPL) tools [5]. The off-the-shelf NPL tools use machine learning-based method that requires a golden training set of adequate annotated clinical text notes. The authors [10] provided an important number of frontal chest X-ray images and image labels (tags) mined from the radiology reports using natural language processing (see Table 1). Fourteen text-minded labels (tags) represent common thoracic pathologies. These extracted tags are namely, Atelectasis, Consolidation, Infiltration, Pneumothorax, Edema, Emphysema, Fibrosis, Effusion, Pneumonia, Pleural_thickening, Cardiomegaly, Nodule, Mass and Hernia.

Table 1. Chest X-ray image and its extracted disease keywords [10]

Radiology report	Extracted keywords	Image
findings: frontal lateral chest x-ray performed in expiration. left apical pneumothorax visible. small pneumothorax visible along the left heart border and left hemidiaphragm. pleural thickening, mass right chest. the mediastinum cannot be evaluated in the expiration. bony structures intact. impression: left post biopsy pneumothorax.	Mass Pneumothorax	

Medical images are pictures that represent the internal structures and functions of an anatomic region [11]. The commonly used medical imaging techniques are Ultrasound, Magnetic Resonance Imaging (MRI), Computed Tomogram Scan (CT Scan) and X-rays [12]. Tagging approach is a representation of semantic interpretations. It affords an efficient management of pictures, such as their search and discoverer [12]. Tagging will facilitate diagnosis of diseases by reducing loosely annotated or unannotated medical images. The tagged medical images will facilitate clustering patients with common diseases and help healthcare providers' interpretations.

Our motivation position encourages the use of succinct medical expressions and terms "Tags". Indeed, suggestions are made to involve physicians in generating succinct and easily readable notes containing essential information [9]. A Tag is a descriptive annotation that represents the commonly used clinical terms. The use of tags will promote sharing medical information efficiently by protecting patients' sensitive information.

The chest X-ray exam is considered as one of the most frequent and cost-effective medical imaging examination [10,21]. This paper focuses on improving interpretation of images (e.g. X-ray images) by suggestion relevant tags as pathologies terms. Therefore, in order to achieve clinically relevant computer-aided detection and diagnosis of medical images, we aim to develop a recommender system of tags, MedicalRecomTags approach, helping diagnosis by suggesting relevant tags to annotate the medical images and improve their interpretation. This approach proposes an advanced tag co-occurrence recommendation by using generated graphs. The graph-based tag recommendation will rely on two graphs, a graph relating different tags (medical diseases terms) and another graph linking the community of patients.

The rest of the paper is organized as follows: Sect. 2 presents related research to tags recommendation. Section 3 describes the proposed approach of the recommendation of tags, called MedicalRecomTags. The experimental results and evaluation are described in Sect. 4. Finally, the conclusion and future directions are delineated in Sect. 5.

2 Related Work

The approach of tagging is one such approach to facilitating organization of images and potentially improve their findability, understandability and discovery [12]. The tagging process can take full advantage of the tag recommendation [22]. Tag recommendation employs several underlying techniques, namely, content-based, tag co occurrence based, matrix factorization based, graph-based, clustering based, L2R based [13].

The tag co-occurrence based method analyzes previously used tags. The recommender system suggests related tags to the user based on the previous user's or other people attributed tags. The recommender system of tags is updated with additional entered or selected tags annotating the object [14]. The proposed interactive method is extended by exploring tag co-occurrences within different categories. Either restricting the tag suggestion to the object of a specific user, or to the community of the user or to explore the whole data collection [15,16].

In addition to the exploration of tags co-occurrences, researchers [16,17] proposed hybrid methods using also the content based method that extract tag candidates from the textual feature of the target object. The content-based item recommendation method, which aims at matching a target user's interests by filtering items similar to the items that the user had rated, annotated or liked previously [18]. The content-based techniques solve the cold start problem when there is an absence of previous tags. However, these techniques have to deal with extracting pertinent terms from a large number of textual content features of the untagged object. They lack novelty since they rely on already existing descriptive terms which may be less useful than the other new diversified tags [13].

The graph-based tag recommendation method relies on the neighbourhood of the target object or user to extract candidates. The nodes of the graph represent the related objects (or users) connected by edges describing their similarity in terms of similar features, including previous tags describing the objects (or the similar tags previously used by users). The exploration of the tag's history of users compared to the target user's previously used tags initiate the collaborative filtering-based method [13]. In this context, the collaborative filtering-based method acts on similarities among users. Therefore, to suggest tags to a user, the method finds similar users and recommend tags used by these users. The authors [20] proposed a hybrid TagCombine algorithm. It predicts tags combining multi-label ranking algorithm. The graph-based methods solve the cold start problem by exploring relationships among the nodes (target objects and/or users).

3 Proposed Approach: MedicalRecomTags

The proposed approach considers the co-occurrence technique to construct the graph-based tag recommendation algorithms. We propose a graph-based model for the recommendation of tags called MedicalRecomTags, where tags are the diseases characterizing the medical images. The tags recommendation aims to guide healthcare providers when they analyze the medical images and prepare their reports that summarize the findings and impressions. Indeed, choosing among the suggested tags to describe a medical image will reduce healthcare providers' cognitive load for diagnosing diseases.

We denote a community of patients P having a set of images I annotated with a set of tags T.

$$P = \{P_1, ..., P_l\}\ ,\ I = \{I_1, ..., I_k\}\ and\ T = \{t_1, ..., t_n\} \\ Where,\ l\ ,\ k\ and\ n\ are\ finite\ numbers. \tag{1}$$

Our method (see Fig. 1) models the rich information of the patient and their annotated medical images to build two graphs (a graph of tags, a graph of the community of patients). To address the challenging issue of weighting the graphs between different types of nodes, we propose a graph model derived from the tripartite relationship among patients, their images and tags. It derives 3 layers, namely the patients, images and tags layers. Besides, the approach considers the extraction of tags based on the co-occurrence method that retrieves the assigned tags from the patient's previously taken medical images. We consider two simple graphs (Graph of patients and tags).

3.1 Preliminaries

A graph G = (V, E) represents a set of nodes V and a set of edges E connecting pair of nodes, where E $\subseteq$ V $\times$ V. There are multiple alternatives to centrality measures (e.g. degree, betweenness, closeness centrality) to represent the strength of node in the entire graph. We choose the weighted degree centrality measure of both undirected graphs of tags and patients. It defines the sum of links' weight that the node has with its neighbours. The degree centrality measures the level of involvement of a node within a network.

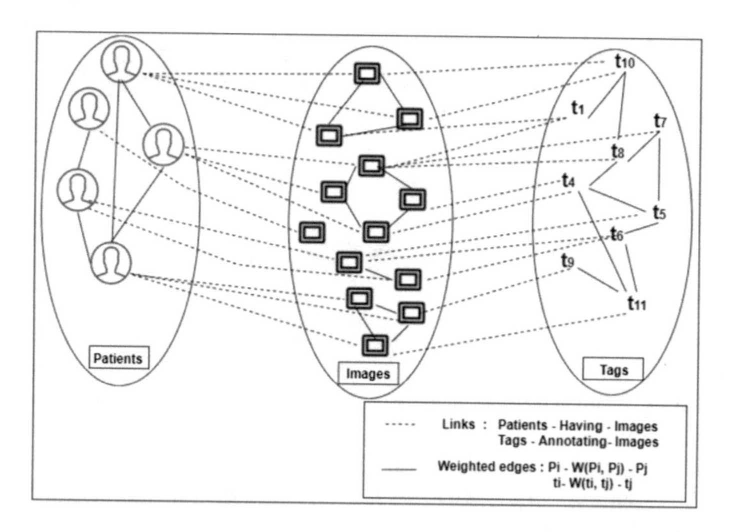

Fig. 1. Tripartite relationship: graph of patients, and a graph of tags related by images

Two undirected weighted graphs are defined, namely patients' network and tags' network, denoted by G_P and G_T. The nodes represent patients in G_P and tags in G_T, tied with weighted edges. Patients are tied with weighted edges connecting two patients that have medical images tagged with common tags. Whereas, tags' ties refer to the common annotated patients and their images.

3.2 Co-occurrence and Graph of Tags

Implicit relationships among tags play an essential role in enhancing the tags recommendation. The tags' community clusters semantically close tags into groups. This semantic relationship considers the association between tags, images and patients. According to the PageRank algorithm, an object is an important source of recommendation when it is tagged by important (active) users [19]. Accordingly, we consider a tag is relevant when it annotates an important number of patient's images. The generated semantic graph of tags is an undirected graph of tags whose nodes are the tags -diseases terms- linked by edges $W(t_i, t_j)$, where $t_i, t_j \in T$.

$$W(t_i, t_j) = W_P(t_i, t_j) \times W_I(t_i, t_j) \tag{2}$$

where:

$W_p(t_i, t_j)$ is the patient based weight;
$W_I(t_i, t_j)$ is the image based weight.

$$W_P(t_i, t_j) = \frac{NP\ having\ images\ annotated\ by\ t_i\ and\ t_j}{Number\ of\ patients\ with\ annotated\ images} \quad (3)$$

$$W_I(t_i, t_j) = \frac{NI\ annotated\ by\ t_i\ and\ t_j}{Number\ of\ annotated\ images} \quad (4)$$

NP is the Number of Patients;
NI is the Number of Images.
Each tag t_i has its weighted degree centrality.

$$w_c(t_i) = \sum_{j}^{n} W(t_i, t_j) \quad (5)$$

where t_i is the focal node, t_j represents all other nodes, with $i \neq j$ and $1 \leq j \leq n$, n is the total number of tags.

Considering a patient $P_i \in P$ who has a set of images $I_{Pi} \subset I$ described by a set of tags $T_{Pi} \subset T$.

The recommendation of tags to annotate an image $i_{Pi} \in I_{Pi}$ can be performed using the Algorithm 1. The algorithm recommends tags of the patient's previous tags (tags co-occurrence recommendation).

Algorithm 1. Tag Recommendation based on the patient's previous tags

1: $P_i \in P$; $I_{Pi} \subset I$; $T_{Pi} \subset T$; ia_{Pi}, $i_{Pi} \in I_{Pi}$
2: Rt_{Pi}, $t_{Pi} \subset T_{Pi}$
3: i_{Pi} : an image from I_{Pi}
4: ia_{Pi} : an annotated image from I_{Pi}
5: t_{Pi} : a set of tags annotating images of P_i
6: Rt_{Pi} : a set of recommended tags
7: **procedure** RecommendationPreviousTags(P_i,i_{Pi})
8: $\quad ia_{Pi} \neq i_{Pi}$
9: $\quad$ **for** each $ia_{Pi} \in I_{Pi}$ **do**
10: $\quad\quad Rt_{Pi} \leftarrow$ list of t_{Pi}
11: $\quad$ **end for**
12: $\quad$ **return** Rt_{Pi}
13: **end procedure**

In order to enhance the recommendation of tags, it is relevant to make use of the graph of tags. The Algorithm 2 describes a Tags' graph based recommendation of tags by suggesting related tags of either the target image or the related tags of the patient's previous tags. Moreover, the graph of tags offers a global view of the strongly related tags so as to solve the cold start problem.

Algorithm 2. Tag Recommendation based on the Graph of tags

```
P_i ∈ P; I_Pi ⊂ I; T_Pi ⊂ T
i_Pi ∈ I_Pi
Relt_Pi, Rt_Pi, t_Pi ⊂ T_Pi
i_Pi : an image from I_Pi
t_Pi : a set of tags annotating images of P_i
Rt_Pi : a set of recommended tags from Algorithm 1
Relt_Pi : a set of related tags
ti_Pi : the target tag from T_Pi
tj_Pi : a set of related tags to ti_Pi
procedure RecommendationGraphTags(P_i,i_Pi,ti_Pi)
    Rt_Pi ← RecommendationPreviousTags(P_i,i_Pi)
    if ti_Pi annotates i_Pi then
        for each tj_Pi ∈ T_Pi And tj_Pi annotating i_Pi do
            ω ← W(ti_Pi, tj_Pi) × w_c(tj_Pi)
            if ω > threshold then
                Relt_Pi ← list of tj_Pi ranked by ω
            end if
        end for
    else if ti_Pi ∈ Rt_Pi then
        for each tj_Pi ∈ Rt_Pi do
            ω ← W(ti_Pi, tj_Pi) × w_c(tj_Pi)
            if ω > threshold then
                Relt_Pi ← list of tj_Pi ranked by ω
            end if
        end for
    else
        for each tj_Pi ∈ T do
            ω ← W(ti_Pi, tj_Pi) × w_c(tj_Pi)
            if ω > threshold then
                Relt_Pi ← list of tj_Pi ranked by ω
            end if
        end for
    end if
    return Relt_Pi
end procedure
```

3.3 Graph of Patients' Community

The community of patients graph is an undirected graph whose nodes are users tied with weighted edges.

Considering two patients P_i, $P_j \in P$, the nodes' weight of these two patients (6) is denoted by $W(P_i, P_j)$.

$$W(P_i, P_j) = \frac{NTC\ annotating\ images\ of\ P_i\ and\ P_j}{Number\ of\ tags\ in\ the\ corpus} \tag{6}$$

NTC is the Number of Tags in Common.

The weight $W(P_i, P_j)$ represents the tag based weight, it is the quotient corresponding to the number of tags in common annotating the distinct medical images of two different patients divided by the total number of existing tags (diseases terms) in the corpus.

$w_c(P_i)$ represent the weighed degree centrality for the patient P_i.

$$w_c(P_i) = \sum_{j}^{l} W(P_i, P_j) \tag{7}$$

where P_i is the focal node, P_j represents all other nodes, with $i \neq j$ and $1 \leq j \leq l$ and l is the total number of patients.

The method of community-based tag recommendation recommends to the healthcare providers the tags assigned to the k most related patients of the target patient's community.

The Algorithm 3 recommends tags of k most related patients to the patient P_i.

Algorithm 3. Tag Recommendation based on the Community of patients

```
P_i ∈ P; I_Pi ⊂ I; T_Pi ⊂ T
P_j ∈ P; I_Pj ⊂ I; T_Pj ⊂ T
t_Pj : a set of tags annotating images of P_j
Relt_Pi : a set of related tags to P_i
procedure RecommendationTagsCommunity(P_i)
    for each P_j ∈ P do
        if W(P_i, P_j) > 0 then
            ω ← W(P_i, P_j) × w_c(P_j)
            for each t_Pj ∈ T_Pj do
                Relt_Pi ← list of t_Pj ranked by ω limit k
            end for
        end if
    end for
    return Relt_Pi
end procedure
```

4 Experimental Results and Evaluation

4.1 Datasets

Our experimental data was taken from the recent available data set [10]. In our experiments we used a total of 1000 patients having 3663 images with 14 pathologies categories considered as tags (The weighted graph of tags represented in Fig. 2). Each disease or pathology "Tag" annotates a patient's image, which consequently, characterizes the patient's electronic health record (see Table 2).

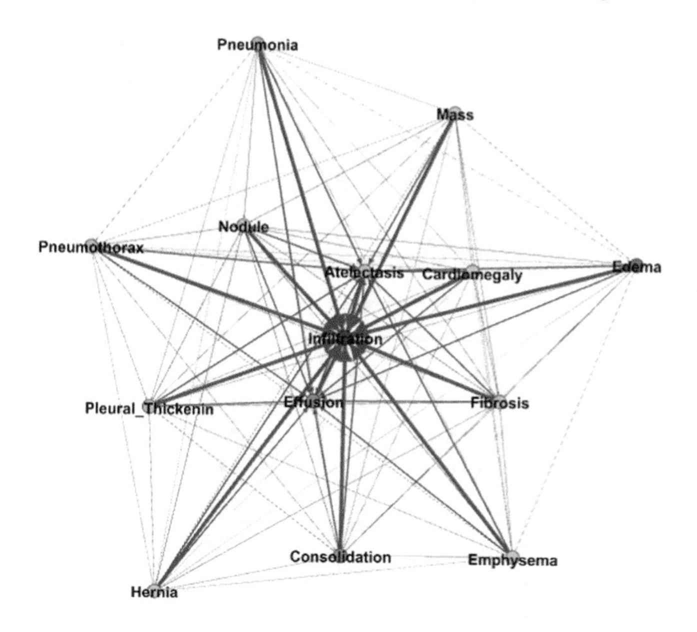

Fig. 2. Graph of tags represented using Gephi

4.2 Results and Evaluation

To evaluate our proposed approach tags recommendations "MedicalRecomTags", we have considered 9 patients to whom the tags recommendations were performed to suggest tags for their X-ray images (10 distinct images).

The evaluation of tag recommendations can be divided into manual or automatic evaluation category [17]. The automatic or offline evaluation considers the previously assigned tags as the ground truth. The images' preassigned tags are the expected answer, true positive, which are the relevant tags for annotating the image. In this case, we are interested in whether the recommender system of tags properly predicts pathologies keywords (tags) to the healthcare providers. The offline evaluation uses the classification accuracy metrics which measure the amount of correct and incorrect classifications as relevant or irrelevant recommended tags. For each patient, we select his previously tags annotating his X-ray image, then generate automatic tags recommendations algorithms (Tag Recommendation based on the Patient's previous tags (Algorithm 1); Tag Recommendation based on the graph of tags (Algorithm 2); Tag Recommendation based on Community of patients (Algorithm 3)) that suggest a set of tags that the health provider will use. The common basic metrics are calculated from the number of tags that are either relevant or irrelevant and either recommended or not. There is four possible outcomes for the recommended tags, as shown in the confusion matrix (see Table 4). The relevant tags are those previous pathologies keywords that are already used to annotate the target X-ray image. The offline metrics used are Precision P, Recall R and F1-measure F (8). These evaluation measures are

Table 2. Number of patients having the disease and number of tagged images for each disease (tag)

Tags	# Patients	# Images
Pneumonia	33	47
Edema	17	60
Pneumothorax	44	139
Hernia	8	23
Mass	61	121
Emphysema	52	95
Consolidation	63	152
Cardiomegaly	79	171
Pleural_Thickening	82	120
Effusion	142	395
Fibrosis	98	141
Nodule	109	162
Infiltration	273	605
Atelectasis	170	350

Table 3. Tag recommendation for the X-ray image

Recommended Tags	Previous Tags	Image
emphysema cardiomegaly fibrosis edema consolidation pleural_thickening infiltration hernia pneumonia nodule pneumothorax mass effusion atelectasis	Mass Pneumothorax	

Table 4. Confusion matrix accumulating the possible results of tag recommendations

	Relevant	Irrelevant
Recommended	True-positive (Tp)	False-positive (Fp)
Not Recommended	False-negative (Fn)	True-negative (Tn)

used to assess how likely the recommendation results meet the ground truth, in other words suggest the relevant previously attributed tags. Precision or true positive accuracy represents the probability that a recommended tag is the relevant tags. Recall or true positive rate represents the probability that a relevant tag is recommended. The best precision and recall are those with the value of 1. The F1-measure combines precision and recall into a single score.

$$P = \frac{Tp}{Tp + Fp}; R = \frac{Tp}{Tp + Fn}; F = \frac{2 \times P \times R}{P + R} \quad (8)$$

Table 5. Evaluation

Relevant tags	Tag recommendation based on								
	Tags graph			Previous tags			Community graph		
	P	R	F	P	R	F	P	R	F
Mass—Pneumothorax	0.666	1	0.8	0	0	-	0.145	1	0.25
Effusion—Fibrosis—Mass—Nodule—Pleural_Thickening	0.571	0.8	0.666	0.5	0.4	0.444	0.385	1	0.555
Atelectasis—Cardiomegaly—Emphysema—Mass—Pneumothorax	0.5	1	0.666	0.25	0.2	0.222	0.384	1	0.555
Atelectasis—Effusion—Infiltration	0.428	1	0.6	0.75	1	0.857	0.231	1	0.375
Effusion—Fibrosis—Nodule—Pleural_Thickening	0.5	1	0.666	0.5	0.5	0.5	0.384	1	0.555
Infiltration	-	0	-	0	0	-	0.083	1	0.154
Atelectasis—Effusion— Pleural_Thickening	-	0	-	0.5	0.666	0.571	0.231	1	0.375
Cardiomegaly—Edema—Effusion—Fibrosis—Infiltration	0.5	1	0.666	0.5	0.4	0.444	0.357	1	0.5263
Atelectasis—Edema—Effusion— Infiltration	0.5	1	0.666	0.5	0.5	0.5	0.333	1	0.5
Consolidation—Effusion—Infiltration—Nodule	-	0	-	0.75	0.75	0.75	0.307	1	0.470

The accuracy measures are presented in the recommender system of tags based on the patient's previous tags, the graph of tags and the community of patients (see Table 5). Obviously, when the evaluation concerns a patient's first taken image, this new patient has never taken an X-ray imaging exam before (i.e. the patient does not have previous annotated X-ray images), the measures scores P and R are equal to zero. In this case, in order to recommend other pathologies or diseases (tags) helping diagnosis, it is pertinent to use both of graph-based recommender system of tags. We notice that the recall is perfectly presenting a good measures' score value which indicates that the proposed approach MedicalRecomTags always recommends the relevant tags that already annotate the target medical image. In general, the scores of the precision, recall and F1-measure are high. The evaluated image in Table 3 is described not only with the previous tags but also with recommended tags coming from the graph based recommender system of tags. However, the healthcare providers' online or manual evaluation is still more accurate to attest the relevancy of the recommender system of tags. The false positive tags might be considered relevant tags which describe other pathologies detected in the X-ray image.

5 Conclusion and Perspectives

The Clinical Decision Support Systems are designed to directly aid in clinical decision making by generating patients specific assessments or recommendations presented to clinicians. We developed a recommender system of tags MedicalRecomTags suggesting relevant diseases (Where tags represent the detected pathologies) to annotate the medical images and improve their interpretation. The recommendations are based on previous images of each patient, based on a graph of the patient's community and a graph relating different diseases (tags). The experimental result has evaluated the effectiveness of our approach. However, we are aiming to proceed with the online evaluation using the healthcare providers feedback. Futures works will focus on strengthening the ties among the network members and expending the patients' community in order to attest the scalability of our method of recommender system of tags "MedicalRecomTags". Furthermore, we aim to consider the mathematical concepts of graph theory to pertinently analyze and define the level of involvement of nodes (patients and tags) within the network. In future perspectives, we will focus on recommending not only tags but also items of interest to healthcare providers and extend the concept of the graph-based recommendation in other application domain such as tourism and education.

References

1. Lin, W., Dou, W., Zhou, Z., Liu, C.: A cloud-based framework for Home-diagnosis service over big medical data. J. Syst. Softw. **102**, 192–206 (2015)
2. Castaneda, C., Nalley, K., Mannion, C., Bhattacharyya, P., Blake, P., Pecora, A., Goy, A., Suh, K.: Clinical decision support systems for improving diagnostic accuracy and achieving precision medicine. J. Clin. Bioinform. **5**(1), 4 (2015)
3. Rosenbloom, S., Denny, J., Xu, H., Lorenzi, N., Stead, W., Johnson, K.: Data from clinical notes: a perspective on the tension between structure and flexible documentation. J. Am. Med. Inform. Assoc. **18**(2), 181–186 (2011)
4. Finn, C.: Narrative nursing notes in the electronic health record: a key communication tool. Online J. Nurs. Inform. (OJNI), **19**(2) (2015)
5. Savkov, A., Carroll, J., Koeling, R., Cassell, J.: Annotating patient clinical records with syntactic chunks and named entities: the Harvey Corpus. Lang. Resour. Eval. **50**(3), 523–548 (2016)
6. Demner-Fushman, D., Chapman, W., McDonald, C.: What can natural language processing do for clinical decision support? J. Biomed. Inform. **42**(5), 760–772 (2009)
7. Moss, J., Andison, M., Sobko, H.: An analysis of narrative nursing documentation in an otherwise structured intensive care clinical information system. In: AMIA Annual Symposium Proceedings, pp. 543–547 (2007)
8. Sinsky, C., Colligan, L., Li, L., Prgomet, M., Reynolds, S., Goeders, L., Westbrook, J., Tutty, M., Blike, G.: Allocation of physician time in ambulatory practice: a time and motion study in 4 specialties. Ann. Intern. Med. **165**(11), 753 (2016)
9. Han, H., Lopp, L.: Writing and reading in the electronic health record: an entirely new world. Med. Educ. Online **18**(1), 18634 (2013)
10. Wang, X., Peng, Y., Lu, L., Lu, Z., Bagheri, M., Summers, R.M.: ChestX-ray8: Hospital-scale chest X-ray database and benchmarks on weakly-supervised classification and localization of common thorax diseases. In: Proceedings of the CVPR, pp. 3462–3471 (2017)
11. Larobina, M., Murino, L.: Medical image file formats. J. Digit. Imaging **27**(2), 200–206 (2013)

12. Chiu, M., Cheng, W., Chu, K., Lin, C., Yeung, S.: Do medical professionals tag images differently from non-medical professionals? an implication of retrieving user-generated images of everyday medical situations. Proc. Assoc. Inf. Sci. Technol. **53**(1), 1–5 (2016)
13. Belm, F., Almeida, J., Gonalves, M.: A survey on tag recommendation methods. J. Assn. Inf. Sci. Tec. **68**(4), 83044 (2016)
14. Garg, N., Weber, I.: Personalized, interactive tag recommendation for flickr. In: Proceedings of the 2008 ACM Conference on Recommender System, pp. 67–74 (2008)
15. Rae, A., Sigurbjornsson, B., van Zwol, R.: Improving tag recommendation using social networks. In: RIAO 2010 Adaptivity, Personalization and Fusion of Heterogeneous Information, pp. 92–99 (2010)
16. Belm, F., Batista, C., Santos, R., Almeida, J., Gonalves, M.: Beyond relevance. ACM Trans. Intell. Syst. Technol. **7**(3), 1–34 (2016)
17. Belm, F., Martins, E., Almeida, J., Gonalves, M.: Personalized and object-centered tag recommendation methods for Web 2.0 applications. Inf. Process. Manag. **50**(4), 524–553 (2014)
18. Musia, K., Juszczyszyn, K., Kazienko, P.: Ontology-based recommendation in multimedia sharing systems. Syst. Sci. **34**(1), 97–106 (2008)
19. Brin, S., Page, L.: The anatomy of a large-scale hypertextual Web search engine. In: Proceedings of the seventh International Conference on World Wide Web 7, pp. 107–117 (1998)
20. Xia, X., Lo, D., Wang, X., Zhou, B.: Tag Recommendation in Software Information Sites. MSR (2013)
21. Guendel, S., Grbic, S., Georgescu, B., Zhou, K., Ritschl, L., Meier, A., Comaniciu, D.: Learning to recognize abnormalities in chest x-rays with location-aware dense networks. CoRR (2018)
22. Qassimi, S., Abdelwahed, E.H., Hafidi, M., Lamrani, R.: Towards an emergent semantic of web resources using collaborative tagging. In: Ouhammou Y., Ivanovic M., Abell A., Bellatreche L. (Eds.) Model and Data Engineering. MEDI: Lecture Notes in Computer Science, vol. 10563, p. 2017. Springer, Cham (2017)

Analytical Approach for Virtual Classification of e-Health Interventions and Medical Data Sources Integration

Cherrat Loubna[1](✉), Khrouch Sarah[2], and Ezziyyani Mostafa[2]

[1] Faculty of Sciences, Chouaib Doukkali University, El Jadida, Morocco
cherratloubna2@gmail.com

[2] Faculty of Sciences and Techniques, Abdelmalek Essaâdi University, Tangier, Morocco
rhksara@gmail.com, ezziyyani@gmail.com

Abstract. This paper aims to helps, facilitate, and improve the efficiency of care, and allows real-time monitoring of patients. In fact, it allows collecting and archiving of heterogeneous medical data in centralized, virtual and secure sources. The main aim of the paper is to improve the efficiency and the quality of care and improve patients' lives through optimal information sharing between doctors and professionals. It also contributes to ensure the continuous monitoring of patients. This innovation in this field of e-health can solve, with a perfect cost control, the challenges related to the health care system. In the second hand this article aims to establish an interactive component at the application layer of the system as "Serious Game" for patients, physicians, professionals, and students in medicine. For physicians and students the device acts as an interactive guide that simulates a medical consultation and can implement all stages of diagnosis, including information gathering, simultaneous notes taking, and physical examination with instruments, so that a doctor would be able to perform a complete assessment of the health state of the patient. Moreover, our solution allows physicians and/or professionals to simulate a whole collaborative training in an educational online game, capable of improving the quality and safety of medical practices. As an example, the solution allows to train professionals in the operating room to avoid all risks before performing a complex surgery. For patients, this component offers schematic solutions that are well adapted to their conditions. Patients learn techniques of cognitive behavioral therapy to address symptoms of depression and become well assisted in their rehabilitation. For instance, patients would be able to deal with negative thinking, solve problems, better plan their activities, and learn how to relax. Our solutions will be applied to two basic application fields.

Keywords: ARCHIMED · Health care system · Medical consultation · Cognitive behavioral therapy · E-health

1 Study and Strategic Coordination

Strategic Coordination

Over the past few years, there has been a rapid growth in the use of ICT in the sector of e-health. These technologies constitute a change in the provision of care as services to

M. Ezziyyani (Ed.): AI2SD 2018, AISC 914, pp. 286–297, 2019.
https://doi.org/10.1007/978-3-030-11884-6_26

the population. E-Health is a relatively recent term, which dates back to at least 1999, and it designates "**all technologies, networks and services of care based on the telecommunication and comprising education programs, collaborative research, consultation and other services offered in the aim of improving the health of the patients**". Focused on the large public, the e-Health covers currently the activities, services, systems, related to health, practices at a distance by means of ICT, for the needs of global health promotion, care, control of epidemics, management and research applied to health care.

1.1 The Basic Components of e-Health

The term e-Health encompasses a range of services or systems, which are on the edge of medicine, health and information technology. It includes:

- **Electronic health records or Medical Record of the patient (DMP):** allows the communication of patient data between different health care professionals (general practitioners, specialists, etc.).
- **E-Prescribing:** gives access to options for prescription, requirements of printing for the patients and the electronic transmission of orders, sometimes from doctors to pharmacists.
- **Telemedicine:** remote physical and psychological treatments, including remote monitoring of functions of patients.
- **E-Health knowledge management:** for example, the epidemiological monitoring or guides to good practice.
- **Virtual teams of health:** composed of health professionals who work together and share information on patients thanks to digital equipment.
- **M-Health or e-Health:** includes the use of mobile devices in the collection of data of patients, providing health information for practitioners, researchers and patients. Real-time monitoring of the vital signs of patients, and the direct provision of care via mobile telemedicine. Examples of m-health products are mobile applications that can help doctors to diagnose. The communicating devices can transmit information (weight, heart rate, etc.) to the physician.
- **Health information systems:** also, often, refer to software solutions for the management of the patient data, the management of working hours and other administrative tasks surrounding the health.

1.2 e-Health and the Private Life

The requirements for the respect of privacy are numerous in an information system, and especially when it comes to information concerning health. One of the factors that are blocking and are to worry about the use of e-health tools is the concern on privacy issues concerning the records of patients, more particularly the DMP (medical record of the patient). This main concern relates to the confidentiality of the data. Examples among others include:

Data Theft: The theft of patient data becomes possible outside the cabinet. There is no way for the patient to realize it. It is an irreversible fact; storage and copying of information is extremely simple with informatics.

- **Centralization:** Centralization of data or access to the latter on a same platform increases the interest of hackers and the gravity of the facts in case of a problem.
- **Sensitivity:** In addition to being part of the individual, the data on the health of a person are worth money for banks, insurance, or a future employer.
- **Security:** If the principle of encryption is infallible in theory, its practical implementation on the other hand is not. All areas of acts of piracy are committed in secure infrastructures.
- **Trust:** We must have faith in the doctor but it also becomes necessary to have confidence in all intermediate computers. This responsibility to protect the data is extended to persons that the patient knows less and has not chosen them.

1.3 The State of the Art of Health in Morocco

A. The actors of health

- **The Legislature:** The health sector is governed by legal texts and it follows that the legislator is a main speaker. It should be noted that all the legal texts are subject to publication in the Official Bulletin detained by the General Secretariat of the Government in compliance with the Moroccan constitution.
- **The ministry of health:** The Ministry of Health is responsible for the development and the implementation of the government policy in the area of health.
- **Ministry of Education:** In Morocco, all the faculties of medicine and pharmacy and dentistry, training institutions, are under the Ministry of Education, Higher Education, executive training and scientific research. Because of this it remains a major player in the health sector.
- **Health care professionals:** They are in direct contact with the patients for consultations, treatments, care, etc. And also, with the scientific research, training and monitoring of future health professionals.
- **The NGOS:** They reinforce the interventions of the Ministry of Health or draw its attention to the topics which are crucial.

All these actors are involved through an infrastructure that covers all the prefectures.

B. The health card of the Country

Morocco remains relatively endowed with offers of care at the level of health care institutions. We have: 4 university hospital centers (CHU): CHU Ibn Sina (Rabat), CHU Ibn Rochd (Casablanca), CHU Hassan II (FES) and CHU Mohamed VI (Marrakech). There are 130 hospitals, including 35 specialized and 65 general practitioners. As to the private clinics, we count about 302. And regarding specialized institutions, we have:

- The National Institute of hygiene,
- A poison control center

- A Pasteur Institute
- A National Laboratory for the control of medicines

The training institutions are many, we can cite among others.

- 4 Faculties of Medicine and Pharmacy in Rabat, Casablanca, Fez and Marrakech.
- A faculty of dentistry in Casablanca.
- Training Institutes in Health care.
- A National Institute of Health administration.

1.4 Economic Benefits and Social Impact

The term e-health refers to all the opportunities that digital systems bring or are likely to bring to the health care field. This represents, as an example in France, a market estimated between 2.5 and 3 billion Euros. The development of new technologies in health is therefore a major challenge for the industry and the economy of the state. Platforms and software are all services which must facilitate the exchange and sharing between professionals in the community. They also aim to improve the conditions of the practice of the profession by an optimization of the coordination of care and an improvement in the involvement of patients in their medical history.

In the area of health, Morocco has embarked on a reform of its health care system which aims to enhance the quality of care and to guarantee access to the whole population. And to do so, Morocco needs to adopt e-health system which offers the citizens access to all of the information, communications and services, as well as a direct communication with the professionals and the health services; the main benefits of the e-health for health professionals are an improvement of the access to systems of clinical decision support to improve the quality of their decision and that of their delivery of services. Besides, it offers access to sources of information that are extremely rich for training continuous professionals. The impact of this project on the socio-economic sector can be summarized into:

- Improves the quality of care and avoid additional costs associated with duplication of treatments and interventions.
- Facilitates access to care particularly in areas of medical desertification.
- Offers home care and rapid home return for a better follow up in a familiar environment.
- Ensures better coordination between professionals.
- Facilitates the elaboration of statistics and the process of making decisions as well as the generalization of care on the totality of the Moroccan territory.
- Gives a global vision on the state of the health of citizens and the adverse effects of the environment on the citizens.
- Permits a quick Check of the progress and the distribution of diseases.
- Ensures an efficiency of health care system (control and reduction of health care costs).
- Allows training of professionals and students.
- Accelerates the capacities of all actors to produce and share data about health in a secure way with a better coordination of care.

1.5 Diseases Application Fields

a. Cancer Diseases
The project will put in place two attractive services for doctors and students of medicine. These two services are:

1. A tool for monitoring and consultation which centralizes all the data of the patients for their real-time monitoring. The doctor is close to the patients and intervenes remotely in case of need.
2. A simulation tool for the realization of complex surgical operations via a serious game. Examples include the "colposcopy" operation made for the uterus and the "endoscopic" operation made on the stomach. This type of operation requires a high precision because it allows determining the status or the severity of the cancer for these two sensitive organs. The proposed tool allows physicians to simulate the operation several times and discover with more details the steps of the operation prior to making it.

b. Autistic Children (in the context of the project)
Autism or more generally: Autistic Spectrum Troubles (TSA) are human development troubles characterized by an abnormal social and communication interaction, characterized by a restricted and repetitive behavior. In order to communicate with people with autism, a confident, funny and effective communication link must be created. To meet this need, the project proposes serious games, training and methods of integration to make the person with autism closer to normal life and facilitates his/her integration. All proposed options (games, tests, training, films, music etc.) represent effective learning tools that can be customized to match the condition of Autistic patients.

2 Work Packages

Generally, the paper goal addresses the reason, principles and functionalities of e-health and health care systems and presents a novel framework for revealing, understanding and implementing appropriate management interventions leading to qualitative improvement and transfer of health resources and health care by electronic means. It encompasses four main work packages:

- WP 1: Heterogeneous Data collection and classification based on context and optimization of the interrogation: **Big data integration, Cloud computing.**
- WP 2: The delivery of health information and the access to medical knowledge, for health professionals and health consumers through the Internet and telecommunications: **Software architecture of a Digital Smart Health Application, System Architecture, functionalities and validation.**
- WP 3: Using the power of IT to improve public health services, e.g. through the education and training of health workers and reviews standards and guidelines for practicing medicine: "**Serious Game**".

- WP 4: The use of remote monitoring and real time surveillance practices in e-health systems management and data communication with the environment: **Design and development of the wireless sensor network and the energy efficient communication protocol**.

In this context the ARCHIMED project aims to help to facilitate and improve the efficiency of care, and allows real-time monitoring of patients. In fact, it allows collecting and archiving of heterogeneous medical data (pharmaceutical, medical imaging, teleradiology & reports, etc….) in a centralized, virtual and secure manner. The main aim is to improve the efficiency and the quality of care and improve patients' lives through optimal information sharing between doctors. It also contributes to ensure the continuous monitoring of patients (those of chronic diseases for instance). This innovation in this field of e-health can solve, with a perfect cost control, the challenges related to the health care system, while ensuring the quality and safety of care for patients. ARCHIMED allows improving the quality of care (well-suited to the profile of the users) and decision-making based on these needs at all stages of patient care, from initial diagnosis to monitoring by doctors, health professionals located in geographically distributed institutions and private doctors. Concrete applications include screening, diagnosis, treatment guidance, surgeries controlling and therapeutic monitoring. The specificity of ARCHIMED is empowered by developing and implementing further innovative components to ensure all phases of medical information processing, mainly the acquisition, storage, classification, retrieval, querying, adaptation, testing, outsourcing, security, safety, data transfer, availability etc.

In the second hand, the ARCHIMED project aims to establish an interactive component at the application layer of the system in the form of a "**Serious Game**" for patients and physicians, professionals and students in medicine (Players). For physicians and students (future doctors), the device acts as an interactive guide that simulates a medical consultation and can implement all stages of diagnosis, including information gathering, simultaneous notes taking, and physical examination with instruments, so that a doctor would be able to perform a complete assessment of the health state of the patient. Moreover, our solution allows physicians and/or professionals to simulate a whole collaborative training in an educational online game, capable of improving the quality and safety of medical practices. As an example, the solution allows to train professionals in the operating room to avoid all risks before performing a complex surgery. The sessions can be replayed and analyzed as many times as needed to enable physicians (and/or students in training) to master the process of interventions, avoid all possible contingencies, manage risks and prevent serious adverse events. One innovation in the solution we propose is that when one (or many) player(s) is (are) not physically present to complete various components of the game, the system automatically offers adaptive and smart replacing agents with all necessary functionalities to automatically interact with the system and the other users. For patients, this component offers schematic solutions that are well-adapted to their conditions. Patients learn techniques of cognitive behavioral therapy to address symptoms of depression and become well-assisted in their rehabilitation. For instance, patients would be able to deal with negative thinking, solve problems, better plan their activities, and learn how to relax. In doing so, patients would be monitored both at the hospital and at home and are more independent and active in their rehabilitation. Our solution is a multiplayer platform: it allows patients to see their progress in the game and use the results from other patients' requests (accomplished quests, past levels …). In addition, the patient does not re-educate himself alone as he deals with other patients or family members. This allows the patient to get out of his isolation thanks to a real innovative and customized working tool. In this feature, the proposed system is connected with different devices: Kinect, touch pad (iPad or Android), mouse and graphic tablets, to ensure extreme and precise adaptability to different motor abilities of the patient during his rehabilitation program.

3 Basic Functionalities of ARCHIMED System and Key Words

Shared services for medical data analysis/Data Center for patients' medical information (DMP)/Reuse of medical results/service-oriented Awareness/Body virtualization and Medical Imaging/Data Analysis and extraction for automatic prediction/Security and safety of online health data/Connecting health care and social information systems/Remote control and monitoring of patients/Telemedicine and mobile collaboration technology.

1. WP1 Heterogeneous Data collection and classification based on context and Optimization of the interrogation
With a multitude of actors in the health field, the studies have demonstrated that the capital information on the medical knowledge doubles every seven years. This explosion of information is not without problems of organization of medical knowledge, which is more accessible to a human mind in its entirety. Therefore, this WP proposes a solution that every citizen can have an electronic medical record which can be used separately both by the patient and doctors to improve the quality of the medical care with the possibility of interactivity with all sources in relation to a high efficiency and in better working conditions. Besides, the introduction of an interoperability frame work systems for e-health with technical conditions, legal financial and organizational functionalities of the health sector will allow relevant statistical and policy analyses. Particularly in the context of epidemiological studies and in the transformation of medical knowledge on a broader spectrum of integrated systems for country decisions and prevention. Thus, the analyses of risk factors determine the steps of diagnostic research and therapeutic strategies. This type of tools is also widespread in all western countries, but it faces now competition from private products which do not offer the same guarantees neither for the functionality nor for the instruments developed by public authorities. This situation calls for vigilance and determination in the conduct of public projects (Fig. 1).

This WP requires a methodical and pragmatic approach which will allow a development of a system for integration and federation of e-Health sources in order to ensure:

- Communication and interaction with each data source as needed.
- Specification of a query, expressed in terms of a user-specified vocabulary (ontology), across multiple heterogeneous and autonomous data sources.

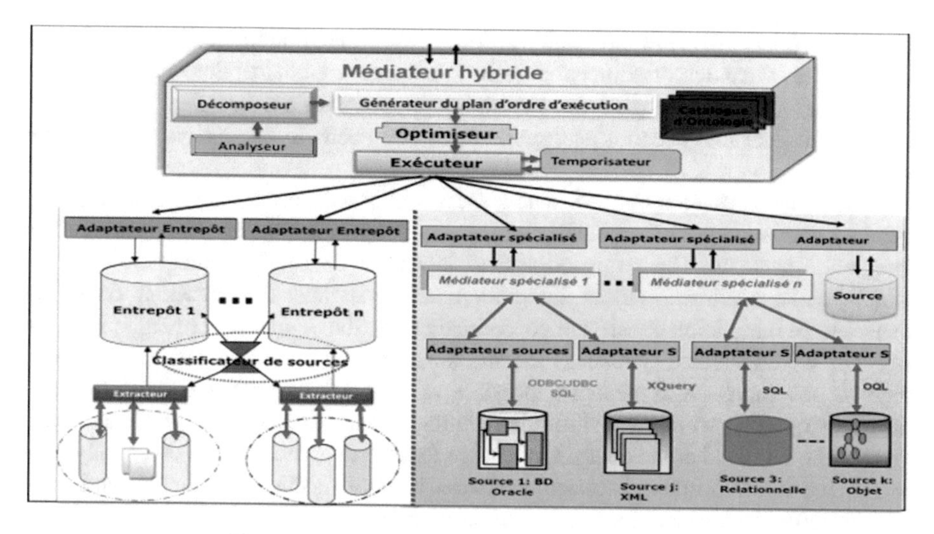

Fig. 1. The hybrid integration system architecture

- Specification of mappings between user ontology and the data-source specific ontologies.
- Transformation of a query into a plan for extracting the needed information by interacting with the relevant data sources.
- Integration and presentation of the results in terms of a vocabulary known to the user.
- Deployment on national scale of the generic services for sharing e-Health documents between health professionals following rule clearances controlled by the patient, and provision of the first on line and secure platform for medical data (history, prescriptions drug, biological test results, radiology reports of hospitalization and consultations etc.…).
- Implementation of new services to patients which offer available information about them (automatic receive results analysis avoiding travel, for example) or the help in their taken load (callbacks, capacity computerized exchanges with their doctor, therapy support programs … etc.).
- Exchange of information and provision of medical products and flexible and reliable services.
- Provision of high availability and mobility 24 H/24 and 7D/7 by making online patient records, securely and reliably.
- Management of the patient's health in order to improve his health and facilitate support by monitoring permanently the state of a patient.
- Make a profound decision on diseases and make a statistical prediction.

Research Issues

The main issues are: (1) How to detect and resolve problems related to heterogeneity? (2) How to effectively find the relevant data sources and generate an optimal execution plan? (3) How to automate the generation of queries? (4) How to reduce the search space for a query? (5) How to classify data sources for integration? (6) How to take into account the semantics of sources? (7) How to make a global optimization for query processing? (8) How to give the possibility to users to express their preferences? (9) How to take into account user preferences and needs in the design of integration system?

The general research context of this section is based on the integration of heterogeneous data sources and especially on the global optimization of interrogation of the integration systems. The proposed system is similar to a hybrid integration system, insofar as it combines virtual integration and materialized integration data. The materialized integration consists in consolidating distributed data, after being pretreated in a single consolidated synthesis base and integrated by topic. Extracting, by queries, parts of the database, it becomes possible to analyze the data and make the best decisions quickly; while in a virtual integration, the data remains in the local sources and will be retrieved at the query. Our choice for hybrid architecture is essentially done to achieve a compromise between freshness of data mediation approach and rapid response time to requests for data warehouse approach.

The use of ontologies in the integration process is an approach that has been successful and is still promising with a large number of researches done in this area. Known by their undeniable contributions to the semantic level, they are addressing the semantic problems to reduce the heterogeneity of the data. Their formal aspect allows, in addition, to automate the integration process, which is a very interesting contribution when dealing with a large number of data sources. That is why we also want that the user of our integration system can be able to query the internal and external data simultaneously using the global ontology of the data integration system. Indeed, to automatically exploit the resources distributed across different data warehouses and mediators, the definition of ontologies and a shared ontology field is required. Given the objectives mentioned previously, the main objective of this WP can be summarized in the following sub-tasks:

Task 1.1: Define hybrid integration Architecture of heterogeneous information sources

In this task we will develop a flexible data integration framework by implementing hybrid integration architecture to overcome the major limitations of virtual and materialized methods when they are used separately. Our first objective is to develop a hybrid multi-mediators functional architecture for our integration system. It is an architecture that responds perfectly to a data integration approach that focuses on the performance and the overall optimization of query processing, which aims to make more relevant and accurate interrogation in the sense where the user can access the parts of the resources that meet his request.

Task 1.2: Global Shared Ontology for hybrid integration system modeling the medical field

One Solution to provide a global optimization query processing is the restriction of the search space using semantic knowledge (ontology) level of integration system. Our objective in this level is to build the global shared ontology for the system that models knowledge about the domain of interest "the medical field" that we have defined for the application integration scenario. We also provide a structuration for the ontologies in our hybrid integration system that meets its functional architecture. The approach we have adopted enables automatic integration of the e-health sources and it also aims to create first the shared ontology of the system and then to extract local ontologies associated with the sources of real data from the different concepts of the global ontology. Each source contains concepts in the pre-existing domain ontology by referring to his local ontology. This is an “a priori” approach that simplifies the design process and reduces the time for the construction of local ontologies.

Task 1.3: Automatic generation of execution order plan for querying the ARCHIMED system

We present our solution to reduce the search space of a query by imposing a partial optimal order for the access to sources by querying the sources most relevant to a given query and by avoiding access to less relevant sources. It is a new method for automatic generation of an optimized execution order plane of sub queries regarding the degree of importance of sources capable of satisfying the user query based on a weight measure associated with each source or concept and the semantic links that connect the concepts of sources. These two criteria are used when querying for assessing the relevance of a response to a query. To ensure the computability of this plan, we will offer a comprehensive mathematical model and an algorithm for the construction of the canonical graph of order execution for the development of an optimal ordered sequence of relevant data sources for a query.

Task 1.4: Optimization of the interrogation process by the combinatorial data warehousing of sources

Another objective concerns the proposal of an efficient method for automatic classification of data sources by combinatorial data warehousing of sources. This is a query optimization approach based on the classification of data sources to integrate into homogeneous groups of sources (local data warehouses), which respond similarly to changes in user requests. The principle of this classification is based on the knowledge of the distance, similarity and coupling function between all pairs of sources to classify and integrate, and a combination of the principles of two classic methods of classification: the hierarchical top-down method and mobile centers method. Unlike optimizers which consider a restricted search space, the optimizer that we will propose, runs sources groups hierarchically and in depth according to the priority of sources. A performance evaluation of the approach through a comparative study on the distribution network overloaded with the proposed solutions will be designed to validate our approach.

Task 1.5: Develop and use cooperatives ontologies for customizing the interrogation process of a hybrid mediator

The last distinctive point of our approach is the use of cooperative ontologies for the improvement of the integration process of the ARCHIMED system. In order to customize the hybrid mediator, we are interested in taking into account profiles and interests of users in the interrogation process to refine and improve in terms of relevance the search results. To achieve this goal, we performed a classification of ontologies into profile ontology and query ontology. These ontologies cooperate with each other in order to take into account changes in the semantics of the data according to user profiles and the operating mode of the integration system. The proposed technique is based on the interaction between dimensions of the profile represented by the search history in the sources integrated by the hybrid mediator and interests of user groups.

Task 1.6: Define a security and privacy model for patient data
ARCHIMED platform must have a national norm of accommodation of document associated with integrated services: confidence, protection, identification, authentication, management clearances and collection of consent. Therefore, this task focuses on the aspect of security and confidentiality of patient data which is an important issue for the development of uses of ICT in the health sector. The services offered must make the regulatory measures of health data treatment, such:

- Each personal health record will be inviolable, that is to say protected against all risks of intrusion during its storage and transfer.
- All the rules and terms of access as well as the governed use of expression consent, the empowerment of the health professionals, identification, authentication, and traceability access ensure to patients the respect of their right to the confidentiality of their personal data and to exercise health professional secrecy.
- Patients and healthcare professionals are confident that the collection and use of health information will only be used legitimately and be uniformed everywhere and every time for everyone. Moreover, this information can be applied everywhere to protect individuals against inappropriate discrimination or harm from intentional misuse.
- Confidentiality and security protections are uniform and they set a high standard throughout the country for fair, reasonable, and uniform health information practices that respect the rights of the individual and the public (storage, transfer or access).
- Confidentiality, privacy, and security laws and regulations are conscientiously enforced, and those who break these laws or ignore these regulations face vigorous prosecution and serious penalties for their offenses.
- Individuals will have the right to access their health information in any setting and with minimal limits, have an understanding of their privacy rights and options for that setting, be notified about all information practices concerning their information and have the right to appropriately challenge the accuracy of their health information.

4 Conclusion

As like as Health fields, in the distributed environment where a query involves across several heterogeneous sources (Clinical, chirurgical, DMP), communication cost must be taken into consideration. In this perspective we describe tow query optimization approach using dynamic programming technique for a given set of integrated heterogeneous sources. The primary objective of the optimization is to minimize the total processing time including load processing, request rewriting and communication costs, to facilitate communication inter-sites and to optimize the time of data transfer from different sites. Moreover, the ability to store the data on centre site, gives more flexibility in terms of

Security/Safety and overload the network. In contrast to optimizers which consider a restricted search space, the proposed optimizer searches the subsets of sources and independency relationship which may be deep laniary or bushy trees. Especially the execution de query can be start traversal anywhere over any subset and not only from a specific one.

The main problem is to maintain a distributed data warehouse, consisting of multiple local data warehouses (sites) adjacent to the collection points, together with a coordinator. In order for such a solution to make sense, we need a technology for the data classification process. We must develop an algorithm for this task. This algorithm translates a set of sources into distributed distinct subsets and generates distributed warehouses, with the following concept: (i) each generated data warehouse performing some computation and communicating the query result to the coordinator, and (ii) the coordinator synchronizing the results and (possibly) communicating with the warehouses. The semantics of the subqueries generated by system ensure that the amount of data that has to be shipped between warehouses is independent of the size of the underlying data at the sites.

The solution allows for a wide variety of optimizations that are easily expressed in the interrogation and thus readily integrated into the query optimizer. The optimization algorithm included in our prototype contribute both to the minimization of synchronization traffic and the optimization of the data processing at the local sites. Significant features of this approach are the ability to perform both distribution-dependent and distribution in dependent optimizations that reduce the data transferred and the number of evaluation rounds.

References

1. Harabagiu, S.A., Miller, A.G., Moldovan, D.I.: WordNet 2: morphologically and semantically enhanced resource. In: Proceedings of Lexical Semantics and Knowledge Representation, SIGLEX 1999 (1999)
2. Heflin, J., Hendler, J., Luke, S.: SHOE: a knowledge representation language for internet applications. Technical CS-TR-4078, Institute for Advanced Computer Studies, University of Maryland (1999)
3. Alasoud, A., Haarslev, V., Shiri, N.: A hybrid approach for ontology integration. In: Proceedings of the 31st VLDB Conference, Trondheim, Norway (2005)
4. Ezziyyani, M.: Conception et Développement, Orienté Domaines d'Application, du médiateur pour l'intégration des systèmes d'information hétérogènes. AXMed: Advanced XML Mediator. Thèse de doctorat de l'université Abdelmalek Essaadi (2006)
5. Ezziyyani, M., Bennouna, M., Essaaidi, M., Cherrat, L.: Mediator of the heterogeneous information systems based on application domains specification: AXMed Advanced XML Mediator. Int. IEEE J. Comput. Sci. Appl. IJCSA, 25–45 (2006)
6. Busse, S., Kutsche, R.D., Leser, U., Weber, H.: Federated Information Systems: Concepts, Terminology and Architectures, Technical report no. 99-9, Technical University of Berlin, April 1999
7. Bernstein, P., Giunchiglia, F., Kementsietsidis, A., Mylopoulos, J., Serafini, L., Zaihrayeu, I.: Data management for peer-to-peer computing: a vision. In: Workshop on the Web and Databases, WebDB 2002 (2002)

MRI Images Segmentation for Alzheimer Detection Using Multi-agent Systems

Kenza Arbai[1(✉)] and Hanane Allioui[2]

[1] Laboratory of Genetics, Neuroendocrinology and Biotechnology, Faculty of Sciences, Ibn Tofail University, BP 133, Kenitra, Morocco
Kenza.Arad@gmail.com

[2] Computer Science Department, Faculty of Sciences Semlalia, Cadi Ayyad University, Bd Prince My Abdellah, BP 2390, Marrakech, Morocco
hananeallioui@gmail.com

Abstract. Neurodegenerative diseases such as Alzheimer's disease (AD), present increasing challenges. Determining the sequence and evolution of the symptoms and pathologies of AD will enable pre-symptom differential diagnosis, and treatment monitoring. Current diagnosis of Alzheimer is made by clinical, neuropsychological, and neuroimaging assessments. In fact, Magnetic Resonance Imaging (MRI) can be considered as the best neuroimaging examination for AD due to the well-defined measurement of brain structures, especially the size of the hippocampus and related regions. Image processing techniques has been used for processing the (MRI) image. Multi-agent Systems (MAS) is a strong paradigm full of complexity that offers promoters solution. We present a MAS solution that aims to automate the search and optimization of image processing. In this survey we propose a three-dimensional (3D) segmentation process based on cooperative MAS.

Keywords: Alzheimer · Neurodegenerative diseases · Multi-agent system · Cooperation · 3D image analysis · Segmentation

1 Introduction

Since the discovery of Alzheimer's Disease (AD), billions of euros have been spent in order to finance researches in that field. However, finding an effective therapy is still in progress. The main symptoms that typify the AD could include the memory damage, decision and problem-solving ability impairment, the luck of visuospatial abilities, difficulties using languages, or sometimes vicious behavior. First, we have to pinpoint that (AD) is a progressive neurodegenerative disease. Considered as the most common cause of dementia Alzheimer's disease (AD) is clinically defined by a set of episodic memory problems and a general decline of cognitive function [1].

In recent decades, (AD) has attracted tremendous attention from the scientific community as it has become the most common type of dementia and therefore represents a huge burden for society, public health, and then for the economy. Alzheimer's disease is characterized clinically by progressive deterioration of memory, and pathologically by histopathological changes including extracellular deposits of

M. Ezziyyani (Ed.): AI2SD 2018, AISC 914, pp. 298–313, 2019.
https://doi.org/10.1007/978-3-030-11884-6_27

amyloid-β (Aβ) peptides forming senile plaques (SP) and the intracellular neurofibrillary tangles (NFT) of hyper phosphorylated tau in the brain, which are commonly regarded as the hallmarks of the disease [2]. The prevalence of AD is expected to increase dramatically as the population around the globe continues to age [3]. And recent pharmaceutical trials have demonstrated that slowing or reversing pathology in Alzheimer's disease is likely to be possible only in the earliest stages of disease, perhaps even before significant symptoms develop. Pathology in Alzheimer's disease accumulates for well over a decade before symptoms are detected giving a large potential window of opportunity for intervention.

Imaging techniques detect subtle changes in brain tissue before significant macroscopic brain atrophy. Current diagnostic techniques often do not permit early diagnosis or are too expensive for routine clinical use. Magnetic Resonance Imaging (MRI) is the most versatile, affordable, and powerful imaging modality currently available, being able to deliver detailed analyses of anatomy, tissue volumes, and tissue state. In this mini-review, we consider how MRI might detect patients at risk of future dementia in the early stages of pathological change when symptoms are mild [4].

Many MRI techniques have been used to understand the underlying pathology in patient populations already diagnosed with AD. Magnetic resonance imaging (MRI) may be considered the preferred neuroimaging test for Alzheimer's disease because it allows accurate measurement of brain structures. Image processing techniques have been used for image processing (MRI) in order to obtain good results making it easier to diagnose cases. New technological trends to optimize processing and calculation, which has a great impact on the image-processing field. The most important part of image processing is image segmentation, which can be defined as a processing technique used to classify and cluster an image into several disjoint parts by grouping the pixels to form a region of homogeneity based on the pixel characteristics [5].

Segmentation techniques encompass a whole range of methodologies used to serve the varied purpose of finding out the Region of Interest in different types of medical images. In medical imaging, segmentation is used for examining different anatomical structures, tissue types and determination of Region of Interest in various images. It facilitates the automatic partitioning of different types of medical images especially AD cases. This step is very crucial in medical imaging because it is after this step that important decisions regarding treatment and surgery planning can be performed [6]. Multi-agent systems (MAS) have been proposed as a new vision paradigm. They use a decentralization of knowledge and behavior: to provide a resolution of segmentation issue. Such task is awarded to more than one agent, operating locally and communicating with others.

In this paper, we develop a platform for multi-agent facilitating the testing of segmentation strategies in order to integrate it into a parallel architecture. We opt for cooperation between different segmentation methods produce the maximum visual cues (regions, edges, points of interest…) to increase the increment of an image processing time. This cooperation allows exploiting the advantages of several techniques to achieve a result more accurate and more faithful than that obtained using a single technique. We present here the approaches to cooperative segmentation into three classes: sequential cooperation, cooperation results and cooperation.

The rest of the paper is divided as follows: At first, we review the characteristics of vision systems that use a multi-agent architecture and its application in segmentation. An overview of techniques for acquiring 3D images will be exposed. Then we will detail the system development and implementing such a mode of cooperation. Moreover, we conclude with a description of our intents to achieve that work.

2 Related Work

2.1 Alzheimer Disease

i. A brief history

In 1948, R. D. Newton was the first one to acknowledge that AD may occur "at any age", by presenting evidence that the rate of cognitive decline occurring in AD varies between patients. He described that the term "Alzheimer Disease" was used when the disease occurred at a relatively young age (now called early-onset AD). When it occurred during old age with rapid progression, it was called "senile dementia", and simply "senility" when the rate of cognitive decline was slow (both conditions are referred to as sporadic AD now). In order to suggest better terminology, Newton proposed to refer to AD as "Alzheimer's dementia", a term which is still frequently used in modern literature [7].

In 1983, the "cholinergic hypothesis" became the dominant force in AD. According to the work of Coyle et al., selective denervation of acetylcholine-releasing neurons, whose cell bodies are localized to the basal forebrain, may occur in AD. These cholinergic neurons innervate the cortical areas and related structures, especially the regions related to cognition and memory. It was suggested that cortical amyloid plaques primarily cluster around the cholinergic terminals, thus leading to retrograde degeneration of the related neurons and cognitive decline [8].

In 1985, Wong et al. [9], have determined that the amyloid beta peptide is the main component of neurotic plaques present in the brain of AD patients. Shortly after, Nukina et al. [10] identified Tau protein as a principal constituent of paired helical filaments (PHF) and neurofibrillary tangles. These findings paved the way for a number of key discoveries which occurred in the years that followed.

The "Vascular hypothesis" proposed that abnormalities in brain microvasculature, occurring as a result of aging, may contribute to AD. It was suggested that beta amyloid may cause accelerated degeneration of brain capillaries. Disturbances in the cerebral blood flow that follow, are likely to result in reduced delivery of both the glucose and oxygen to cerebral neurons. Energy deprivation and the resultant ischemia produces tissue damage which causes inflammation and may eventually result in neurofibrillary tangle formation [11].

In 2011, recent evidence suggests that cholinergic hypothesis clearly has its flaws. However, very few things in science are sufficiently "polished" when first proposed. An excellent review by Contestabile on the history of the cholinergic hypothesis points towards the advances this theory led to in AD research [12]. One of the most recently introduced hypotheses is termed "dendritic hypothesis" and is partly based on "synaptic dysfunction" hypothesis [13]. Since the identification of synapse as a possible site of AD-related damage, additional scientific effort was put towards identifying the role the dendrites play post-synoptically.

ii. Diagnosis of AD

In clinical areas, the AD diagnosis is based on medical history, physical and neurological examinations, and neuropsychological evaluation. AD clinical diagnosis has an accuracy of 70–90% relative to the pathological diagnosis, with greater accuracies being achieved in specialty settings such as memory disorder clinics [14]. Once the patient's cognitive damage has an atypical clinical course or is suspected to be due to other etiologies in addition to AD, the diagnosis of a possible AD dementia is mentioned. Generally, patients with AD have normal results on physical and neurological examinations [15]. The AD diagnosis relies on clinical-neuropathological assessment. Neuropathological results on autopsy examination remain the standard for AD diagnosis. The clinical diagnosis of AD is correct approximately 80%–90% of the time.

- **Clinical signs** they are noticed by a lowly progressive dementia.
- **Neuroimaging** that comprises a set of tools, which include different types of magnetic resonance imaging such as functional magnetic resonance imaging (fMRI), Magnetic Resonance Spectroscopy (MRS), Arterial Spin Labeling (ASL), and radiotracer imaging such as positron emission tomography and single photon emission computed tomography [16].
- **Neuropathological results** which includes Microscopic β-amyloid neurotic plaques, intra neuronal neurofibrillary tangles (containing tau protein), and amyloid angio-pathy at postmortem examination. The plaques should stain positively with β-amyloid antibodies and negative for prion antibodies, which are diagnostic of prion diseases. The numbers of plaques and tangles must exceed those found in age-matched controls without dementia.
- **Cerebrospinal fluid** (CSF) test can be represented by decreased Aβ amyloid 42 and increased tau.

Establishing the diagnosis of Alzheimer disease relies on clinical-neuropathological assessment. Neuropathological findings on autopsy examination remain the gold standard for diagnosis of AD. The clinical diagnosis of AD (prior to autopsy confirmation) is correct approximately 80%–90% of the time (Table 1):

Table 1. Diagnosis of AD

Clinical signs	Slowly progressive dementia
Neuroimaging	Gross cerebral cortical atrophy on CT or MRI
Neuropathological findings	Microscopic β-amyloid neurotic plaques, intra neuronal neurofibrillary tangles (containing tau protein), and amyloid angiopathy at postmortem examination
Cerebrospinal fluid (CSF)	Decreased Aβ amyloid 42 and increased tau

In our case, our interest is to study the part of neuroimaging, so we offer a platform for multi-agent facilitating the testing of segmentation of MRI images of a case of AD.

iii. Memory problems

It is necessary to describe what happens in normal ageing and understand what can go wrong and gives rise to abnormal conditions such as dementia. Ageing can be distinguished in terms of biological, social and psychological disciplines, but there is often a great overlap and interaction between them. Memory can also be affected [17], sometimes because of a fail of receiving information correctly or sometimes because it can no longer be effectively encoded or stored [18]. The effect of ageing on memory, particularly episodic memory [19], is very often one of the first of the cognitive functions to be noticed by others and can cause considerable distress to the individual and to relatives, close friends and careers. Deterioration in memory functioning is characteristic of dementia [20] but it can also indicate other dysfunctions which should always be considered in any assessment. Memory can be divided to several categories such as:

- Long-term memory allows one to remember a familiar telephone number from day to day and year to year [21].
- Short-term memory, now elaborated into the concept of working memory [22] is the system which allows one to remember a new telephone number while one is dialing it, so long as one is not distracted.
- Semantic and episodic memory: Different types of knowledge appear to be stored differently, episodic memories are for particular events, while semantic memories are context-free facts.
- Declarative and procedural memory may include some types of sensory stimuli. Generally, older people can learn as much as younger people, but more time is needed for them to achieve the same level of learning as they cannot process and 'absorb' information quickly.

iv. Phases of Alzheimer disease

Alzheimer's disease will vary slightly in appearance according to personality. Emotional, behavioral and cognitive changes will also vary, but generally there is three phases that describe the disease level (Table 2):

v. Image processing and Alzheimer's Disease

Brain imaging/neuroimaging is based on different techniques in order to directly or indirectly analyze the structure, function and pharmacology of the nervous system. Brain imaging falls into two broad categories:

- Structural imaging, to treat the structure of the nervous system, as well as the diagnosis of intracranial diseases.
- Functional imaging, to diagnose metabolic diseases and lesions at a finer scale (such as Alzheimer's disease), but also for research in neurological and cognitive psychology and the construction of brain-computer interfaces.

Table 2. Alzheimer disease phases

1st phase	It's usually characterized by difficulties in recalling recent events, and a tendency to forget where objects have been placed. Names of people and places, previously familiar, may be poorly recalled and a general disorientation persists
2nd phase	Known as the 'confusion phase'. Increasingly poor attention span and a decline in generalized intellectual performance are seen with a deteriorating memory. Disorientation in place, word-finding difficulty and other changes to speech may be seen Complex tasks are performed with difficulty, sometimes in a clumsy or inaccurate manner and often the skills the person learned last will be lost first. Lack of interest in news and surroundings follows relatively quickly and can be extremely distressing to family and friends
3rd phase	The 'dementia phase', is characterized by a lack of purpose in the person's behavior which appears disjointed and sometimes bizarre. Remaining intellectual and self-care abilities require constant supervision as people in this phase undergo further deterioration in memory capacity, calculating ability (dyscalculia) and aspects of language are severely affected and eventually lost Constant assistance is required for self-care skills such as grooming, dressing, and toileting and for feeding. A progressive physical wasting can also be seen which will mean help with walking. Sometimes one or two years of life will follow in an almost vegetative state until death

Many techniques have a relatively low resolution, including hundreds of thousands of neurons in a single voxel. Many functions also involve multiple parts of the brain, meaning that this type of claim is probably both unverifiable with the equipment used, and generally based on an incorrect assumption about how brain functions are divided. In some cases, the brain mapping techniques are used for commercial purposes, lie detection, or medical diagnosis in ways which have not been scientifically validated [23]. Indeed, the complexity of neuroimaging data sets allows researchers to examine properties of collective neural activities, that's why image segmentation is a relevant field.

2.2 Image Segmentation

i. Segmentation of 2D/3D images

Segmenting an image is usually one of the major and most challenging steps in the pipeline of image analysis. One classical and promising approach is to consider segmentation as a classification task, where the aim is to assign to each pixel the label of the objects it belongs to [24]. In fact, defined as one of the first steps leading to the analysis, the segmentation divides the image into meaningful regions that have a sense for a specific task. For that, image segmentation, can be classified using several approaches: outline, region, or classification.

The outline-based approaches, are characterized by taking into account only the information on the outlines. So to be able to detect more interesting objects, this approach is always non-satisfying. So, other properties should be considered, to improve the image processing results. Other approaches consist to grow a set of selected points in the image. These are the approaches by regions [25]. A homogeneity criterion is selected to increase the regions. When several regions meet, their boundaries define the contours of the final region. The classification methods [26] uses collected information, and proceed a matching pixel-class property as color, texture, etc. Spatial information may also be considered.

Many methods exist according to these three approaches, but each one specializes in one type of image (textured, uniform, etc.), which limits its application fields. The problem of the efficiency and the accuracy remains whole for the image. Facing this difficulty in the segmentation, it is necessary to adapt the locally methods on the image to obtain a precise global segmentation, through using cooperation, or competition. The agent paradigm is a "natural" response to the implementation of this adaptation.

ii. Multi-agent approaches in image segmentation

According to Ferber, an agent can be a physical or virtual entity that can act, perceives its environment (in a partial way) and communicate with others; it is autonomous and has the abilities to achieve its goals and tendencies. It is in a multi-agent system that contains an environment, objects and agents (the agents being the only ones to act), relations between all the entities, a set of operations that can be performed by the entities and the changes of the universe in time and due to these actions [27].

The use of multi-agent systems and precisely the agents located in the picture constitute a framework well adapted to the segmentation problems. Indeed, the agents constitute a natural framework for expressing local adaptation in the environment (image) or cooperation between different approaches. The interaction between several behaviors, leads to a new feature, such as image segmentation [28].

iii. Recent studies

In the medical imaging field, many studies have taken place; the following table summarizes the comparison between the results obtained by some researcher's approaches and non-oriented agent segmentation methods (Table 3):

Research in multi agent systems do not cease to evolve, from day to day tomorrow a new approach revolutionizes the technological world, so necessarily there are other works that have adopted the MAS for the segmentation of medical images including cerebral, in this tables on tried to cite just a few examples from year to year.

3 The Proposed Approach

Digital image processing allows an algorithm to avoid problems such as the buildup of noise and signal distortion occurring in analog image processing. When expressing the data feature extraction of the interesting objectives, image segmentation, using multi agent systems, is to transform the data set of the features of the original image into tighter and general data set. The system we are developing is a tool to analyze the contribution of cooperative agents with the objective:

Table 3. Comparison table for the recent studies in image segmentation using MAS

Researchers	Year	Image type	Results meet non-agent methods
Spinu et al. [29]	1996	Muscle cell and MRI	Optimal solution
Boucher et al. [30]	1998	Living cells	Adaptable method and the result contain rich information
Germond [31]	2000	MRI of brain	The mean quality percentage is 96%
Duchesnay [32]	2001	192 × 192 Images including both medical and non-medical one	The approach is completely autonomous, does not required priori information
Richard [33]	2004	MRI of brain	Adaptation to intensity; non-uniformity and noise
Benamrane et al. [34]	2007	MRI of brain that contains tumors	Good success in image includes heterogeneous, local and repartee information
Chitsaz et al. [35]	2013	A cranial CTscanner with an image size 512 × 512	The average accuracy is more than 91% for each region in the images. And computation time of all datasets is less than 8 s
Arsene et al. [36]	2015	MRI cerebral image	Reduce the complexity of the parallel programs
Nachour et al. [37]	2016	MRI images	More information in the combined region and edge detection while preserving the edges to the same degree as the regions
Sauwen et al. [38]	2017	MRI images	User-defined voxel selection is applied to initialize pathological sources of the NMF analysis, and to exploit knowledge about the spatial location of the tumor to remove false positives in a post-processing step

- Facilitate the information integration;
- Integrate the concept of texture in the characterization of the researched objects;
- Adopt a truly multi-agent approach for AD detection;
- Minimize the computation time while maintaining ergonomic.

Several segmentation techniques-based agents have been presented in the literature and have shown interest of these distributed approaches in the sharing of process of segmentation or the combination of techniques (contour based or region). The multi-agent system (MAS) presented is intended to make the extraction process of fusion of the results following the cooperation and competition behavior associated with specific agents.

3.1 The System Components

The proposed system is divided into three parts:

1. The Data, Part contains the observable aspect (image) and the non-observable (information produced after treatment).
2. The active part, which consists of different agents working for one common goal: to segment the image.
3. The Knowledge Part contains the different procedures and methods used in image processing (segmentation and analysis) and information concerning the search for target objects in the image (Fig. 1).

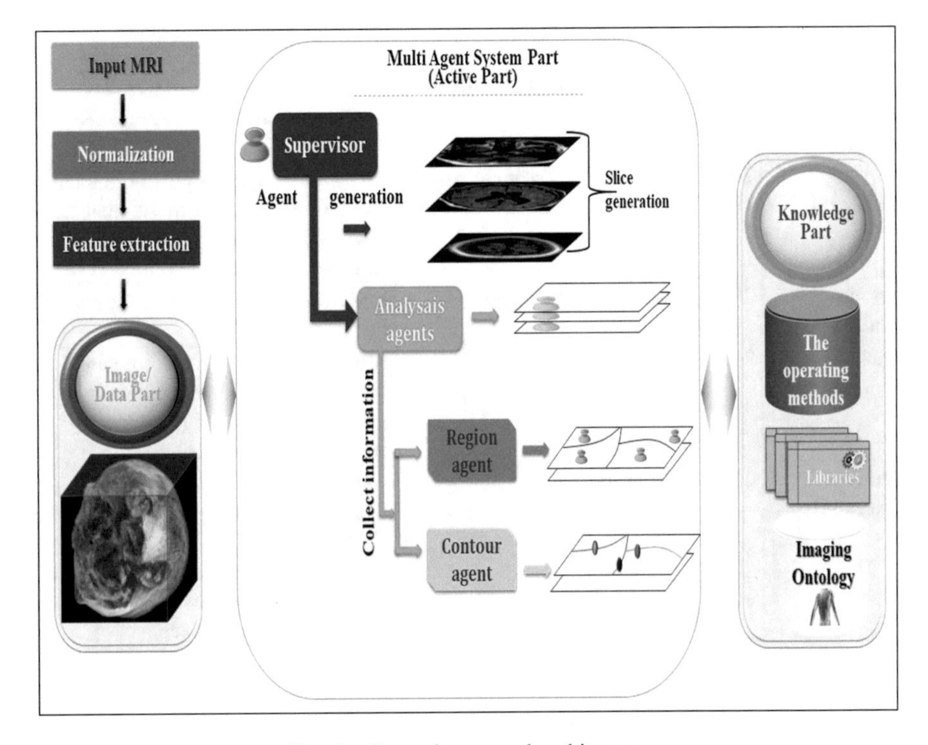

Fig. 1. General proposed architecture

In application, we introduced an agent named 'Supervisor Agent', who will manage all the activities in the system, and serve as the primary interface. It enables the following tasks: Receiving the image to be processed, generate slices (called image-slices) and analysis agents (one agent per slice), and manage the operation of agents and the results of the segmentation.

That agent also creates the environment in which the agents of segmentation part will be deployed. The environment will be a structure representing the image slices sources in addition to a space to place the data generated from their visual cues (extracted segmented images and objects).

3.2 System Organization

By cooperative method, we mean that (Meta) heuristics, executed in parallel as agents, have the ability to share information at various points throughout a search [39]. Our architecture falls into the area of distributed systems, where a number of agents work together to cooperatively to obtain a common aim. Agents can abandon their goals to meet the needs of others to ensure better cooperation using different types: (i) Confrontation: proceeding by fusion of data/results; (ii) Increase: simple addition of the skills of agents; (iii) Integration: decompose the solution a problem into sub tasks to schedule.

In fact, different types of agents located in an image slice are implemented (Table 4):

Table 4. Types of the agents located in an Image slice

The supervisor	-The supervisor places an 'analysis' agent on each image-slice, then retrieves the results of the analysis (map contours, uniform zones and textured areas as well as seed points) -It will place the segmentation agents (regions and contours) in the image grid lines -Wait until all agents have finished their perception of their visual marks -Wait for the message ' end' from agents
Analysis agent (AA)	The analysis agent will perform an image processing and produce global parameters of segmentation with seed points. Analysis agents use many techniques and methods, for global analysis of an image, in order to accomplish his tasks
Segmentation agent (SA)	A segmentation agent (region or contour) constructs its own criteria of segmentation, using the parameters of the analysis agent. The region agent(SAr) is intended to capture a homogeneous region around its initial seed. It has a homogeneity standard, it will use to mark the pixels and also to negotiate a fusion with these best neighbors. The interactions between region agents will lead to an image segmentation. The contour agent(SAc), in turn appropriates a border region between agents using the seed points of transition

At the end of the images-slices segmentation, a cognition relationship can be established between the agents of consecutive slices to determine the regions (contours) in common. The operation is to build a 3D object through its regions and contours in the slices. Generally, an automatic segmentation method is difficult to conceive. Indeed, several factors involved: the nature of the various areas of the image (textured, uniform…), the shooting conditions (pose, light…), Scanning defects ("noise" introduced by the hardware) and especially the huge loss of information due to the 3D to 2D projection (which is a problem of interpretation even for simple geometric objects) [40]. The segmentation agent is distributed according to his working methodology in two types: region and an outline the segmentation agent is distributed according to his working methodology into two types: the region and the outline. Its principal role is to segment and interpret the assigned region. Furthermore, the implementation of an outline/region cooperation, is one of the most interesting aspects regarding the processing of image sequences, and how launch agents in the following image of the sequence, depending on what is taking place in the current one.

4 Experimentation and Results

The clinical diagnosis of AD is supposed to be correct 75% to 90% of the time [41]. According to Shadlen et al. [42] accuracy is highest for neurologists specializing in memory disorders and lowest for general practitioners, who has a tendency to over diagnose Alzheimer's disease. The clinical accuracy also tends to be lower for older patients who often have mixed pathology rather than a single cause of dementia [43]. The only clinical means of establishing a definite diagnosis is by microscopic examination of brain tissue as there are no laboratory tests and neither sophisticated imaging techniques nor detailed neuro-psychological evaluation that can specify Alzheimer's disease categorically [44]. However, this work's goal is improving the RMI images analysis to offer a primary report for neurologists.

The basic systems used in conventional image processing favor the definition of an object that one seeks to achieve, minimize the response time and offer real-time reports on the processed image. Various software and platforms have been tested to evaluate the performance of the mechanism presented in this article. The use of MAS allows us to have more detailed analyzes in the special areas we choose. A conflict of interest is created when two potentially conflicting agents may induce a professional actor to make a decision and/or act in a manner that harms or may harm the interests of a stakeholder.

We used data from The National Alzheimer's Coordinating Center (NACC), which was established in 1999, maintains a cumulative database including clinical evaluations, neuropathology data when available, and now MRI imaging. NACC invites researchers throughout the AD community to take advantage of this valuable resource. With NACC's MRI selection preview system, we were able to download a sample of up to 10 images.

In our proposed system, an agent is implanted into a 3D environment. Thus, it acts and interacts with others. Interactions between agents and the environment can be asynchronous or synchronous. In one hand, in the asynchronous case, at first, an agent has to send a read message to his environment in order to know resources status, then the environment replies with the appropriate response. In the other, in a synchronous case, the messages exchange could be avoided, so the run time would be reduced.

In a parallel or distributed processing, an image slice is a huge shared resource of a concurrent system. A recurrent access by agents to the areas can become a problem that limits system performance and scalability. A given agent competes with different opponents and the results obtained have an impact on its current analyses. Adopting a working agent as the basic unit of behavior simulation in the environment (image), the proposed system attempts to consider directly the real mechanisms behind behavioral actions at the individual level, placing perception, communication, cooperation, negotiation, and behavioral action under one simulation.

In this work, we discuss the approach to computational model agent behavior by combining results obtained from behavioral analysis in the studied slices. We presented an improved version of the MAS image processing. The results are shown in the following figures (Figs. 2 and 3):

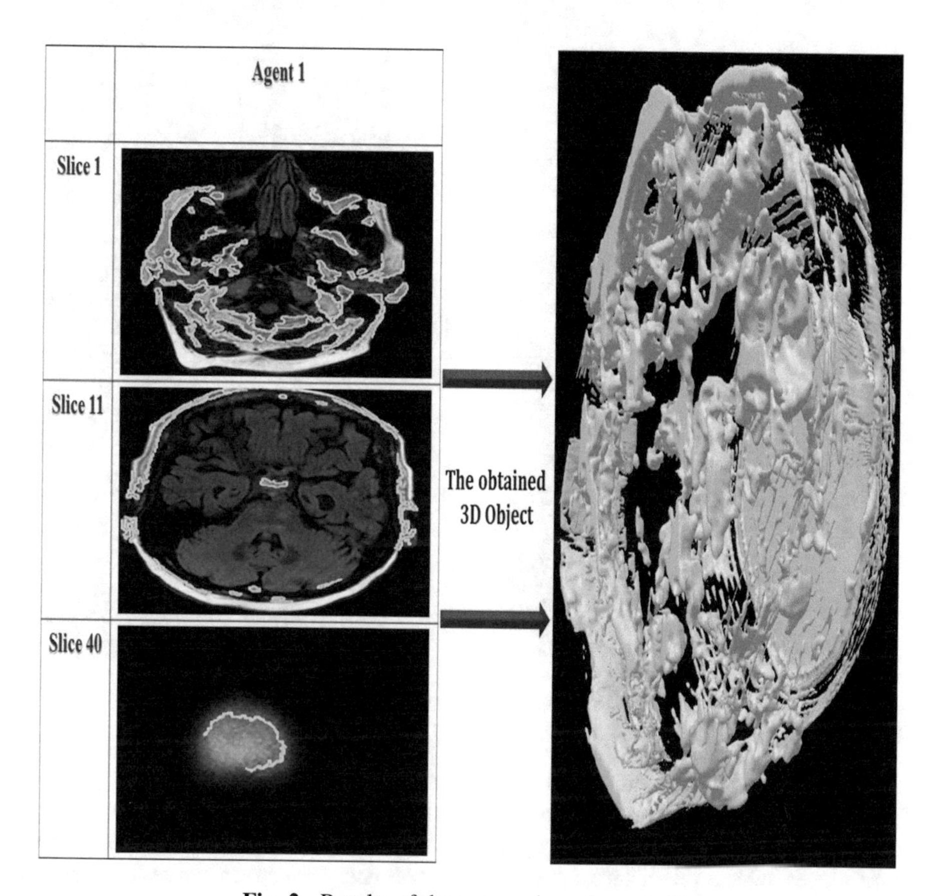

Fig. 2. Results of the progression of agent n°1

The entries for this agent are several slices. The agent n°1 begins with a series of data preprocessing steps, including binary masks of the brain and ventricle, correction of non-uniformity, scaling and intensity normalization. The pre-processed brain slices are then checked; from the germs the regions are formed. This agent, offers a good quality of visualization of the detected objects, as well as the reconstruction of the 3D object.

The agent progression found several absences of this object in the slices, it's work progression didn't obtain a continuous object in all the slices. However, these potential benefits need to be weighed against the fact that changes in results from one agent to another may be more likely than measurements of the whole brain to be analyzed correctly, also to perform different tests.

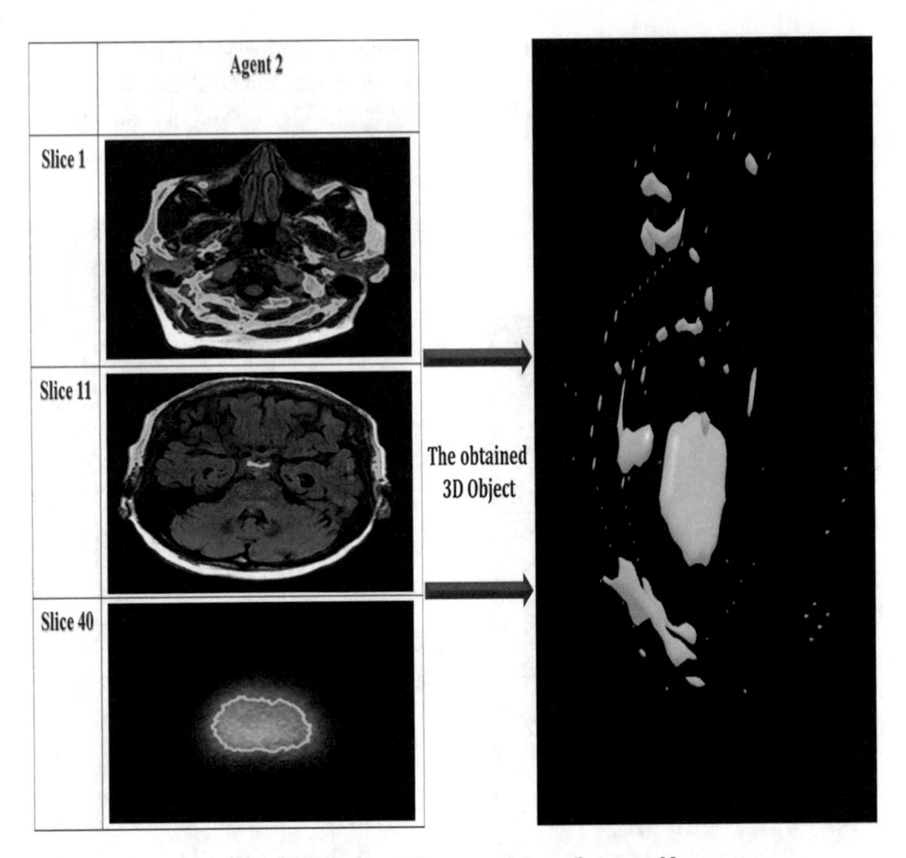

Fig. 3. Results of the progression of agent n°2

After several tests, we noticed that a large number of similar regions were grouped, fewer segments were generated, and a better subjective coherence of the image objects could be perceived. Segmentation algorithms in existing software will typically work with images whose characteristics are in the outlines. In a given context, a custom similarity task performed from an agent, obtained from a single slice, can be generalized for an integer number of slices, so that the supervisor can easily compare the results obtained and produce the requested reports.

5 Conclusion

In this paper, we developed a novel 3D approach to segment MRI images, in order to offer a preliminary diagnosis of AD. we presented a new method for 3D object segmentation, based on the use of a combined multi-agent system, a supervised classification approach and a region growing method. The multi-agent architecture presented provides a richer approach for the image segmentation by region merging (in 3D). The proposed method can advance the research on automated brain structure segmentation as well as offer a powerful and effective tool for more neuroimaging and neuroscience studies, where accurate segmentation of brain structures is essential. In fact, we extend our proposed method to solve the problem for detecting the small object in the images. As well as shown in the experimental results we have satisfied segmentation results. For the millions suffering, this new direction for AD research is one that ought to be taken.

Major efforts are underway to develop disease-detection agents for Alzheimer's disease (AD); In the future, it will be important to perform quantification of serial regional volume changes and to correlate atrophy rates with neuro-pathologic changes in different diagnostics, also we aim to follow the evolution of patients and compare the results obtained in different periods.

References

1. Citron, M.: Alzheimer's disease: strategies for disease modification. Nat. Rev. Drug Discov. **9**, 387–398 (2010)
2. Dong, S., Duan, Y., Hu, Y., Zhao, Z.: Advances in the pathogenesis of Alzheimer' s disease: a re-evaluation of amyloid cascade hypothesis. Transl. Neurodegener. **1**, 18 (2012)
3. Varghese, T., Sheelakumari, R., James, J.S., Mathuranath, P.: A review of neuroimaging biomarkers of Alzheimer's disease. Neurol. Asia **18**(3), 239–248 (2013)
4. Knight, M.J., McCann, B., Kauppinen, R.A., Coulthard, E.J.: Magnetic resonance imaging to detect early molecular and cellular changes in Alzheimer's disease. Front. Aging Neurosci. **8**, 139 (2016)
5. Khan, A.M., Ravi, S.: Image segmentation methods: a comparative study. Int. J. Soft Comput. Eng. (IJSCE) **3**(4) (2013). ISSN : 2231-2307
6. Khare, P., Mittal, N.: Analysis of medical image segmentation techniques. Int. Bull. Math. Res. **2**, 188–193 (2015)
7. Newton, R.D.: The identity of Alzheimer's disease and sinile dementia and their relationship to senility. J. Ment. Sci. **94**(395), 225–249 (1948)
8. Coyle, J.T., Price, D.L., DeLong, M.R.: Alzheimer's disease: a disorder of cortical cholinergic innervation. Science **219**(4589), 1184–1190 (1983)
9. Wong, C.W., Quaranta, V., Glenner, G.G.: Neuritic plaques and cerebrovascular amyloid in Alzheimer disease are antigenically related. Proc. Natl. Acad. Sci. U.S.A. **82**(24), 8729–8732 (1985)
10. Nukina, N., Ihara, Y.: One of the antigenic determinants of paired helical filaments is related to tau protein. J. Biochem. **99**(5), 1541–1544 (1986)
11. de la Torre, J.C., Mussivand, T.: Can disturbed brain microcirculation cause Alzheimer's disease. Neurol. Res. **15**(3), 146–153 (1993)
12. Contestabile, A.: The history of the cholinergic hypothesis. Behav. Brain Res. **221**(2), 334–340 (2011)
13. Cochran, J.N., Hall, A.M., Roberson, E.D.: The dendritic hypothesis for Alzheimer's disease pathophysiology. Brain Res. Bull. **103**, 18–28 (2013)
14. Barnes, D.E., Yaffe, K.: The projected effect of risk factor reduction on Alzheimer's disease prevalence. Lancet Neurol. **10**, 819–828 (2011)
15. Camicioli, R.: Distinguishing different dementias. Can. Rev. Alzheimer's Dis. Other Dement. **9**, 4–11 (2006)

16. Paulus, M.P.: The role of neuroimaging for the diagnosis and treatment of anxiety disorders. Depress Anxiety **25**(4), 348–356 (2008)
17. Freidl, W., Schmidt, R., Stronegger, W.J., Reinhart, B.: The impact of sociodemographic, environmental, and behavioural factors, and cerebrovascular risk factors as potential predictors of the mattis dementia rating scale. J. Gerontol. **52**(2), 111–116 (1997)
18. Small, G.W., La Rue, A., Komo, S., Kaplan, A., Mandelkern, M.A.: Predictors of cognitive change in middle-aged and older adults with memory loss. Am. J. Psychiatry **152**(12), 1757–1764 (1995)
19. Nyberg, L., Backman, L., Erngrund, K., Olofsson, U., Nilsson, L.G.: Age differences in episodic memory, semantic memory, and priming: relationships to demographic, intellectual, and biological factors. J. Gerontol. **51**(4), 234–240 (1996)
20. Morris, R.G.: Recent developments in the neuropsychology of dementia. Int. Rev. Psychiatry **6**, 85–107 (1994)
21. Baddeley, A.D.: Working memory. Science **255**, 556–559 (1992)
22. Mitrushina, M., Uchiyama, C., Satz, P.: Heterogeneity of cognitive profiles in normal aging: implications for early manifestations of Alzheimer's disease. J. Clin. Exp. Neuropsychol. **17** (3), 374–382 (1995)
23. Satel, S., Lilienfeld, S.O.: Brainwashed: The Seductive Appeal of Mindless Neuroscience. Basic Books, New York City (2015). ISBN 978-0465062911
24. Machairas, V., Baldeweck, T., Walter, T., Decencière, E.: New general features based on superpixels for image segmentation learning, February 2016. https://hal.archives-ouvertes.fr/hal-01276132
25. Shapiro, L.G., Haralick, R.M.: Computer and Robot Vision, vol. 1. Addison-Wesley, Boston (1992)
26. Chardin, A.: Modèles énergétiques hièrarchiques pour la résolution des problèmes inverses en analyse d'images, France (2000)
27. Ferber, J.: Les Systèmes Multi-agents: vers une Intelligence Collective. InterEditions, Paris (1995)
28. Mazouzi, S., Guessoum, Z., Michel, F., Batouche, M.: An agent-based approach, for range image segmentation. In: Jamali, N., Scerri, P., Sugawara, T. (eds.) Massively Multi-agent Technology. LNAI, vol. 5043, pp. 146–161. Springer, Heidelberg (2008)
29. Spinu, C., Garbay, C., Chassery, J.: A multi-agent approach to edge detection as a distributed optimization problem. In: Proceedings of the 13th International Conference on Pattern Recognition, Austria, vol. 2, pp. 81–85 (1996)
30. Boucher, A.: A society of goal-oriented agents for the analysis of living cells. Artif. Intell. Med. **14**(1–2), 183–196 (1998)
31. Germond, L.: A cooperative framework for segmentation of MRI brain scan. Artif. Intell. Med. **20**(1), 77–93 (2000)
32. Duchesnay, E.: An agent-based implementation of irregular pyramid for distributed image segmentation. In: Proceedings of the 8th International Conference on Emerging Technologies and Factory, France, pp. 409–415 (2001)
33. Richard, N., Dojat, M., Garbay, C.: Automated segmentation of human brain MR images using a multi-agent approach. Artif. Intell. Med. **30**(2), 75–153 (2004)
34. Benamrane, N., Nassane, S.: Medical image segmentation by a multi-agent system approach. In: Proceedings of the 5th German Conference on Multiagent System Technologies, Germany, pp. 49–60 (2007)
35. Chitsaz, M., Seng, W.C.: Medical image segmentation using a multi-agent system approach. Int. Arab J. Inf. Technol. **10**(3), 222–229 (2013)

36. Arsene, O., Dumitrache, I., Mihu, I.: Expert system for medicine diagnosis using software agents. Expert Syst. Appl. **42**, 1825–1834 (2015)
37. Nachour, A., Ouzizi, L., Aoara, Y.: Multi-agent segmentation using region growing and contour detection: syntetic evaluation in MR images with 3D CAD reconstruction. Int. J. Comput. Inf. Syst. Ind. Manag. Appl. **8**, 115–124 (2016)
38. Sauwen, N., et al.: Semi-automated brain tumor segmentation on multi-parametric MRI using regularized non-negative matrix factorization. BMC Med. Imaging BMC Ser. – Open Incl Trusted **17**, 29 (2017)
39. Martin, S., Ouelhadj, D., Beullens, P., Ozcan, E., Juan, A.A., Burke, E.K.: A multi-agent based cooperative approach to scheduling and routing. Eur. J. Oper. Res. **254**, 169–178 (2016)
40. Singh, M., Duggirala, M., Hayatnagarkar, H., Balaraman, V.: A multi-agent model of workgroup behaviour in an enterprise using a compositional approach (2016)
41. Sadgal, M., El Faziki, A.: Une architecture mult-agents Basée Sur la Catégorisation dans le Traitement d'images. In: International Conference on Image an Signal Processing, Agadir, 3–5 May 2001, pp. 608–617 (2001)
42. McKhann, G.M., et al.: The diagnosis of dementia due to Alzheimer's disease: recommendations from the national institute on aging-Alzheimer's association workgroups on diagnostic guidelines for Alzheimer's disease. Alzheimer's Dement. **7**(3), 263–269 (2011)
43. Shadlen, M., Larson, E.: Evaluation of cognitive impairment and dementia. In: Basow, D. (ed.) Up To Date, Waltham (2010)
44. Dickson, D.W.: Neuropathology of Alzheimer's disease and other dementias'. Clin. Geriatr. Med. **17**(2), 209–228 (2001)

Alzheimer Detection Based on Multi-Agent Systems: An Intelligent Image Processing Environment

Hanane Allioui(✉), Mohamed Sadgal, and Aziz El Faziki

Computer Science Department, Faculty of Sciences Semlalia,
Cadi Ayyad University, Bd Prince My Abdellah, BP 2390, Marrakech, Morocco
hananeallioui@gmail.com, {sadgal,elfazziki}@uca.ma

Abstract. Nowadays, robust image processing and intelligent systems have gained much popularity and importance in several fields o studies; Consequently, the use of Multi-agent systems (MAS) has been adopted as a strength paradigm for analyzing images. Since, medical image segmentation faces multiple obstacles, the use of MAS has proved precious benefits to accomplish many tasks such as quantification of tissue volumes, medical diagnosis, anatomical structure studies, treatment planning, etc. Currently, diagnosis of Alzheimer Disease (AD) can be made by different methods, neuroimaging assessments are the most used one. Meanwhile, Magnetic Resonance Imaging (MRI) offers well-defined measurement of brain structures, it has been considered as one of the best neuroimaging examination for AD. For this reason, MAS adopt the decentralization of knowledge and behavior in order to provide a powerful resolution of segmentation issues. We briefly describe a framework for Agent Based modeling (ABM) which is designed to 3D image processing especially Alzheimer MRI analysis, and highlights its important characteristics: agent behavior, perception, interactions, cooperation, and negotiation.

Keywords: Agent Based Modeling · Multi agent systems · Image analysis · 3D image processing · Segmentation · Cooperation · Negotiation · Neuroimaging · Alzheimer · Neurodegenerative diseases

1 Introduction

Thanks to technological progress, several research fields have been advanced, so as neuroimaging. Intelligent medical image processing award special interest to brain markers of serious cerebral illness including Alzheimer disease (AD). Considered as the most common neurodegenerative disease, AD is a major public health problem that is becoming increasingly important as life expectancy increases [1]. Indeed, a neuropathological confirmation of amyloid plaques and neurofibrillary tangles is necessary for the definitive diagnosis of AD [2]. MRI offers strong support for diagnosis and monitoring of AD progression. Opposing to the relatively more advanced stages of

M. Ezziyyani (Ed.): AI2SD 2018, AISC 914, pp. 314–326, 2019.
https://doi.org/10.1007/978-3-030-11884-6_28

Alzheimer's disease, quantification of damaged brain regions and the study of structural changes during the early stages of Alzheimer's disease or during normal clinical stages is a major challenge.

Currently, magnetic resonance imaging (MRI) is the most multipurpose, the most used and the most powerful imaging technique. MRI can provide detailed analyzes of anatomy, and tissue volumes. With its ability to provide accurate measurements of brain structures, MRI can be considered as an important test for Alzheimer disease. For MRI processing various techniques have been used to obtain good results, which facilitates the diagnosis of cases. This justifies the importance of the phase of image segmentation which is a processing technique used in order to classify and group an image into several separated parts by grouping the pixels to form a homogeneity region based on the characteristics of the pixels [3].

In an image, the segmentation process aims to obtain significant information in the regions of interest in order to help in annotating of the object scene [4]. The segmentation of brain images is a particularly important problem and one of the most difficult to study in the field of image analysis and processing. In the case of diagnosis of AD, it is sought to detect and locate particular areas in an image. Knowledge of these areas is then used to establish a pre-clinical or predictive diagnosis. Thus, there is a growing need to find effective ways to provide AD detection, and follow-up of cases. For these reasons, Intelligent systems are considered as a new way to interact between medical staff and technology. Moreover, it is important to mention that these technologies must allow the performance of the imaging system, ensure an autonomous functioning without disturbing the people's environment, and making easier their daily activities.

In the world of intelligent and dynamic systems, the agent [5] paradigm has a progressive importance, since its participation makes it possible to meet the objectives and requirements of the developed systems. Moreover, Multi-agent systems (MAS) have been proposed as a new computer vision pattern. They provide a powerful high-level tool and aim to support their environment using the knowledge and behavior decentralization aiming to ensure a good resolution for segmentation issues.

In this work, we discuss the approach to computational model agent behavior by combining results obtained from behavioral analysis in the studied slices. We presented an improved version of the MAS image processing. We present a method for 3D object segmentation, based on the use of a combined multi-agent system, a supervised classification approach and a region growing method. The multi-agent architecture presented provides a richer approach for the image segmentation by region merging (in 3D).

The rest of this paper is divided as follows: At first, we present a brief review the vision systems based on multi-agent architecture and its application in image segmentation. Then we will detail the system development and implementing while highlighting the cooperation and negotiation approach. Moreover, we conclude with a description of our intents to achieve that work.

2 Related Works

2.1 Image Processing and Alzheimer's Disease

Being defined as a chronic neurodegenerative disease, Alzheimer's disease AD worsens with time [6]. The experts have defined different stages in order to describe the evolution of the capacities of a person with Alzheimer's disease until an advanced stage. AD, this irreversible and progressive brain disorder, is able to destroys slowly memory and thinking abilities and eventually decreases the ability to perform the simplest tasks. The part of brain which is responsible for the formation of memories is damaged first. As the neurons die, additional parts of the brain are damaged one after the other until total brain tissue weakening in the final phase of AD.

Brain imaging or neuroimaging techniques allow doctors and researchers to have a clear idea about brain activities or anomalies. Today, many techniques have become more common quickly. Generally, brain imaging techniques are classified in two basic categories:

- Structural imaging studies the structure of the nervous system, as well as facilitates the diagnosis of intracranial diseases.
- Functional Imaging can diagnose diseases and metabolic lesions at a finer scale (such as Alzheimer's), but also provides strong support for research in neurological and cognitive psychology and the construction of brain-computer interfaces.

In the field of imaging, there are a large number of brain imaging techniques, but they have a relatively low resolution. Thus, many studies also have technical problems such as small sample size or inadequate calibration of equipment, which means they cannot be duplicated. Sometimes, brain mapping techniques are used for commercial purposes, such as the detection of lies or medical diagnosis in a way that has not been scientifically validated [7].

2.2 Image Segmentation

Prior literature image segmentation is really huge, due to the key role that segmentation plays in image analysis, and computer vision systems. Image segmentation defines the process of separating or grouping different fragments of an image [8]. Numerous methods have been adopted to segment an image. One of the classical approaches considers segmentation as a classification task, in order to assign to each pixel the label of the objects to which it belongs [9]. Actually, segmentation is one of the primary phases of image processing. It provides an exact partition of the image into different regions. For this, the classification of image segmentation is done according to several approaches: thresholding, graphs, contour, region, clustering …

The thresholding method is considered as the simplest method of image segmentation. This method is based on a pixel-level or more precisely a threshold value, to turn a gray-scale image into a binary image. The key idea is that, the thresholds are derived from the radiographs instead of the (reconstructed) image [10]. Otherwise, clustering algorithms can be categorized according to their cluster model. One of most used clustering algorithm is k-means clustering. It is simple and computationally faster than the hierarchical clustering. And it can also work for large number of variable. But it produces different cluster result for different number of cluster [11].

More performance was implemented using different region-based segmentation methods. Region growing method has been widely used for image segmentation [12], and in particular medical image applications. It is a region-based segmentation in which pixels are segmented by grouping similar neighboring pixels of seed points [13]. However, two major problems plaguing the traditional region growing algorithms: first the difficulties to select the appropriate initial seed automatically, second, the noises and regions with holes form [14]. Region merging is a process in which sub-regions are fused together to produce a meaningful reduced. Another developed field of image processing is contour-based models design a gradient stop function to accurately segment object boundaries in high quality images, while they are more sensitive to image noise and boundaries presenting weak gradient magnitude [15].

2.3 Multi-agent Importance in Image Segmentation

In the last decade, the quality of segmentation algorithms has increased, either at the level of automatic or manual segmentation, due to the advanced number of the used techniques. the 3D concept has become more interesting, so the appropriate method for image segmentation has become unavoidable [16–19]. The 3D segmentation [20, 21] experienced a significant development, especially with the technical evolution of the materials, as well as areas of use. In fact, the integration of MAS has ensured better flexibility by increasing robustness against slow changes in the systems used.

Most of these proposed approaches are often sensitive to initialization and may require quite long execution times. The methods based on the concept region are fuzzy approaches that associate germs to the object to be segmented and build for each of the seed points, a connectivity map by aggregation of image points (or voxels in 3D). Even approaches that have adopted MAS, they have exploited only a few properties, either by setting up autonomous agents each one of them performs a specific task, or a set of agents cooperating together to perform a segmentation task.

The resolution of different operational problems can deploy MAS technology [22]. However, MAS is a rich paradigm in terms of properties that can be exploited correctively to meet the needs of image segmentation, and especially to cope with annoyances encountered. Facing these limits encountered by the various approaches, that they carry according to each one of them on object detection, sensitivity to initialization, or rather long execution times, a way to bring innovation can be the development of hybrid methods, which necessarily lead to greater complexity.

Typically, these mentioned approaches aimed at improving classical algorithms by introducing the distribution notion as a parallelism by taking into consideration certain hypotheses such as communication by messages [23]. However, facing with the need to handle a significant number of the exchanged messages, most of the earlier approaches reported communication problems. From now on it is essential to overcome the difficulty of looking for specific functions, to ensure the solution emergence. In our approach, we aim to solve this problem based on the collective decision-making of all agents, using coalition and negotiation mechanisms.

3 The Proposed Approach

3.1 Objectives

Our work consists on developing a performant platform for image segmentation technologies in an important real-world application scenario (Alzheimer detection), covering the following issues:

- Adopt an agent-oriented approach to facilitate AD detection in the early stages.
- The development of a new Intelligent imaging system based on multi-agent systems: the main aim is improving the segmentation's performance, in order to make easier the determination pf brain injuries or tumors.
- The development of a multi-agent architecture, which provides a high-level framework for intelligent information fusion and management.
- The appropriated use of virtual organizations of agents for the overall management.
- Control systems for high-level sensor data management.
- Study the cooperative situation between agents, and the conflict ones.
- Focus on negotiation techniques and extending the system proposed.

The use of agents facilitates the combination of new image region fusion techniques to the platform. Cooperation allows the dynamic grouping of specialized agents, which provides a strong basis region merging techniques.

3.2 The Multi-agent Approach

Generally, the cooperative approaches concept consists of combining many techniques to get the best output for particular application. In such approaches, the complementarity of region growing, and contour techniques information is taken into account to reach a more precise segmentation that is faithful to the desired real objects. Our proposed system is presented in the Fig. 1; it consists of the flowing steps:

- After inserting the image, it undertakes a pre-processing phase;
- Elimination of the noise, and super-pixelization of the image to have a primary map of the regions, for the distribution of the seed points;
- Position of agents in seed points;
- Each agent is seeking neighboring pixels which are similar to his seed point;
- Agents coordinate task advances each time;
- Contour agents and region agents cooperate to obtain reliable segmentation results;
- In case of conflict situation, agents negotiate in order to solve the faced segmentation problem;
- After these operations, the segmentation data are extracted, evaluated, and validated in order to obtain correct segmented image, and all needed statistics.

In multi-agent systems, agents provide a more flexible and autonomous approach to coordinate their knowledge and activities, in order to model the problem to be solved, and this may involve cooperation or competition among different groups of agents. Agent environment is constructed, so agents have the responsibility to segment the input image. Each agent starts by using an input image and superpixel values for each

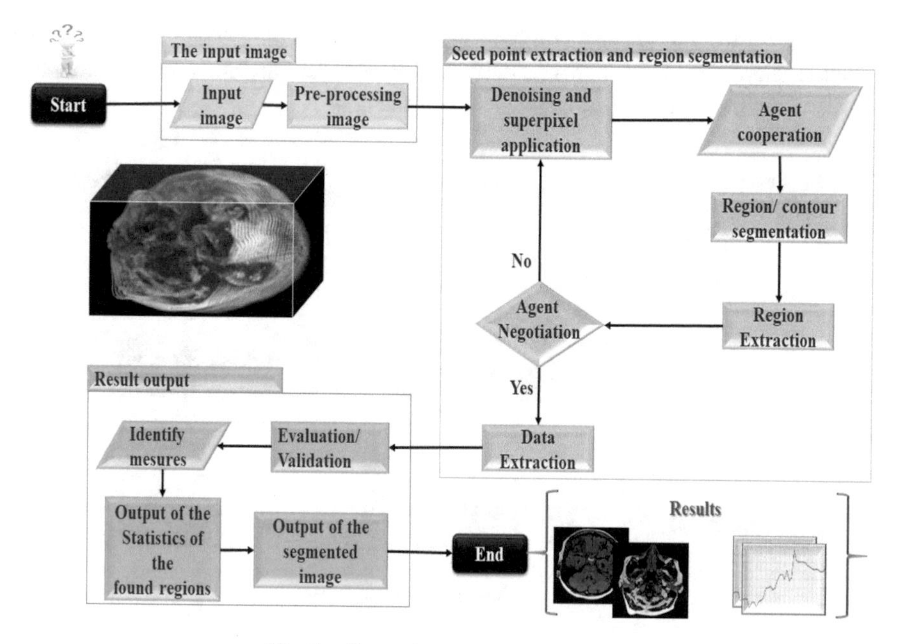

Fig. 1. General proposed architecture

region which is given priori-knowledge. The region agent needs the following information: a unique identifier, a list of neighboring agents, and the list of neighboring agents which verify the current merging situation. At every behavior end, the region agents and contour agents send an information message to other agents in order to ensure a good control of the system, and to help finding the right result for everyone.

3.3 Description of Agent Behavior

An agent is described as any entity, which is able to perceive its environment through sensors and change it by means of actuators [24]. complex software system can be treated as a collection of many agents. Intelligent systems have the ability to decide at run-time what to do and how to do it. A critical question is how this decision-making process is implemented. Increasingly, multi agent systems have being used within the several domains. Naturally, there is concern that these systems are reliable, efficient and - most of all - safe. for this reason, we have to study agent behaviors.

The MAS consensus with its dynamic topology highlights MAS's collective behavior with being very complex and cannot be easily analyzed by traditional approaches. The possibility to consider multiple agents is very suitable for complex and distributed problems, probably including complicated behaviors, that are very difficult to be solved by classical centrally programmed entities. As an intelligent distributed approach, a multi-agent system has several characteristics like:

– MAS usually contains a set of heterogeneous agents with their own skills, data and abilities for acting and interacting.

– The agents usually share a common goal, then the whole system must be able to divide the tasks to be performed by the agents, taking into consideration their processing capabilities (Fig. 2).

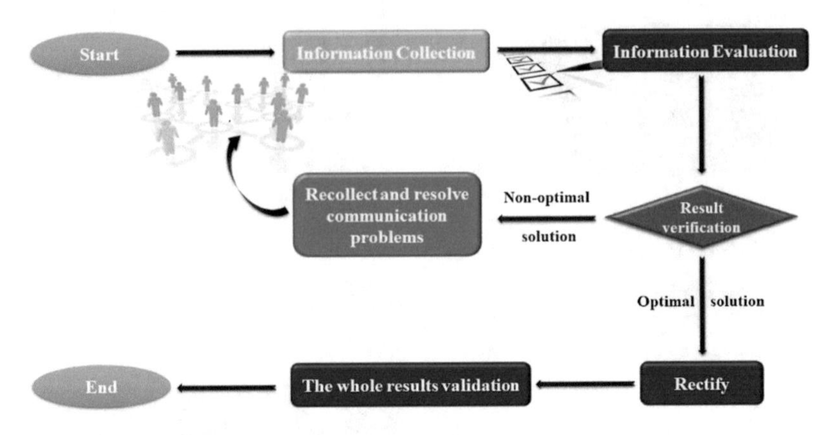

Fig. 2. The general behavior

The general behavior of the agents is described in a way that the information resulting from the work of the agents will be collected, verified, and then validated, and in the case of presence of problem or of detection of a non-optimal solution, the process carried out is moving towards a negotiating behavior. An agent can run a sequence of several behaviors described as below:

- Region marking: each agent marks a region, that corresponds to its primitive, in a shared environment. Then, each agent stores different types of information in a local database. Each region agent stores photometric and image features extracted.
- Exploration: each agent is exploring the shared environment around its territory to discover its neighbors in the image.
- Merging: Once agents are connected with each other's, each region agent tries to find out similar neighbors to merge with.
- Cooperation: In order to improve the quality of the fusion results, agents cooperate with each other.
- Reproduction: each agent creates a new agent in the next segmentation level.

3.4 Inter Agent Communication

Once created an agent is in perception of its environment in order to discover the new criteria allowing him to pursue his tasks. While segmentation progressing, agents communicate using different ways (Fig. 3):

During image processing, many agents could be in competition situation; in that case, there is a need to define a communication protocol that allows them to solve their conflicts in order to reach a cooperative agreement. This protocol is called negotiation.

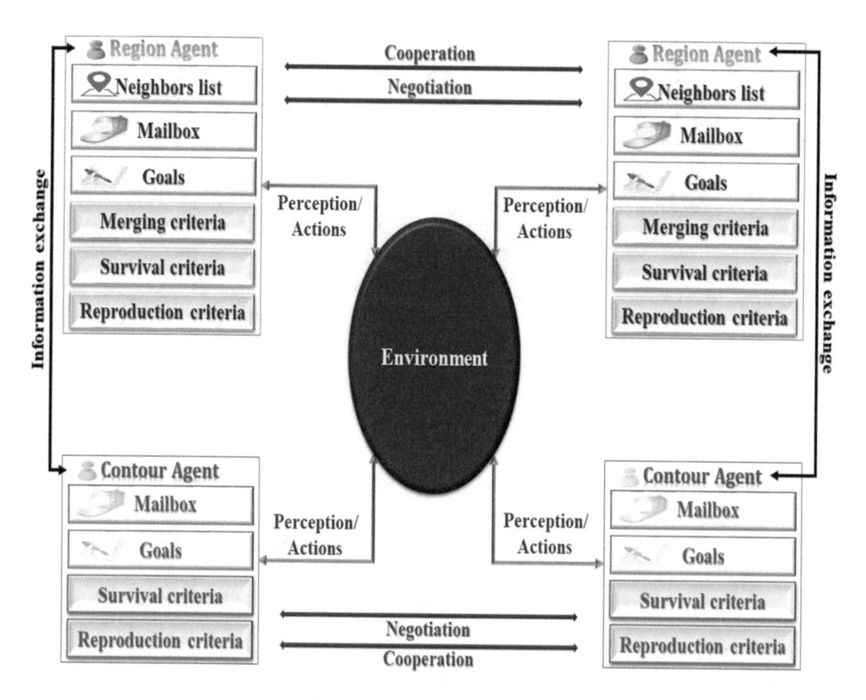

Fig. 3. Inter agent communication

An agent-based negotiation system is used to evaluate the capability of analyzing the risk associated in the inter agent communication. Our architecture makes agents in charge of getting the transmitted messages from neighbors, and then sending them to supervisor who defines the appropriate set of functions that define the actions or moves to be done at each seed point during the negotiation process.

4 Experimentation and Results

4.1 Acquaintance Relationship

Manipulating 3D data can sometimes be the more complicated task of image analysis compared to 2D data. In order to segment a 3D object, the easiest way is to make sets projected data, whose analysis agents are exclusively responsible. Following the directive of the Supervisor, once the slices have been segmented, analysis can be performed. The segmentation agent will project its region (or outline) on adjacent slices knowledge and establish a relationship with agents who have in their area (or outline) the same homogeneity criteria, found in its projections.

The main idea is to build a 3D object, including all the segmented objects in each image-slice, based on their projections on the segmented slices. Any Segmentation agent of the slice i must first build its region or contour in its slice. At the end of this operation, it will seek to establish the relationship of acquaintance with the Agents of adjacent slices. Each agent of the slice i seek its contacts in the slice $i - 1$ and $i + 1$.

There is an acquaintance between the agent Ak and Am if and only if there is an intersection of zones or contours (geometric projections) between slice i and j (j = i − 1 or j = i + 1) Zone (Za) of acquaintance is the common area (Fig. 4).

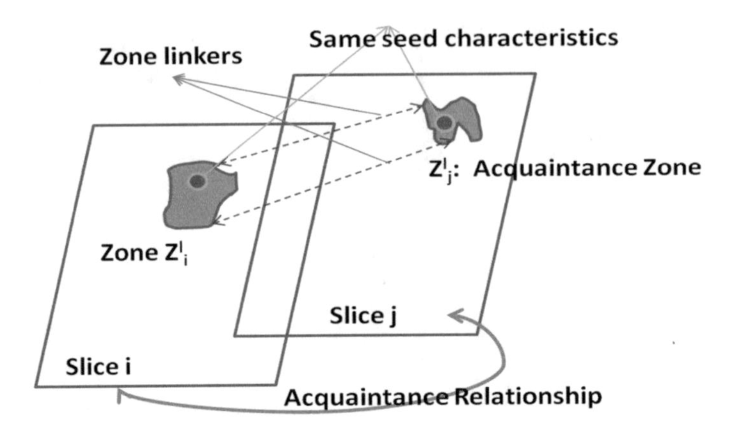

Fig. 4. Acquaintance relationship

An object is constructed by grouping a series of encountering zones, throughout the studied volume, for example from the slice Slice i i + p:

$$O1 = Zli \cup Zli + 1 \cup \ldots \cup Zli + p$$

Zlj is the cutting of object Ol represented by a region of agent in the slice j.

Among all potential objects, we need to filter out those who are the most significant by using a set of well-defined criteria. For example, first determine the minimum number (Nm) of slots used by the object. In the case of maintenance of Ol, it is necessary that $p \geq Nm$.

4.2 Imaging Test

The used data are from The National Alzheimer's Coordinating Center (NACC). NACC was established by the National Institute on Aging/NIH (U01 AG016976) in 1999 to facilitate collaborative research. Using data collected from the NIA-funded Alzheimer's Disease Centers (ADCs) across the United States, NACC has developed and maintains a large relational database of standardized clinical and neuropathological research data. In partnership with the Alzheimer's Disease Genetics Consortium (ADGC), the National Cell Repository for Alzheimer's Disease (NCRAD), and the NIA Genetics of Alzheimer's Disease Data Storage Site (NIAGADS), NACC provides a valuable resource for both exploratory and explanatory Alzheimer's disease research. NACC data [25] are freely available to all researchers (Fig. 5).

We compared the results of agents by crossing different slices to explore areas of the brain and detect brain abnormalities. We carried out several tests in order to have reliable results, we found that after the end of the tasks of the agents, a large number of

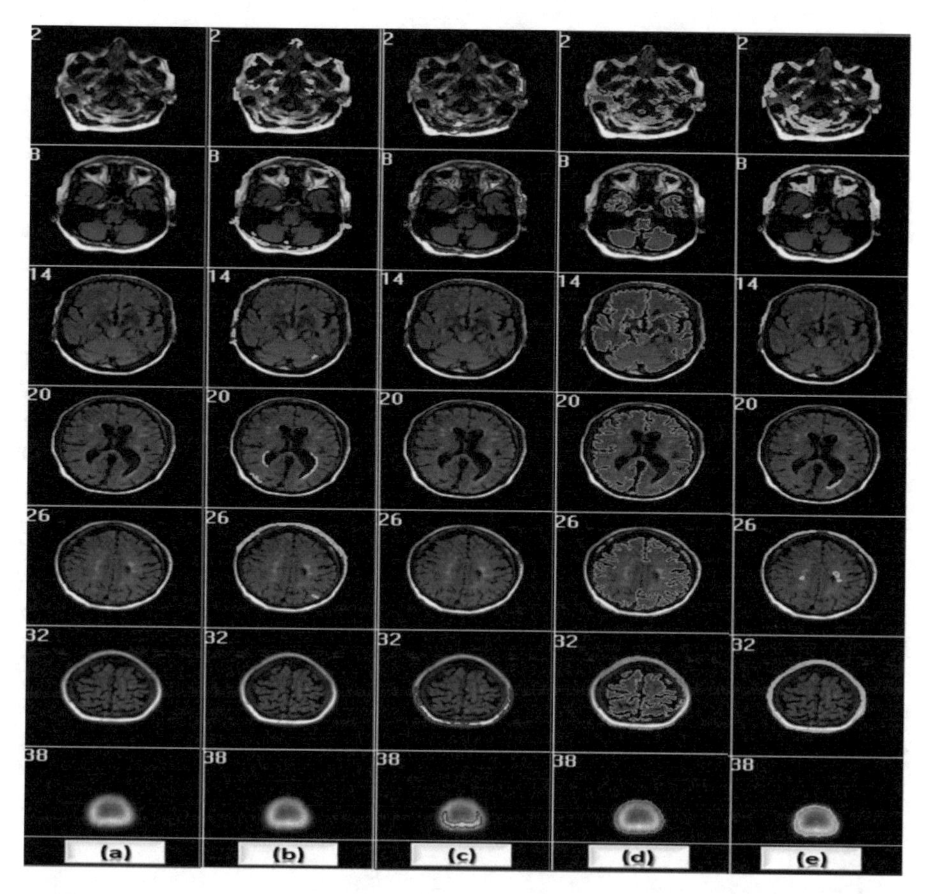

Fig. 5. Comparison of segmentation results using MAS analysis for 7 level slices, case of 4 agents. (a) original image. (b), (c), (d) and (e) are agents 1, 2, 3, 4 results respectively.

similar regions were regrouped, therefore fewer segments were generated, which ensures a better subjective coherence objects perceived in the image. Another interesting finding is in terms of knowledge transfer, in the sense that using a MAS model for RMI image segmentation, with both different global and local goals structure and different object appearance, can help better analyze previously unseen brain areas. So that physicians can predict AD in earlier stages. These test show that our MAS is able to detect small structures and excludes most of the contour pixels belonging to blood vessels and some artifacts. In fact, the results obtained by the system remain important structures different from normal brain.

4.3 Discussion

The proposed system is composed of a set of autonomous agents. The agents have the ability to preserve the system, to receive task requests, to extract the information they need from the image, and to it in order to perform a specific segmentation task. Thus, each agent has its own sensors and behaviors, as well as reactions over the image. Each agent perceives information from the image and/or the other agents, then acts by sending messages to the system. These actions form the agent behavior. Each behavior may include several tasks (exploring neighbors, merge, cooperation, negotiation, reproduction, …) depending on the state of the agent, which can be changed by itself, or by another agent to respond to the system needs. Agents can negotiate with other agents so an important amount of messages is exchanged while the system execution. In fact, the ability of a single agent is not enough, all agents must interact with each other in order to achieve the global purpose for solving a problem, planning, searching, decision-making and learning [26].

The data we tested are downloaded from NACC database is both a strength and a possible weakness of our study. Our ability to robustly classify MRI images with very possible impairment provides encouragement for future development of this approach as a diagnostic tool for Alzheimer detection. Otherwise, it is important to highlight that our hypotheses were proved using Multi-agent system to obtain robust cooperative segmentation that can provide a confident brain analysis and a powerful AD predictive tool.

To achieve this work, we had to use a single clinician MRI images for validation due to practical difficulties in finding more experienced clinicians in contouring Alzheimer disease based on MRI imaging. Comparison against multiple clinician cases MRI images may be part of our future studies. Currently, the process of segmentation is still depending on the performance of the used machines for test. The majority of the time is spent in loading the images and waiting he end of tasks of all agents. Since we are working in a sensitive medical field, we aim to limit the number of messages exchanged to ensure system flexibility, and to study the rules of the MAS. Agents must respect a specified number of rules in terms of the overall activities and behaviors.

5 Conclusion

This paper presents an MRI images segmentation system for Alzheimer disease detection based on cooperative techniques that can be used for automatic detection as well as classification of AD later. The multi-agent architecture presented provides a strong approach for the image segmentation by technique cooperation: region merging (in 3D) and contour segmentation.

The proposed approach offers the optimum results with very less computational efforts. This explain the efficiency of our proposed system in recognition and segmentation of the Alzheimer disease images. Another advantage of using this method is that AD can be identified at early stage or the initial stage. To improve the obtained results more clinical data would be tested, taking into consideration physician opinion.

References

1. Fan, Y., Wu, X., Shen, D., Resnick, S.M., Davatzikos, C.: Yong, detection of prodromal Alzheimer's disease via pattern classification of MRI. Neurobiol. Aging **29**(4), 514–523 (2008)

2. Braak, H., Braak, E., Bohl, J., Bratzke, H.: Evolution of Alzheimer's disease related cortical lesions. J. Neural Transm. Suppl. **54**, 97–106 (1998)
3. Khan, M., Ravi, S.: Image segmentation methods: a comparative study. Int. J. Soft Comput. Eng. (IJSCE) **3**(4), 84–92 (2013)
4. Padmavathi, G., Subashini, P., Sumi, A.: Empirical evaluation of suitable segmentation algorithms for ir images. IJCSI Int. J. Comput. Sci. **7**(4), 22 (2010)
5. Wooldridge, M., Jennings, N.R.: Agent theories, architectures, and languages: a survey. In: ECAI 1994: Proceedings of the Workshop on Agent Theories Architectures, and Languages on Intelligent Agents, Amsterdam, The Netherlands, pp. 1–22 (1995)
6. Burns, A., Iliffe, S.: Alzheimer's disease. BMJ **338**, b158 (2009). https://doi.org/10.1136/bmj.b158. PMID 19196745
7. Satel, S., Lilienfeld, S.O.: Brainwashed: The Seductive Appeal of Mindless Neuroscience. Basic Books, New York (2015). ISBN-13 978-0465062911
8. Singh, V., Misra, A.K.: Detection of plant leaf diseases using image segmentation and soft computing techniques. Inf. Process. Agric. **4**(1), 41–49 (2017)
9. Machairas, V., Baldeweck, T., Walter, T., Decencière, E.: New general features based on superpixels for image segmentation learning. In: 2016 IEEE 13th International Symposium on Biomedical Imaging (ISBI) (2016). https://doi.org/10.1109/ISBI.2016.7493531
10. Batenburg, K.J., Sijbers, J.: Optimal threshold selection for tomogram segmentation by projection distance minimization. IEEE Trans. Med. Imaging, 676–686 (2009). https://doi.org/10.1109/tmi.2008.2010437
11. Dhanachandra, N., Manglem, K., Chanu, Y.J.: Image segmentation using k-means clustering algorithm and subtractive clustering algorithm. In: Eleventh International Multi-Conference on Information Processing (IMCIP 2015). Procedia Computer Science, vol. 54, pp. 764–771 (2015)
12. Zucker, S.W.: Region growing: childhood and adolescence. Comput. Gr. Image Process. **5** (3), 382–399 (1976)
13. Wei, C.H., Chen, S.Y., Liu, X.: Mammogram retrieval on similar mass lesions. Comput. Methods Programs Biomed. **106**(3), 234–248 (2012)
14. Rouhi, R., Jafari, M., Kasaei, S., Keshavarzian, P.: Benign and malignant breast tumors classification based on region growing and CNN. Expert Syst. Appl. **42**, 990–1002 (2015)
15. Niu, S., Chen, Q., de Sisternes, L., Ji, Z., Zhou, Z., Rubin, D.L.: Robust noise region-based active contour model via local similarity factor for image segmentation. Pattern Recogn. **61**, 104–119 (2016)
16. Qian, Y., Gao, X., Loomes, M., Comley, R., Barn, B., Hui, R., Tian, Z.: Content based retrieval of 3D medical images. In: eTELEMED 2011: The Third International Conference on eHealth, Telemedicine, and Social Medicine (2011). ISBN 978-1-61208-003-1
17. Strzelecki, M., Lee, M.: Analysis of three-dimensional magnetic resonance human liver images. IETE J. Res. **57**(3), 237–245 (2011)
18. Airan, R.D., Foss, C.A., Ellens, N.P., Wang, Y., Mease, R.C., Farahani, K., Pomper, M.G.: MR-Guided delivery of hydrophilic molecular imaging agents across the blood-brain barrier through focused ultrasound. Mol. Imaging Biol. **19**(1), 24–30 (2017)
19. Henriet, J., Lang, C.: Introduction of a multiagent paradigm to optimize a case-based reasoning system designed to personalize three-dimensional numerical representations of human organs. Biomed. Eng. Appl. Basis Commun. **26**(5), 1450060 (2014)
20. Pitiot, A., Delingette, H., Thompson, P.M., Ayache, N.: Expert knowledge-guided segmentation system for brain MRI. NeuroImage **23**, S85–S96 (2004)
21. Shattuck, D.W., Mirza, M., Adisetiyo, V., Hojatkashani, C., Salamon, G., Narr, K.L., Poldrack, R.A., Bilder, R.M., Toga, A.W.: Construction of a 3D probabilistic atlas of human cortical structures. NeuroImage **39**, 1064–1080 (2008)

22. Coelhoa, V.N., Cohen, M.W., Guimaraes, F.G., Coelho, I.M., Liu, N.: Multi-agent systems applied for energy systems integration: state-of-the-art applications and trends in microgrids. Appl. Energy **187**, 820–832 (2017)
23. Yokoo, M.: Algorithms for distributed constraint satisfaction problems: with review. Auton. Agents Syst. Multi-Agent **3**, 198–212 (2000)
24. Russell, S.J., Norvig, P.: Artificial Intelligence: A Modern Approach, 3rd edn. Prentice Hall, Upper Saddle River (2014)
25. Center, The National Alzheimer's Coordinating. https://www.alz.washington.edu
26. Liu, L., Zhou, L.-L., Bao, H.-F.: Remote sensing image segmentation algorithm based on multi-agent and fuzzy clustering. In: 2017 2nd International Conference on Environmental Science and Energy Engineering (ICESEE 2017) (2017)

Author Index

M. Ezziyyani (Ed.): AI2SD 2018, AISC 914, pp. 327–328, 2019.
https://doi.org/10.1007/978-3-030-11884-6

Printed in the United States
By Bookmasters